ESSENTIALS OF

ORAL HISTOLOGY
AND EMBRYOLOGY

A Clinical Approach

evolve

To access your Instructor Resources, visit:

http://evolve.elsevier.com/Avery/oralhistology/

Evolve Student Learning Resources for Avery/Chiego: Essentials of Oral Histology and Embryology: A Clinical Approach, 3/e offers the following features:

- **Web Links**
  Links to websites related to text content provide additional resources and further reading

- **Crossword puzzles**
  Interactive crosswords challenge your knowledge of key terms from the book

- **Drag-and-drop exercises**
  These challenging activities allow you to practice attaching labels to correct areas of images from each chapter to identify important features of oral histology and embryology

ESSENTIALS OF
ORAL HISTOLOGY AND EMBRYOLOGY
A Clinical Approach

THIRD EDITION

JAMES K. AVERY, DDS, PhD

Professor Emeritus of Dentistry, School of Dentistry
Professor Emeritus of Anatomy, Medical School
University of Michigan
Ann Arbor, Michigan

DANIEL J. CHIEGO, JR., MS, PhD

Associate Professor, School of Dentistry
Department of Cariology, Restorative Sciences and Endodontics
University of Michigan
Ann Arbor, Michigan

MOSBY

ELSEVIER

MOSBY
ELSEVIER

11830 Westline Industrial Drive
St. Louis, Missouri 63146

ESSENTIALS OF ORAL HISTOLOGY AND EMBRYOLOGY:
A CLINICAL APPROACH
Copyright © 2006, 2000, 1992 by Mosby, Inc

ISBN 9780-323-03339-8
ISBN 0-323-03339-3

Notice

ISBN 9780-323-03339-8
ISBN 0-323-03339-3

Publishing Director: Linda Duncan
Executive Editor: Penny Rudolph
Associate Developmental Editor: Julie Nebel
Publishing Services Manager: Melissa Lastarria
Project Manager: Rich Barber
Design Manager: Bill Drone

Printed in Canada

Last digit is the print number: 9 8 7 6 5 4 3 2 1

PREFACE

The central purpose of this textbook is to educate students in the dental professions with an explanation of the structures related to histology of the masticatory apparatus. The fields of head and neck embryology and histology are of utmost importance in the study of dental practice and dental hygiene. Oral histology is paramount to the understanding of dental pathology, so connecting these fields of study provides an explanation for the cause-and-effect nature of dental conditions and resulting treatment choices. To undertake the best treatment for the patient, one must first understand what is normal to gain better awareness of the abnormal.

The third edition of *Essentials of Oral Histology and Embryology: A Clinical Approach* is therefore designed as the basic science information text to help in the comprehension of the microscopic anatomy of the oral and facial tissues. Chapter 2 of this edition, "Structure and Function of Cells, Tissues, and Organs," has been especially revised to provide more essential information about these building blocks of the body's systems. Other areas of the book, including Suggested Reading and Self-Evaluation Questions at the end of each chapter, have been updated with new information. As with previous editions of the text, an effort has been made to position explanatory diagrams and illustrations as close as possible to their accompanying textual descriptions. In addition, most illustrations are now presented in color to enable students to better correlate structure with function by observing histology as they would view it in reality. We believe that the use of so many detailed photographs, drawings, and diagrams will allow a greater ease in understanding the numerous theoretical and clinical concepts presented here.

Another key to learning the content of this text effectively is possessing a thorough grasp of the sometimes complicated terminology used in the fields of histology,

embryology, and oral anatomy. The third edition now includes a list of Learning Objectives and Key Terms at the beginning of each chapter. Learning Objectives list the main ideas discussed in each chapter and what the student can be expected to know by reading its content, thus allowing readers and instructors to set goals for comprehension and engage in more directed learning at the outset of the chapter. The *Key Terms* are listed alphabetically and are then bolded where they are discussed in the text, where the reader will find a contextual explanation of that term. The Glossary at the end of the book provides definitions for these key terms that will allow students to use them in their clinical vocabulary with confidence.

Special features such as the *Consider the Patient* boxes and *Clinical Comment* boxes are continued in this edition. *Consider the Patient* boxes demonstrate the applicability of the book's concepts by presenting the reader with situations and patient questions relevant to the current chapter discussion that could occur in clinical practice. Each box has a coordinating *Discussion* box at the end of the chapter that provides common answers to the questions or possible recommendations and explanations for certain conditions, thereby preparing students for how they would respond to similar situations in real life and opening the door to further discussion of other possible solutions. Additional *Clinical Comment* boxes placed throughout this edition offer clinical tips and notes of interest pertaining to chapter content.

The most drastic change in this third edition is the inclusion of an Evolve website that accompanies and enhances the textual material. This website, available at the URL listed on the inside front cover of this book, contains multiple online learning resources to aid the student and instructor alike in their efforts to cover the content of the book. The weblinks listed connect readers to up-to-date articles and current information on the Internet, whereas the Electronic Image Collection provides them with an opportunity to study the histology and embryology pictures from the text up close. Interactive learning activities and a comprehensive test bank encompassing all aspects of oral histology and embryology further challenge students' knowledge of the material and prepare them for clinical experience. Composed with extensive input from Penny Rudolph, Executive Editor, and Julie Nebel, Associate Developmental Editor, who also provided guidance on the book, these online extras promise to make the third edition of *Essentials* an invaluable asset to classroom learning and individual study alike.

ACKNOWLEDGMENTS

Essentials of Oral Histology and Embryology has been a lifetime project of the senior author, and I am grateful for the numerous suggestions of and thoughtful interactions with involved students observed in the many years that this book has been in use. This new edition of *Oral Histology and Embryology* is enhanced by the addition of a close associate, Dr. Daniel J. Chiego, Jr. In the past, he made many helpful suggestions for revisions, and in agreeing to co-authorship of this edition, he became responsible for updating much of the text and making numerous contributions.

A textbook does not survive without illustrations, and this book has a large number of these. Alayne Evans contributed many of the original drawings in the previous edition. In addition, Chris Jung, medical illustrator at the University of Michigan, has contributed several drawings and diagrams in both the second and third editions. His contributions were expanded in this edition as some new drawings were added in the earlier chapters. I also want to remember Pauline Steele for her efforts in editing the last edition and who made immeasurable contributions in the past to this text.

James K. Avery

TABLE OF CONTENTS

ESSENTIALS OF
ORAL HISTOLOGY
AND EMBRYOLOGY

A Clinical Approach

DEVELOPMENT AND STRUCTURE OF CELLS AND TISSUES

CHAPTER OUTLINE

LEARNING OBJECTIVES

After reading this chapter the student will be able to:
- describe the cell and how it divides
- discuss the origin of tissue, the ovarian cycle, and development of the embryonic disk
- describe the various tissues of the human body and some of the adverse factors such as environmental stress and hereditary and dietary factors that may affect development of these tissues

KEY TERMS

Absorption
Agranulocytes
Anaphase
Angioblasts
Angiogenic clusters
Appositional

Assimilation
Astral rays/asters
Basophils
Blastocyst
Cartilage
Cell cycle

Centrioles
Centromere
Cerebellum
Cerebral hemispheres
Chondroblasts
Chromatids

KEY TERMS—cont'd

Chromosomes
Conductivity
Cytoplasm
Cytosol
Deoxyribonucleic acid (DNA)
Dermatome
Dermis
Ectodermal
Elastic or fibrous cartilage
Embryonic disk
Embryonic period
Endochondral bone development
Endodermal
Endometrium
Endoplasmic reticulum (ER)
Eosinophils
Epidermis
Epiphyseal line
Epithelium
Equatorial plate
Erythrocytes
Excretion
Fetal period
Fibroblasts
Fluid
Foramen ovale
Forebrain, midbrain, and hindbrain
Frontal, temporal, and occipital
    lobes
G1 phase, G2 phase

Gastrointestinal tract
Gene expression
Genetic mechanisms
Golgi apparatus, complex
Granulocytes
Growth
Growth factors
Hemoglobin
Hyaline cartilage
Implantation
Induction
Intercalated disks
Intercellular material
Interstitial
Interstitial growth
Intramembranous bone formation
Irritability
Leukocytes
Lymphatic system
Lymphocytes
Lysosomes
Melanocytes
Mesenchymal cells
Mesodermal
Metaphase
Metaphysis
Microtubules
Mitochondria
Monocytes
Morula

Myotome
Neural plate, tube
Neuroblasts
Neurons
Neutrophils
Nuclear envelope
Nuclear pores
Nucleolus
Nucleus
Organizer
Osteoblasts
Plasma
Plasma membrane
Pons
Proliferative period
Prophase
Reproduction
Respiration
Ribonucleic acid (RNA)
S phase
Sclerotome
Smooth muscle cells
Somites
Spindle fibers
Striated voluntary muscles
Telophase
Umbilical system
Visceral mesoderm
Vitelline vascular system
Zygote

OVERVIEW

The smallest unit of structure in the human body is the cell, composed of a nucleus and cytoplasm. The nucleus contains **deoxyribonucleic acid (DNA)** and **ribonucleic acid (RNA),** the fundamental structures of life. The cytoplasm functions in absorption and cell duplication, in which organelles perform specific actions. The cell cycle is the time required for the DNA to duplicate before mitosis. This chapter discusses the four stages of mitosis: prophase, metaphase, anaphase, and telophase. Also described are the three periods of prenatal development: proliferative, embryonic, and fetal. The fertilization of the ovum in the distal uterine tube, zygote migration, and the zygote's implantation in the uterine wall are discussed. In addition, the origin of human tissues—ectoderm, mesoderm, and endoderm—is presented, followed by the differentiation of tissue types, such as those of ectodermal origin, epithelium and skin with its derivatives, and the central and peripheral nervous systems. This chapter also delineates development of the mesodermal components involving connective tissues of the body, such as fibrous tissue, three types of cartilage, two types of bone, three kinds of muscles, and the cardiovascular system. The reader will better comprehend the origin, development, organization, and structure of the various cells and tissues of the human body.

CELL STRUCTURE AND FUNCTION

The human body is composed of cells, intercellular substance (the products of these cells), and fluid that bathes these tissues. Cells are the smallest living units capable of independent existence. They carry out the vital processes of **absorption, assimilation, respiration, irritability, conductivity, growth, reproduction,** and **excretion.** Cells vary in size, shape, structure, and function. Regardless of function, each cell has a number of characteristics in common with other cells, such as **cytoplasm** and a **nucleus,** which contains a **nucleolus.**

However, some cell characteristics are related to function. A cell on the surface of the skin, for example, serves best as a thin, flattened disk, whereas a respiratory cell functions best as a cuboidal or columnar cell to facilitate adsorption with mobile cilia to move fluid from the lung to the oropharynx. Surrounding each cell is the **intercellular material** that provides the cell with nutrition, takes up waste products, and provides the body with form. It may be as soft as loose connective tissue or as hard as bone cartilage or teeth. **Fluid,** the third component of the body, is the blood and lymph that travel throughout the body in vessels or the tissue fluid that bathes each cell and fiber of the body.

Cell Nucleus

A nucleus is found in all cells except mature red blood cells and blood platelets. The nucleus is usually round to ovoid, depending on the cell's shape. Ordinarily a cell has a single nucleus; however, it may be binucleate, as are cardiac muscle cells or parenchymal liver cells, or multinucleate, as are osteoclasts and skeletal muscle cells. The nucleus is important in the production of DNA and RNA. DNA contains the genetic information in the cell, and RNA carries information from the DNA to sites of actual protein synthesis, which are located in the cell cytoplasm. The nucleus is bound by a membrane, the **nuclear envelope,** which has openings at the **nuclear pores.** This envelope is composed of two phospholipids layers similar to the plasma membrane of the cell. The pores are associated with the endoplasmic reticulum that forms at the end of each cell division. The nucleus contains from one to four nucleoli, which are round, dense bodies constituting the RNA contained in the nucleus. Nucleoli have no limiting membrane (Fig. 1-1).

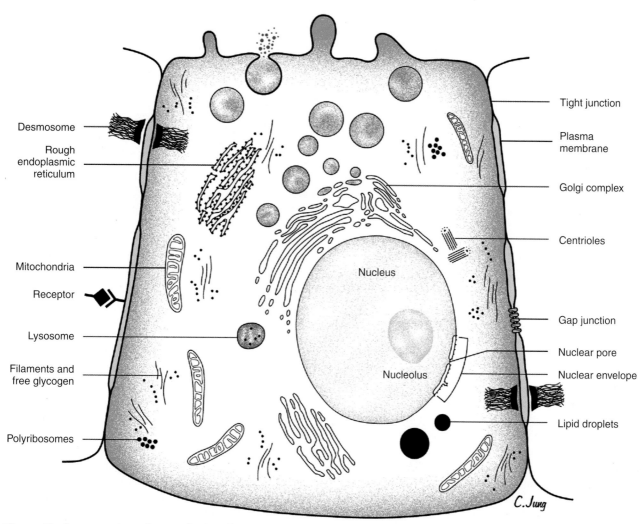

Fig. 1-1 Nucleus, rough surface endoplasmic reticulum, mitochondria, Golgi apparatus, centrioles, and gap junctions as viewed by electron microscopy. Cells communicate with each other to regulate organization, growth, and development.

Cell Cytoplasm

Cytoplasm contains structures necessary for adsorption and for creation of cell products. The **cytosol** is the part of the cytoplasm that contains the organelles and solutes. The cytosol uses the raw materials brought into the cell to produce energy. It also functions in the excretion of waste products. These functions are carried out by the **endoplasmic reticulum (ER)**—parallel membrane-bound cavities in the cytoplasm that contain newly acquired and synthesized protein. Two types of ER, smooth surfaced and granular or rough surfaced, can be found in the same cell. Rough-surfaced ER is caused by ribosomes on the surface of the reticulum and is the site at which protein production is initiated. Proteins are vital to the cell's metabolic processes, and each type of protein is composed of a number of different amino acids linked in a specific sequence. Amino acids form protein-containing groups, which, in turn, form acids or bases.

Ribosomes are particles that translate genetic codes for proteins and activate mechanisms for their production. They can be found as separate particles in the cytoplasm, clustered, or attached to the ER membranes. Ribosomes are nonspecific as to what type of protein they synthesize. The type is dependent on the messenger RNA (mRNA), which carries the message directly from the DNA of the nucleus to the RNA in the ER. This molecule attaches to the ribosomes and gives orders about the formation of the amino acids.

The ER transports substances in the cytoplasm. The ER is connected to the Golgi apparatus via small vesicles. The **Golgi apparatus** or **complex** helps sort, condense, package, and deliver proteins arriving from the ER. The Golgi apparatus is composed of cisternae (flat plates) or saccules, small vesicles, and large vacuoles. From here the secretory vesicles move or flow to the cell surface, where they fuse with the cell membrane and the plasmalemma and release their contents by exocytosis.

Lysosomes are small, membrane-bound bodies that contain a variety of acid hydrolase and digestive enzymes to help break down substances both inside and outside the cell. They are in all cells except red blood cells but are prominent in macrophages and leukocytes.

Mitochondria are membrane-bound organelles that lie free in the cytoplasm and are present in all cells. They are important in generating energy, are a major source of adenosine triphosphate (ATP), and therefore are the site of many metabolic reactions. These organelles appear as spheres, rods, ovoids, or threadlike bodies. Usually the inner layer of their trilaminar bounding membrane inflects to form transverse-appearing plates, the cristae (see Fig. 1-1). Mitochondria lie adjacent to the area that requires their energy production.

Microtubules are small tubular structures in the cytoplasm that are composed of the protein tubulin. These structures may appear as singles, as doublets, or as triplets. They probably function as structural and force-generating elements and relate to cilia (motile cell processes) and to centrioles in relation to mitosis. They have cytoskeletal functions in maintaining cell shape. **Centrioles** are short cylinders appearing near the nucleus. Their walls are composed of nine triplets of microtubules. Centrioles are microtubule-generating centers and are important in mitosis, self-replicating before mitosis begins.

Surrounding the cell is the **plasma membrane** or plasmalemma, which envelops the cell and provides a selective barrier that regulates transport of substances into and out of the cell. All membranes are composed mainly of lipids and proteins with a small amount of carbohydrates. The plasma membrane also receives signals from hormones and neurotransmitters. In addition, cells contain proteins, lipids, or fatty substances that provide energy in the cell and are important components of cell membranes and permeability. Carbohydrates are also important in cells as the most available energy component in the body. These carbohydrates may exist as polysaccharide-protein complexes, glycoprotein complexes, glycoproteins, and glycolipids. Carbohydrate compounds are important in cell function and for development of cell products, such as supportive tissues and body lubricants.

Genetic mechanisms help a cell to develop and maintain a high degree of order. The ability is dependent on the genetic information that is expressed within the cell. The basic genetic processes in the cell are RNA and protein synthesis, DNA repair, and replication and genetic recombination. These processes produce type proteins and nucleic acids of a cell. These genetic events are relatively simple compared with other cell processes.

CELL DIVISION

Cell Cycle

Cell division is a continuous series of discrete steps by which the cell component divides. This function is related to the need for growth or replacement of tissues and is partly dependent on the length of the cell's life. Continually renewing cells line the gastrointestinal tract and compose the epidermis and the bone marrow. A second type of cell is part of an expanding population—the cells of the kidney, liver, and some glands. The third type of cell does not undergo cell division or DNA synthesis. An example is the neurons of the adult nervous system. For a somatic cell to undergo cell division, it must pass through a **cell cycle,** which ensures time for DNA genetic material in the daughter cells to duplicate that of the parent cell. However, in a sex cell, ovum, or spermatozoon, the process of meiosis occurs, in which a reduction division of chromosomes in the daughter cell takes place. The result is that half as many chromosomes are in the daughter cell as are in the parent cell. Through meiosis, after fertilization of the ovum by the male chromosomes, the original (diploid) number of chromosomes is regained. The duration of the cell cycle in somatic cells is now known (Fig. 1-2). After mitosis, the cells enter the reduplication or **G1 phase** of the interphase, the initial resting stage. This is followed by the **S phase**, in which DNA synthesis is completed. Next the cell enters the **G2 phase** or quiescent phase of the post-DNA duplication and proceeds into the mitotic stages of prophase, metaphase, anaphase, and telophase (Fig. 1-3). The cell then reenters and remains in the interphase stage until duplication resumes the mitotic process of developing two daughter cells identical to the parent cells.

CLINICAL COMMENT

Development of the embryo and fetus is a genetically well-coordinated series of events that defines the beginning of life. Initial events associated with fertilization determine the sex of the forming embryo, XX for female and XY for male.

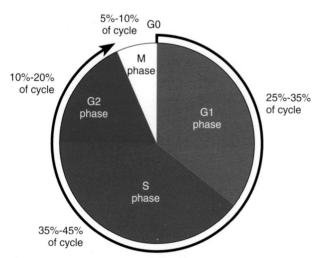

Fig. 1-2 Periods of cell cycle indicate relative time needed for each phase. G1 is the reduplication phase, or resting phase, which takes about 6 to 8 hours. In the S phase, DNA duplication takes place in 8 to 10 hours. The G2 phase is the postduplication phase, which takes about 4 to 6 hours. In the M phase, mitosis takes about 35 to 40 minutes. These figures are for cultured mammalian cells. The total is 18 to 24 hours for these four stages of cytokinesis. Other types of cells can have a longer or shorter cell cycle.

Mitosis

Before mitosis the cell exists in the interphase, as seen in Figure 1-3, *A*. The first step of mitosis is **prophase,** in which four structural changes occur (Fig. 1-3, *B*). The chromatin thread of the nucleus thickens into rodlike structures called **chromosomes.** Each chromosome then splits, forming two **chromatids.** These chromatids line up along the central area of the cell, called the **equatorial plate.** Each chromatid pair is attached to a spherical body called a **centromere.** The centriole pair duplicates, and the chromatids accompany the centrioles' migration to the opposite ends of the cell. Those fibers not formed between the migrating centrioles are **spindle fibers** and those that form around the centrioles are **astral rays** or **asters** (Fig. 1-3, *C*). At this time the nucleolus disappears and its components become attached to the chromatids. Finally, the nuclear envelope breaks down and changes into granular elements, such as the ER (Fig. 1-3, *D*).

Chromatids have moved to the cell center by the **metaphase** stage. They are arranged along an equatorial plate at right angles to the long axis of the spindle (Fig. 1-3, *E*). The two chromatids of each chromosome become attached centrally at the equatorial plate to a centromere. These chromatids then split at the centromere into two sets of chromosomes.

In **anaphase,** the daughter chromosomes move to the opposite poles of the cell with the full complement of 46 at each end (Fig. 1-3, *F* and *G*). This is thought to occur by movement of the chromosomal microtubules that attract the chromatids toward the poles. A constriction begins to appear around the midbody of the cell (Fig. 1-3, *G*).

In **telophase,** the chromosomes detach from the chromosomal microtubules and the microtubules disintegrate. The chromosomes next elongate and disperse, losing their identity and regaining the chromatin thread appearance. Both the nucleoli within the nucleus and the nuclear envelope then reappear. As each nucleus matures, the cleavage furrow deepens in the midcell until the two daughter cells separate (Fig. 1-3, *H*).

Meiosis

Meiosis is the process of reduction of the number of chromosomes to half the normal number in the germ cells to allow fusion of the male and female germ cells. There are two cell divisions in meiosis. In the first meiotic division, the chromosomes divide equally with pairing of the homologous chromosomes and the appropriate synthesis of DNA. In the second meiotic division, the DNA is not synthesized, and three of the daughter cells divide into polar bodies that become inactive; the one remaining germ cell containing half the amount of DNA pairs with the germ cell of the

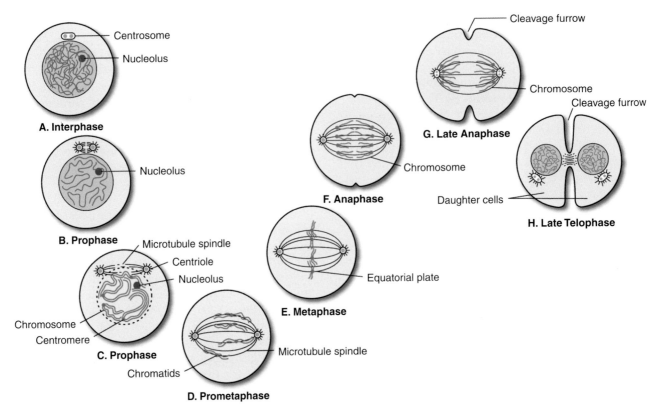

Fig. 1-3 Mitosis of somatic cell. The continuous process of cell division is shown. Mitosis is replication of parent chromosomes and distribution of two sets of chromosomes into two separate and equal nuclei. Stages are as follows: **A,** Interphase, resting cell. **B** and **C,** During prophase, chromatin thread shortens and thickens and becomes chromosomes, which then split into pairs of chromatids. Nuclear membrane disappears, and centrioles appear and begin migration to opposite poles of cell. **D,** In prometaphase, or early metaphase, chromatid pairs attach to centromere and line up in equatorial plate of cell. **E,** Metaphase occurs when centromeres and chromatids line up in middle of cell. Centrioles are at opposite ends of cell and attach to chromosomes by mitotic spindles. **F,** Anaphase is a division and movement of completed identical sets of chromatids (chromosomes) to opposite ends of cells. **G,** In late anaphase, identical sets of chromosomes have reached opposite ends of the cells as cleavage begins. **H,** In telophase, a nuclear membrane reappears, nucleoli appear, and chromosomes lengthen and form chromatin thread. Mitotic spindles disappear, and centrioles duplicate so that each cell has completely identical properties.

opposite sex. This pairing of the XY chromosomes of the male and female germ cells provides the needed mature somatic cell.

Apoptosis

Apoptosis, or programmed cell death, is the fragmentation of a cell into membrane bound particles, which are then eliminated by phagocytosis by specialized cells. Cell death is the usual accompaniment of embryonic growth and differentiation. It is a means of eliminating transient and obsolete tissues. Thus, cell death, as well as histogenesis and morphogenetic movement, accomplishes the final form of the structure. Cell death typically occurs at sites during folding or invagination of tissues.

Cell death is a useful way of eliminating tissues or organs that provided a function during early embryonic life, for example the tadpole tail and gills.

Adult stem cells (Fig. 1-4) are found in hematopoietic cells in bone marrow and have the multipotent capacity to form a number of cell types. Stem cells have been found in the dental pulp as well as the brain, muscle, skin, intestinal tract, and blood vessels. It is the hope of the future that these cells will be able to replace damaged, dead, or malfunctioning tissue. It has recently been reported that damaged corneal cells of the eye can be replaced with bits of oral epithelium utilizing the patient's own stem cells to aid in the healing process and in restoring vision.

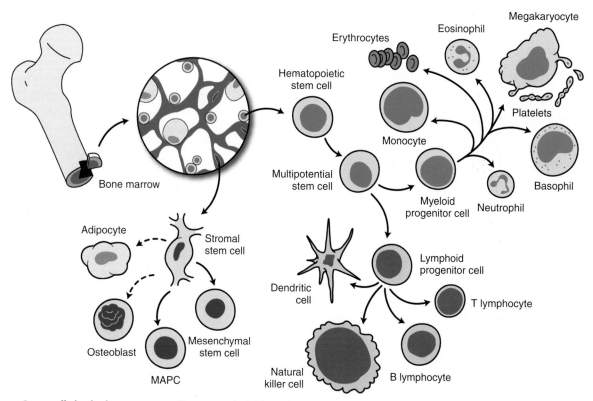

Fig. 1-4 Stem cells in the bone marrow (hematopoietic) have been studied extensively. These cells can differentiate into blood and immune cell lines. Other stem cells in the bone marrow are stromal stem cells, and they have been reported to be able to differentiate into fat and bone cell precursors. Other stem cells have been discovered in the brain, eyes, skin, muscle, dental pulp, blood vessels, and gastrointestinal tract.

 CLINICAL COMMENT

All cells have a limited lifetime. For example, the life span of a white blood cell is only a few hours to a few days. Red blood cells live approximately 120 days before they are ingested by macrophages. Surface-covering cells—such as those of the skin, hair, or nails— renew as they are replaced as do cells lining the respiratory, urinary, and gastrointestinal tracts. Other cells in the body—such as those of the liver, kidneys, and thyroid gland—do not normally renew after maturity unless they are injured.

ORIGIN OF HUMAN TISSUE

Epithelial Mesenchymal Interaction

The following are several definitions that are important to understanding the basic processes of early development.

Induction

Induction is the process in which an undifferentiated cell is instructed by specific organizers to produce a morphogenic effect.

Cell Differentiation

The **organizer** is the part of an embryo that influences another part to direct histologic and morphologic differentiation. Chemical substances called **growth**

factors induce cells to initiate specific cellular processes including DNA synthesis in a specific temporal and spatial manner.

Periods of Prenatal Development

Implantation and enlargement of the blastocyst, which contains the embryonic tissue, occur rapidly in the **proliferative period,** which lasts for 2 weeks. During this time, fertilization, implantation, and formation of the embryonic disk take place. After the second week, this mass of cells begins to take the form of an embryo, so the period of 2 to 8 weeks is termed the **embryonic period.** During this period, the different types of tissue develop and organize to form organ systems. The heart forms and begins to beat by the fourth week, and the face and oral structures develop during weeks 4 to 7. The embryo takes on a more human appearance in the eighth week and moves into the **fetal period,** which extends until birth (Fig. 1-5). During this period, the tissues that developed in the embryonic stage enlarge, differentiate, and become capable of function.

Consider the Patient

An expectant mother has reason for concern about the health of her baby. She asks whether tests are available to find out if her baby is healthy. She wants to know what the tests would reveal and if any risks are involved. (See discussion at end of chapter.)

Ovarian Cycle, Fertilization, Implantation, and Development of the Embryonic Disk

The origin of tissue begins with fertilization of the egg, or ovum, which occurs when sperm contact the egg in the distal part of the uterine tube (Fig. 1-6). The fertilized egg then grows and is termed the **zygote.** The cell mass produces a ball of cells (the **morula**) in the uterine tube. The morula grows and begins migration medially to the uterus, which it reaches at the end of the first week. The uterine cavity meanwhile prepares for the arrival of the fertilized ovum. The uterine lining **(endometrium)** thickens, and capillaries and glands develop to nourish the ovum. Estrogen and progesterone control this cyclical event (Fig. 1-7). The morula increases in size and is termed a **blastocyst.** As the blastocyst swells, it becomes hollow and develops a small inner cell mass. When this blastocyst or zygote reaches the uterine cavity, it attaches to the sticky wall of the uterus and becomes embedded in its surface. The cells of the zygote digest the uterine endometrium, permitting deeper penetration. This process is known as **implantation.** If no fertilized ovum reaches the uterine cavity, the development of capillaries and glands is terminated by menstruation (Fig. 1-8).

Two small cavities develop on either side of the inner cell mass. They reach each other in the center, where a small disk (the **embryonic disk**) is formed (Fig. 1-9). The embryonic disk becomes the embryo, composed of the common walls of the two adjacent sacs. One sac is lined with **ectodermal** cells, which will form the outer body covering **(epithelium).** The other sac is lined with

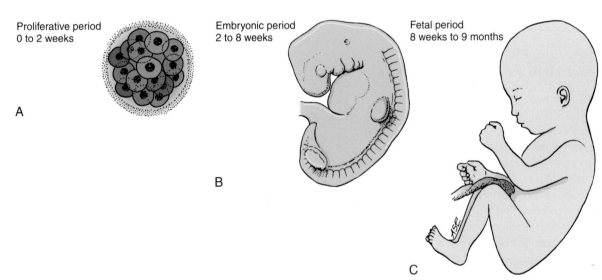

Fig. 1-5 **The developing human passes through three periods of growth. A,** Proliferative period: the first 2 weeks when cell division is prevalent. **B,** Embryonic period: from the second to the eighth weeks. **C,** Fetal period: from the eighth week to birth.

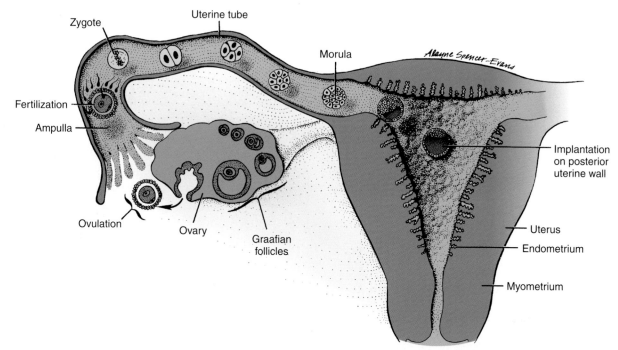

Fig. I-6 Schematic diagram of the uterus and uterine tubes reveals the path of sperm to the distal tube, in which fertilization of the newly appearing ovum from the adjacent ovary occurs. The resultant zygote travels to uterus while undergoing cleavage, and implantation occurs on seventh day after conception.

Fig. I-7 Implantation of a fertilized ovum (zygote) in wall of uterus. Outer cells of trophoblast digest uterine cells to implant. An embryoblast develops within cell mass. As the mass expands, a surrounding cavity is formed.

endodermal cells. On the dorsal surface of the embryonic disk, the ectoderm forms the **neural plate,** whose lateral boundaries elevate to form a **neural tube** that will become the brain and spinal cord (Fig. 1-10). The endodermal cells also form a tube, which will become the **gastrointestinal tract.** As this tube elongates, it anteriorly develops outpouchings that form the pharyngeal pouches, lung buds, liver, gallbladder, pancreas, and urinary bladder (Fig. 1-11).

Next, cells develop between the ectodermal and endodermal layers in the embryonic disk. This area becomes the **mesodermal** layer. These cells will develop into the

CLINICAL COMMENT

Environmental teratogens may affect the development of normal cells, tissues, organs, or organ systems. A defect in the development of a group of cells is considerably less damaging than a defect in an organ or organ system. The smaller and less complex the development, the less extensive the problem created. Development is also related to timing. Tissues are most susceptible to defective development when they begin to differentiate in the embryonic period (2 to 8 weeks).

Fig. 1-8 Cyclical events of ovulatory cycle.
Top, Endocrine changes: ovulation is controlled by estrogen and progesterone. *Center,* Ovarian changes: the ovum matures, is expelled from ovary on fourteenth day, and if fertilized, becomes implanted in uterine wall 7 days later. *Bottom,* Uterine changes: uterine wall thickens and prepares for implantation each month. If implantation does not occur, uterine wall erodes with loss of blood vessels and gland ducts (menstruation).

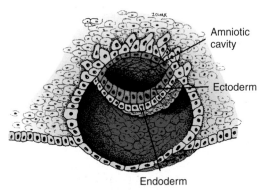

Fig. 1-9 Second small cavity lined with ectoderm develops *(amniotic cavity).* The other cavity (yolk sac) is lined with endoderm. The two cell layers contact in the center to form an area of ectoderm and endoderm for embryonic disk.

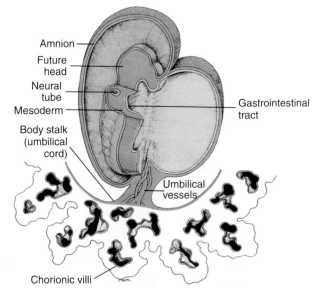

Fig. 1-10 A 3-week human embryo, viewed from the ventral-lateral aspect, illustrating an elongating gastrointestinal tube and a dorsally located neural tube.

muscles, skeleton, and blood cells of the embryo (Fig. 1-12). Mesodermal cells also accompany the elongating digestive tube and support its walls with muscle growth. This enables function and assists in the formation of organs arising from the developing gastrointestinal tube. From these three layers—ectoderm, mesoderm, and endoderm—develop all tissues of the body, as well as the complex organs (see Fig. 1-12).

DEVELOPMENT OF HUMAN TISSUES

Epithelial Tissue

The skin is a dual organ that has an **epidermis,** a surface cell layer that develops from the surface of ectodermal cells, and a **dermis,** which arises from the underlying

mesoderm. The dermis originates in the **somites,** the masses of mesoderm that lie on either side of the neural tube. From this mesoderm come both the dermis of the epithelium and the visceral mesoderm that covers the yolk sac and later becomes the gastrointestinal tract (Fig. 1-13). Therefore, all the muscles functioning in peristalsis of the intestines arise from this mesoderm.

Initially, the embryo is covered with a single layer of ectodermal cells (Fig. 1-14, *A*). By 11 to 12 weeks, this ectodermal layer of epithelium thickens into four layers. From the basal layer of cells come the more superficial

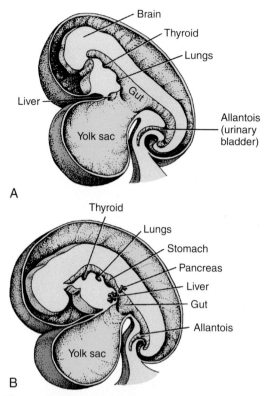

A

B

Fig. 1-11 Further development of the gastrointestinal tract. A, At 4½ weeks and **B,** at 5 weeks. Outpouchings of the intestinal tube form gastrointestinal organs.

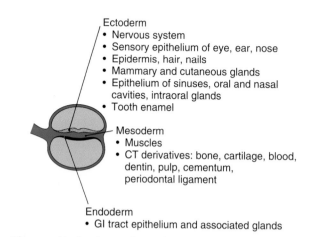

Ectoderm
- Nervous system
- Sensory epithelium of eye, ear, nose
- Epidermis, hair, nails
- Mammary and cutaneous glands
- Epithelium of sinuses, oral and nasal cavities, intraoral glands
- Tooth enamel

Mesoderm
- Muscles
- CT derivatives: bone, cartilage, blood, dentin, pulp, cementum, periodontal ligament

Endoderm
- GI tract epithelium and associated glands

Fig. 1-12 Derivatives of ectoderm, mesoderm, and endoderm germ layers.

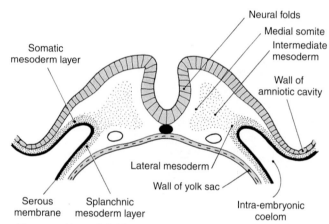

Fig. 1-13 Neural folds and somites in transverse section at approximately 20 days after conception. Medial somite *(mesoderm)* forms the axial skeleton that surrounds neural tube. Intermediate mesoderm forms striated muscle of body, and lateral mesoderm forms dermis of the epithelium of the body wall *(somatic)* and gastrointestinal tract *(splanchnic).*

cells of the epithelium (Fig. 1-14, *B*). Later, **melanocytes** invade and pigment the skin. At birth, the skin may show varying degrees of keratinization. Hair, teeth, nails, and mammary, sebaceous, and salivary glands all develop from a combination of epidermal and dermal cells. This development occurs when epithelial cells proliferate, invade the underlying dermis, and finally differentiate into glands or teeth, with both the epidermis and dermis contributing to each of these structures.

Epithelial-mesenchymal interactions are the necessary interactions of an epithelium and underlying mesenchyme that determine the terminally differentiated tissue. There are many examples of this process including tooth and salivary gland induction and differentiation during development.

Nervous System

Brain and spinal cord

The neural folds appear during the third prenatal week. The lateral edges of the neural plate begin to elevate as folds arising dorsally (see Fig. 1-9). These folds represent the first change in shape of the embryo's body from the flat sheet of cells (see Fig. 1-8). These folds reach the midline, first in the cervical region, and then the neural tube closes both anteriorly and posteriorly (Fig. 1-15). When the anterior tube closes, it shows three dilations that form the primary brain vesicles, the **forebrain, midbrain,** and **hindbrain** (Fig. 1-16, *A*). The neural tube bends forward just behind the midbrain and backward behind the hindbrain (Fig. 1-16, *C* and *D*). The **cerebral hemispheres** develop from the forebrain vesicles. The midbrain is a pathway from the cerebral cortex to centers in the **pons** and **cerebellum** of the hindbrain. The fifth cranial nerve develops in the midbrain (Fig. 1-16, *B* to *D*). The cerebral hemispheres of the forebrain develop into the **frontal, temporal,** and **occipital lobes.**

Fig. 1-14 Development of the skin. A, At 4 weeks and **B,** at 36 weeks. Initial layer of epithelial cells thickens into multiple layers, and underlying connective tissue becomes dermis. Dermis and epithelium combine to become skin.

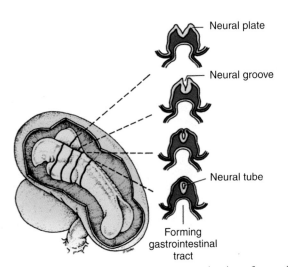

Fig. 1-15 *Left,* Dorsal view of closing neural tube of 3-week human embryo. Closure occurs initially in the dorsal area, then anteriorly and posteriorly. *Right,* Transverse sections of neural folds appear anteriorly, and those of closed neural tube are in the midbrain region.

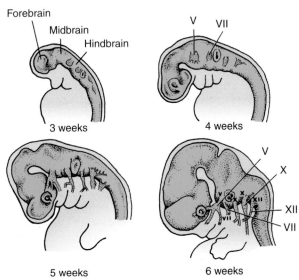

Fig. 1-16 Development of cranial nerves. A, 3 weeks; **B,** 4 weeks; **C,** 5 weeks; **D,** 6 weeks. At 3 weeks, the forebrain has enlarged, and sensory vesicles are laterally located. At 4 and 5 weeks, the forebrain has bent forward, and cranial nerves have grown into tissues they innervate. At 6 weeks, the anterior brain has enlarged and bent back on the posteriorly located cerebellum.

Cranial nerves

The ventricles of the brain are continuous and connect posteriorly with the spinal cord. The walls of the neural tube are lined with neuroepithelium. As these cells proliferate, they differentiate into **neuroblasts** and become the white and gray matter of the spinal cord. Neuroblasts are primitive nerve cells that develop into adult nerve cells called the **neurons.** These cells do not divide further. Along the surface of the developing brain and spinal cord, neural crest cells form the sensory system of the dorsal root ganglia of the cranial and spinal nerves (Fig. 1-17). The neural crest cells also contribute to tissues of the face, such as cartilage, muscles, teeth, and ligaments.

Fig. 1-17 Migration pathway of neural crest cells from neural folds to the developing face.

Connective Tissue

Connective tissue proper

Connective tissue develops from the somites as fibroblasts migrating from either side of the neural tube (see Fig. 1-13). Early in formation, the ventromedial part of the somite differentiates into the **sclerotome,** the dorsolateral part becomes the **dermatome,** and a third division becomes the intermediate mesoderm or **myotome.** The medial sclerotome differentiates into **mesenchymal cells,** which become **osteoblasts, chondroblasts,** and **fibroblasts.** A large part of the embryonic skeleton develops from these cells. Dermatome cells form the dermis, the subcutaneous tissue, and the **visceral mesoderm,** which supports the endoderm of the gastrointestinal tract, as well as a system of mesenteries that stabilize and support the gastrointestinal tract (Fig. 1-18). Also, connective tissue arises from the somites, providing supporting connective tissues, bones, cartilage, tendons, and ligaments. The tendons connect the muscles to the skeleton as they develop. Connective tissue also functions as capsules of glands and the supporting tissues within them.

Blood and lymphatic tissues

Blood is a specialized connective tissue that is composed of seven liters of fluid and cells in the body. The blood contains formed elements that are the red blood cells or **erythrocytes,** white blood cells or **leukocytes,** and blood platelets suspended in a liquid termed **plasma.**

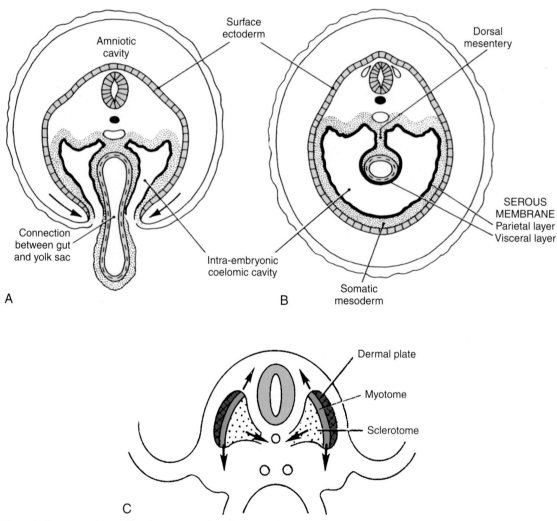

Fig. 1-18 **Cross sections of embryo. A** and **B** illustrate the yolk sac's role in development of the gastrointestinal tube. The developing body wall is growing ventrally, closing the ventral opening. **C,** Contributions of somite to skin, muscles, and cartilage. Cartilage forms a support for the spinal column *(sclerotome),* which surrounds neural tube. Contribution of somitic mesoderm *(dermal plate)* to the body wall seen in **B.** Muscles arise from intermediate mesoderm *(myotome).*

The red blood cells are most numerous (5×10^3 per mm³), and they carry oxygen from the lungs by means of a substance termed **hemoglobin** and also carry carbon dioxide from the cells of the tissue to the lungs by both the hemoglobin of the red blood cell and the plasma of the blood. Thus, blood is a pathway for conducting blood cells throughout the body. The white blood cells or leukocytes are few compared with the red (6,500 to 10,000/ml) and function in defending the body against bacteria. The leukocytes only travel in the blood vessels from their site of origin to the area of infection where they leave the blood vessel, migrating between the endothelial cells to travel in tissue spaces to the site of infection. Three types of **granulocytes** exist: **neutrophils, eosinophils,** and **basophils,** and two types of **granulocytes** and **agranulocytes: lymphocytes** and **monocytes.** The neutrophils (polymorphonuclear leukocytes) are the most numerous of the white blood cells, representing 60% to 70%, and function in destroying bacteria that invade the tissue spaces. The platelets are small, disk-shaped cell fragments carried in the blood and originate from megakaryocytes in the marrow spaces. There are 300,000 to 350,000 platelets in 1 mm³ of blood; they function to limit hemorrhage to the endothelium of the vessel.

The **lymphatic system** is composed of the lymph nodes, thymus and the spleen as well as the vessels that carry the lymph throughout the body. The lymphatic system is a protective mechanism as the immunologic defense of the body. The lymphoid system destroys bacteria, viruses, and invasive microorganisms. The lymphatics are made up of the innate and the adaptive immune systems. The cells that constitute the innate and adaptive immune systems are the B cells, the T cells, the NK cells, and macrophages, and they are all formed in the bone marrow. The T cells migrate to the thymus to become immunocompetent. The thymus consists of a cortex and medulla and is composed of epithelia and reticular cells and macrophages. The medulla consists primarily of thymocytes that are immunocompetent T cells. Throughout the lymphatic vascular system are lymph nodes that act as filters for all bacteria or substances foreign to the body. The lymph nodes are composed of a cortex and a medulla, the cortex is composed of lymph nodules and the medulla is composed of lymph sinuses interposed with cords of lymph cells. The spleen is the other lymphatic organ and is composed of a cortex and the hilum where the blood vessels enter and exit. The spleen functions in T- and B-cell formation and also in blood formation if the need arises.

Cartilage and bone

The initial skeletal component in the embryo is **cartilage.** Cartilage cells arise from the sclerotome and migrate to surround the notochord and spinal cord, which form the spinal column (see Fig. 1-18, *C*). The skeleton develops in the same segmental pattern as the muscles do (Figs. 1-19 and 1-20). Chondroblasts also form cartilage in the appendages, the cranium, and the face, which first appear in the fifth prenatal week. Cartilage cells undergo both **appositional** (exogenous) and **interstitial** (endogenous) growth (Fig. 1-19, *B*).

Apposition of new layers of cartilage occurs on the surface of cartilage, and interstitial growth involves the proliferation and expansion of the cells within the matrix (Fig. 1-19, *B*). A supportive cartilage skeleton is produced rapidly to support the soft tissues of the growing embryo. Later, most of this same cartilage skeleton is replaced by bone, which offers more rigidity and strength as muscles attach to it, making movement possible (Fig. 1-19, *C*). Most cartilage appears clear and glasslike and is called **hyaline cartilage.** Cartilage may

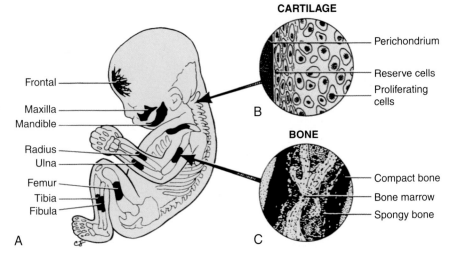

Fig. 1-19 Embryo's skeleton **(A)** illustrating development of cartilage and bones. **B,** Cartilage development by both surface apposition and internal interstitial growth. **C,** Endochondral bone development in the shaft of a long bone.

Frontal
Maxilla
Mandible
Radius
Ulna
Femur
Tibia
Fibula

A

CARTILAGE

Perichondrium
Reserve cells
Proliferating cells

B

BONE

Compact bone
Bone marrow
Spongy bone

C

also contain elastic fibers and be termed **elastic** or **fibrous cartilage.** The intervertebral disks, for example, are fibrous cartilage, but the external ear contains elastic cartilage. Cartilage combines the properties of elasticity and strength.

Bone replaces cartilage by a process termed **endochondral bone development** (Fig. 1-21). In this case a small blood vessel enters the cartilage shaft (diaphysis), the cartilage calcifies and disintegrates in the center, and a marrow space is formed (Fig. 1-21, *B*). New bone develops on the surface of cartilage spicules that border the marrow space (Fig. 1-21, *C*). Small blood vessels enter the head of the long bones, and secondary ossification centers appear, repeating the process that took place in the shaft of the long bone (Fig. 1-21, *D*). During the growth period a developing cartilage disk remains in the neck of each long bone and bone forms on either side. This disk is known as the **epiphyseal line** and will remain as long as the bone is forming. The wider part of the diaphysis adjacent to the epiphyseal line is known as the **metaphysis** (Fig. 1-21, *D*). Cartilage develops and expands by **interstitial growth,** which is growth within the cartilage matrix by each cartilage cell enlarging and forming matrix around each cell. New bone forms along the cartilage margins of the epiphyseal line. After bone replaces the epiphysis, cartilage is limited to covering the heads of long bones, the nasal septum, the ears, and a few other sites.

Direct transformation of connective tissue into bone may also take place. In this case, collagen fibers of connective tissue organize into closely knit meshwork, and this matrix gradually calcifies into bone by a process termed **intramembranous bone formation** or membranous bone formation (Fig. 1-22). It is much simpler for bone cells to organize in this manner and to form

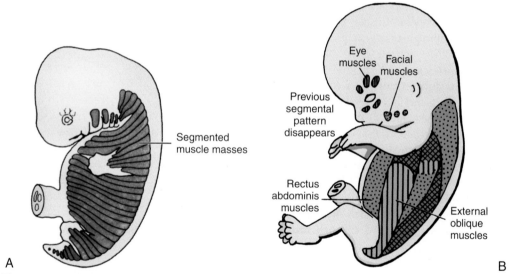

Fig. 1-20 A, Primitive myotome in skeletal muscle formation in an embryo. **B,** Differentiation of skeletal muscle by enlargement of fibers and attachment to bony skeleton to become functional units. The previous segmental pattern disappears.

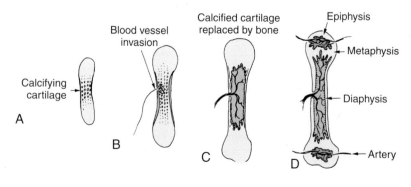

Fig. 1-21 Schematic diagram of endochondral ossification as seen in developing long bones of the body. A, Original hyaline cartilage is calcified in the center of the diaphysis. **B,** A blood vessel invades the center of the shaft. **C,** Marrow space appears in the center of the shaft, and bone forms around the diaphysis. **D,** Bone formation continues in the shaft, and secondary ossification sites appear in the heads *(epiphysis)* of the bones. A disk of cartilage remains between bone forming in the head and the shaft (epiphyseal line).

spicules of bone through coalescence with neighboring spicules until a bony plate is formed. The bones of the face and cranium develop in this manner.

DNA transcription is an example of **gene expression.** Transcription generates mRNAs that carry information for protein synthesis, as well as transferring ribosomal and other RNA molecules that have structural and catalytic functions. RNA molecules synthesize RNA polymerase enzymes, which make an RNA copy of a DNA sequence.

Muscle

By the tenth prenatal week, muscle cells (myoblasts) have begun migrating from the myotome, following a segmental pattern similar to that of the bony skeleton (see Figs. 1-19 and 1-20). They gradually differentiate into elongated, multinucleated muscle fibers, which are specialized cells with the property of contractility. In this manner, muscle is able to provide motion on the basis of structural and functional characteristics.

Muscle is divided into three types: skeletal, smooth, and cardiac. Later, these skeletal muscles lose their segmental pattern of development as they acquire insertion on skeletal elements. These muscle fibers become the **striated voluntary muscles,** which divide into groups that supply the dorsal and ventral parts of the limbs and provide both the deep and superficial muscle fibers (see Fig. 1-20, *B*). These muscles are called striated because they have lines across them that are the contraction sites that cause the muscles to function.

Muscle cells also migrate to the gastrointestinal tract and support the trachea, bronchi, urogenital tract, and larger blood vessels. These muscle cells develop and become oriented in the direction in which their contractility will be exerted. They are termed **smooth muscle cells** and are under the control of the autonomic nervous system, not under conscious control as are skeletal muscles. The blood vessels that develop in the head region, limbs, and body wall gain their muscular coat from local mesenchyme.

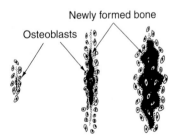

Osteoblasts   Newly formed bone

Fig. 1-22 Membranous bone formation that takes place in connective tissue. Initial membranous sites grow by apposition of new bone on their surfaces.

Cardiovascular System

The cardiovascular system originates from cells termed **angioblasts,** which arise from **angiogenic clusters** from the visceral mesoderm located in the walls of the yolk sac during the third week of prenatal life (Fig. 1-23). As these cells separate into clusters, the outer cells organize into a series of elongating tubes and the inner cells become blood cells (Fig. 1-24). For the first few weeks, nutrition moves from the yolk sac to the embryo through the developing **vitelline vascular system** (Fig. 1-25). The entire blood vascular system within the embryo is created in the same manner with longitudinal growth of vessels and the appearance of blood cells within them. As vessels begin to develop in the embryo, they, in turn, form a vascular network connected to the placenta. Because it traverses the umbilical cord, this network is termed the **umbilical system** (see Fig. 1-25). Through this umbilical system, nutrition and oxygen are conducted to the embryo, and carbon dioxide and wastes to the placenta. By the fourth week, the heart begins to beat. This vascular system takes over the functions as

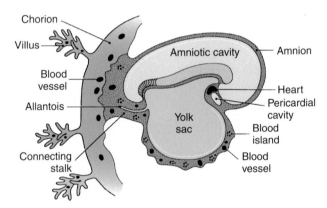

Chorion
Villus
Blood vessel
Allantois
Connecting stalk
Amniotic cavity
Amnion
Heart
Pericardial cavity
Blood island
Blood vessel
Yolk sac

Fig. 1-23 Origin of blood cells and blood vessels in walls of yolk sac, placenta, and body stalk in a 2½-week-old embryo.

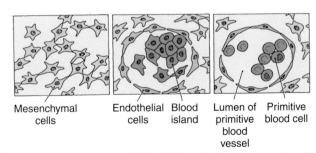

Mesenchymal cells
Endothelial cells
Blood island
Lumen of primitive blood vessel
Primitive blood cell

Fig. 1-24 Appearance of blood islands from mesenchymal cells in the location noted in Figure 1-22. The more peripheral cells form capillary walls, and the inner cells form red blood cells. The tubes or capillaries then lengthen.

the vitelline system expires because the yolk sac has nothing more to contribute (see Fig. 1-25).

Other mesenchyme cells migrate into the pericardial area to function in the development of heart tubes, and these cells later differentiate into cardiac muscle.

Fig. 1-25 Development of blood vascular system in an embryo. *1,* In the yolk sac, vitelline circulation develops, persisting for only a few weeks until this nutritional source is exhausted. *2,* The umbilical system develops in the umbilical cord, supplying the embryo and fetus with oxygen and nutrients until birth.

Two angiogenic cell clusters initially form the straight bilateral endocardial heart tubes, which fuse during the third week. They then enlarge and bend back on themselves (Fig. 1-26). As the great vessels that bring blood to the heart enlarge and become more extensive, the heart grows and internal partitioning begins. An opening persists between the right and left atria **(foramen ovale)** until birth. As the heart tube enlarges and twists during development, strands of muscle take on the arrangement of parallel fibers. Like striated muscle, cardiac muscle fibers are also striated and have an array of specialized junctional complexes between adjacent cells called **intercalated disks.** The myofibrils on either side of these disks exert contraction through the interaction of these many cells. Cardiac muscle is thus not under conscious control and begins to beat during the fourth week. Umbilical circulation then becomes active in transporting oxygen and nutrition from the placenta.

CLINICAL COMMENT

The human placenta is often considered in terms of its function in exchanging fetal oxygen and carbon dioxide. It also exchanges nutrients and electrolytes, such as proteins and carbohydrates. The placenta produces hormones, such as progesterone and estrogen, which can help maintain pregnancy. It also produces a lactogenic hormone that gives the fetus first priority on circulating maternal blood glucose.

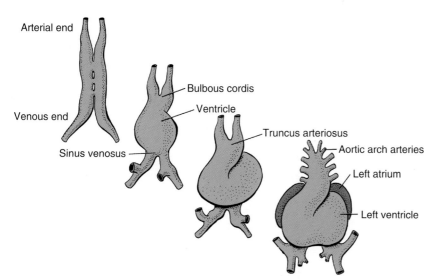

Fig. 1-26 Development of the four-chamber heart from fusion of two bilateral endocardial heart tubes. Tubes fold laterally into a single tube, which is next divided by internal septa into a four-chamber heart.

Developmental Abnormalities

Developmental defects may be environmental or hereditary. Most developmental defects are usually an interaction between environmental and hereditary factors. Not much can be done to reduce hereditary factors in humans. However, we have learned a great deal about dietary and stress factors and when they may affect development. For example, we know the developing human is least susceptible to teratogens during the proliferative period, which is the first 2 to 3 weeks after conception. Because of multiple cell mitosis, compensation may occur. However, the third through the eighth weeks are the most critical time in development because this is the period of differentiation. During this time, the embryo tissues and organs are developing into specific structures. Serious malformations may arise during this period. The fetal period from 8 weeks until birth is a declining period of susceptibility. Only minor defects may occur during this period.

Hereditary causes of abnormalities may result from either genetic or chromosomal abnormalities. Many chromosomal abnormalities may result from an increase or a decrease in number from the normal number of chromosomes (46) in humans.

Genetic abnormalities can perpetuate from one generation to the next. Abnormal development may be caused by expression of defective genes, which may be dominant or recessive. A dominant gene expresses itself whether it is on one member of the pair of homologous chromosomes or both pairs. A recessive gene expresses itself only when it is present on both members of the homozygous chromosomes. An example of a dominant genetic abnormality is dentinogenesis imperfecta, which results in defective dentin formation. Some examples of autosomal recessive genetic disorders include sickle cell disease and cystic fibrosis. There are also sex (X-linked) recessive defects including hemophilia and Duchenne's muscular dystrophy.

SELF-EVALUATION QUESTIONS

1. What is the smallest unit of structure, and what are its eight functions in the body?
2. Name the structures found in cell cytoplasm, and describe their functions.
3. Name the cells that do not undergo division.
4. Describe changes in the embryonic disk during the third and fourth prenatal weeks.
5. Define the cell cycle and describe the activities that occur in the G1 and G2 phases.
6. What is the significance of the angiogenic clusters found in the vitelline and umbilical vascular systems?
7. What develops from the gastrointestinal tract?
8. Describe the characteristics of the three prenatal periods.
9. Name three types of cartilage, and describe where they are in the human body.
10. Name and describe three types of muscle fibers.

 Consider the Patient

Discussion: Two diagnostic tests are available. Amniocentesis is the withdrawal of a small amount of amniotic fluid; it reveals genetic disorders and age of the fetus. Fetal ultrasound reflects body tissues to the video monitor; it reveals abnormal or normal development, vitality, sex, and fetal age. Neither test causes tissue damage. Ultrasound would be the choice in this case.

Suggested Reading

Avery JK, editor: *Oral development and histology,* ed 3, Stuttgart, 2002, Thieme Medical.

Carlson BM: *Human embryology and developmental biology,* ed 3, St. Louis, 2005, Mosby.

Hart TC, Marazita ML, Wright JT: The impact of molecular genetics on oral health paradigms, *Crit Rev Oral Biol Med* 11:26-56, 2000.

Moore KL: *The developing human,* ed 7, Philadelphia, WB Saunders, 2003.

Nishida, et al.: Corneal reconstruction with tissue engineered cell sheets composed of autologus oral mucosal epithelium, *N Engl J Med* 351:1187-1196, 2004.

Sadler TG, editor: *Langman's medical embryology,* ed 9, Baltimore, 2004, Lippincott Williams & Wilkins.

Sperber GH: *Craniofacial development,* Hamilton, Canada, 2001, BC Decker.

Tortora GJ: *Principles of human anatomy,* ed 7, New York, 1995, Harper Collins.

2

STRUCTURE AND FUNCTION OF CELLS, TISSUES, AND ORGANS

CHAPTER OUTLINE

Overview

Cells and Tissues

  Epithelial Tissue

  Neural Tissue

  Connective Tissue

    Cartilage

    Bone

    Blood

    Lymphocytes

Muscle Tissue

Organs and Organ Systems

  Integumentary or Skin

    System

  Neural System

  Skeletal System

  Digestive System

  Respiratory System

  Vascular System

Lymphatic System

Muscular System

Endocrine System

Urinary System

Reproductive Systems

Special Senses

Self-Evaluation Questions

Consider the Patient Discussion

Suggested Reading

LEARNING OBJECTIVES

After reading this chapter the student will be able to:

- discuss how the various tissues of the body build on one another
- describe the components of specific organ systems such as the skin and its accessories, the digestive system, the respiratory system, the vascular system, the lymphatic system, the endocrine system, the urinary system, the reproductive system, and the special senses
- list general functions of each of these organ systems

KEY TERMS

Actin

Afferent (sensory) system

Autonomic nervous system

Axon

Axon terminals

Cancellous bone

Cardiac muscle

Cell body

Central nervous system

Compact bone

Connective tissue proper

Cytoplasm

Dendrite

Dense, loose, loose connective

  tissue with special properties

Dermis

Ear

Efferent (motor) system

Elastic cartilage

Endomysium

Epidermis

Epimysium

Equilibrium

Fibrous cartilage

Hyaline cartilage

Myosin

Neuroglia

KEY TERMS—cont'd

Neurons	Pseudostratified	Stratified epithelium
Olfactory organ	Simple epithelium	Sympathetic and
Perikaryon	Skeletal or voluntary muscle	parasympathetic
Perimysium	Smooth or involuntary muscle	Taste modality
Phagocytic	Somatic nervous system	

OVERVIEW

This second chapter describes the structure and function of the body's primary tissues: epithelial, neural, connective, and muscle. Chapter 1 presented information about how these tissues developed. This chapter continues with a description of the tissues and of how they function in making up organs and organ systems. This chapter initially describes cells and tissue types, and their structure, location, and function in the body. For example, simple squamous epithelium lines the blood vascular and respiratory systems, the kidney, most glands, and the intestine. Stratified squamous epithelium, on the other hand, covers the body and is the lining of the mouth, the pharynx, larynx, vagina, anus, and part of the urinary bladder.

Neural tissue is the next tissue type considered. Both the **central nervous system** (CNS), which is composed of the brain and spinal cord, and the nerves and their ganglial, which comprise the peripheral nervous system, are described. The basic structural unit of the nervous system is the neuron. Along with the supporting neuroglial cells, this tissue forms a communication network. The two properties of a neuron are its irritability and conductivity, both of which enable neurons to react and respond to stimuli. The third tissue type discussed is connective tissue, characterized by its abundant matrix and composed of fibers and amorphous substance. This tissue is classified according to associated cells, fibers, location, and function. Connective tissue proper consists of loose and dense connective tissue and loose connective tissue with special properties. Two other specialized types of connective tissue are cartilage and bone. Three types of cartilage are described—hyaline, elastic, and fibrous—followed by both cancellous (spongy) and compact (dense) bone. A fourth type of connective tissue is blood and lymph that function to carry oxygen and nutrients to the body tissues and to carry carbon dioxide to the lungs, where it is eliminated.

The three types of muscle—striated, voluntary smooth, and cardiac involuntary—are described according to cell shape, matrix, and their functions in the body. Organ systems are then described to illustrate how tissues combine to carry out specialized functions in the human body. These organ systems are integumentary, digestive, respiratory, vascular, lymphatic, endocrine, urinary, reproductive, and special senses. Correlative tables help explain this information. These descriptions are meant only as an introduction to tissues of the human body; for more complete information, refer to a comprehensive textbook of histology.

CELLS AND TISSUES

Epithelial Tissue

Epithelial tissue is composed of different layers. One is a superficial layer of closely packed sheets of cells covering the external surface of the body. Another, the dermis, is the connective tissue layer of the skin underlying the epithelial tissue. A much thinner layer of epithelial tissue also lines the internal cavities of the body and the tubes that drain glands and carry blood throughout the body. Most epithelium has the capability of cell renewal by mitosis of the basal cells, and the rate of renewal is dependent on the location of the epithelium in the body. For example, human buccal mucosa (Fig. 2-1) renews in 10 to 14 days, whereas the junctional epithelium of the gingiva renews in 4 to 6 days.

The dermis is closely associated with the epidermis and has an interdigitating relationship with it in some areas. Because epithelium does not contain blood vessels, the skin depends on vessels located in the connective tissue of the dermis. The vessels are in close proximity, nourishing the skin and playing an important part in its function of thermal regulation. Nerves also exist in the dermis, and some penetrate the epithelial cells to function as receptors. Sweat glands, hair follicles and their associated sebaceous glands, and erector pili muscles are located in the dermis and subcutaneous tissue. Ectoderm is the source of the epithelial lining of some internal organs, but not of all epithelial-lined surfaces. For example, the epithelial lining of the alimentary canal is of endodermal origin. The epithelial lining of the peritoneal cavity and the endothelial lining of blood vessels are from mesoderm. Epithelium is described according to cell shape and cell arrangement in one or more layers. Some cells form a single layer known as **simple epithelium.** Epithelium with all cells in contact with the basal lamina, but not with the surface, is known as **pseudostratified.** The type consisting of several cell layers with only the basal cell layer in contact with the basal lamina is known as **stratified epithelium** (Fig. 2-2). Further modifications are based on cell shape. For example, the surface cells may be flattened, as in keratinized stratified squamous epithelium of the palm of the hand (see Fig. 2-2).

Dermis   Basal cells   Superficial cells

Fig. 2-1 Stratified squamous nonkeratinized epithelium from the oral cavity. Darker stained cells are basal cells. These are dividing to form more superficial layers. As the cells develop in the basal layer, they gradually migrate to the surface and are then lost by attrition.

Fig. 2-2 Stratified squamous keratinized epithelium. This epithelium is distinctive in that its surface layers are dead and non-nucleated, and cell contents are filled with keratin. This skin is located on the palms of the hands and soles of the feet.

TABLE 2-1 CLASSIFICATION OF EPITHELIA

Cell type	Cell shape	Cell modifications	Characteristics	Location
Simple				
1. Squamous				
a. Endothelial	Spindle			Lines heart, blood, and lymph vessels
b. Mesothelial	Oval to polygonal			Lines pleural, pericardial, and peritoneal cavities
2. Cuboidal	Cube		Cilia may appear	Kidney, glands, respiratory passages
3. Columnar	Rodlike		Microvilli, cilia may appear	Most glands, small intestines, respiratory passages
4. Pseudostratified	Rodlike with thin section		Cilia, stereocilia	Respiratory passages, male reproductive organs
Stratified				
1. Squamous	Polyhedral		Intercellular bridges	Covering of the body, mouth, pharynx, vagina
2. Columnar	Columnar cells on cuboidal or columnar on columnar			Oropharynx, larynx
3. Transitional	Cube to pear		Distension causes cell flattening	Urinary passages, bladder

Epithelial membranes function in one or more of the absorptive processes: contractility, digestion, secretion, excretion, protection, and sensation. Table 2-1 illustrates the classification of epithelia by cell type, cell shape, cell modifications, characteristics, and location.

Neural Tissue

Neural tissue is a second type of tissue. Nerve tissue arises from neuroepithelial cells, which are highly organized areas for reception and correlation. The nervous system carries out numerous functions with only two principal types of cells, which are the **neurons** and the **neuroglia.** Neurons are the nerve cells that receive and conduct impulses and regulate muscle and gland activity. Neuroglial cells are the supporting cells of the nervous system. Each neuron consists of three parts. The first part is the **cell body** or **perikaryon,** which contains the nucleus and the **cytoplasm.** The cytoplasm contains a chromatophilic substance or rough endoplasmic reticulum (RER). The function of the RER, as in other cells, is protein synthesis. Sensory ganglia are swellings associated with each of the spinal nerves containing unipolar or pseudounipolar ganglion cells held together with a connective tissue capsule. These ganglia are called dorsal root ganglia of the spinal cord (Fig. 2-3). Ganglia associated with the cranial nerves include the trigeminal, facial, glossopharyngeal, and hypoglossal cranial nerves.

Proteins travel from the perikaryon into the second part of the neuron, the **axon,** which is a long, thin singular process that varies in length from a few millimeters to several feet or more. The axon conducts nerve impulses away from the nerve cell body. It terminates by branching into **axon terminals** or synaptic end bulbs (Fig. 2-4). Axons outside the CNS are protected and insulated by a myelin sheath, which is a multilayer of phospholipid produced by the neurilemma (Schwann's

cells). The third component of the neuron is the **dendrite,** usually multiple, which receives impulses and conducts these impulses to the cell body (Fig. 2-5).

Neuroglial cells carry out the functions of support. These are 5 to 50 times more numerous than neurons. Neuroglial cells protect and support nerve cells, and some are even **phagocytic,** meaning that they ingest bacteria.

Connective Tissue

Connective tissue varies in its proportion of cells, fibers, and intercellular substance and its location in the body.

Fig. 2-3 Nerve cells of a ganglion composed of neuronal cell bodies with singular nucleoli. A sensory ganglion of a spinal nerve appears as swelling of a nerve; these are called dorsal root ganglia.

Fig. 2-4 A nerve fiber surrounded by a myelin sheath and a Schwann cell. Myelin insulates the nerve axon and is produced by Schwann's cells. The axon is a single thin process capable of transmitting impulses to other neurons. Impulses are received by the dendrites and travel to the cell body and then the axon terminals, where they may contact dendrites of an adjacent nerve cell.

⬚ CLINICAL COMMENT

Oral infections can cause pain, tenderness, swelling, and enlarged lymph nodes. Pain is due to the response of a nerve receptor and its transmission to the brain, with corresponding efferent response to both autonomic and somatic systems. This results in a change in vascular tone, causing swelling. Lymph nodes enlarge as defense cells proliferate and become active, filtering and destroying the bacteria and their products in the local lymph nodes.

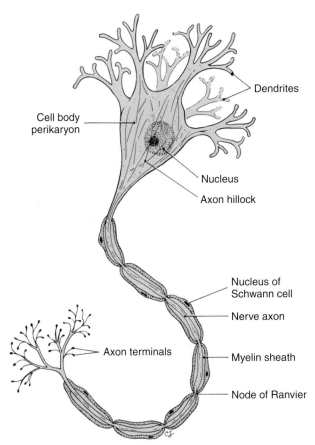

Fig. 2-5 Diagram of a nerve cell and its processes. Myelin insulates the axon and is produced by Schwann's cells. Impulses received by the dendrites travel to the cell body and then to the axon terminals, where they may contact the dendrites of an adjacent nerve cell.

Fig. 2-6 Appearance of loose areolar connective tissue. Observe the collagen and elastin fibers and numerous fibroblasts seen in loose connective tissue.

Fig. 2-7 Appearance of dense regular connective tissue. Large bundles of collagen fibers appear in longitudinal section, with a few pale-stained fibroblasts interspersed between them. The faint banding of these collagen fibers cannot be seen at this magnification.

Connective tissue proper is classified as **loose** (Fig. 2-6), **dense** (Fig. 2-7), or **loose connective tissue with special properties.** It functions in tissue support, and protection of the body parts, in areas of fluid exchange and storage of adipose (fat) tissue. The ligaments that attach bones and the tendons that attach muscles to bones are forms of dense connective tissue.

Cartilage

The three types of cartilage are **hyaline** (Fig. 2-8), **elastic** (Fig. 2-9), and **fibrous** (Fig. 2-10). These are known as specialized connective tissues. Hyaline cartilage is the most common type of cartilage and is present in the nose, the tracheal rings, the larynx, the articular rings and bronchi, the ventral ends of the ribs, and the articulating surfaces of the long bones. The elastic cartilage has abundant elastic fibers in its matrix and functions in the epiglottis, in the cuneiform cartilage of the larynx, and in the auditory canal and tube. Fibrous cartilage contains

bundles of collagen fibers associated with either hyaline cartilage or dense regular connective tissue. It is located in the vertebral disks and intervertebral areas, the insertion of some tendons, and the pubic symphysis.

Bone

Bone is calcified connective tissue. Although it is one of the harder connective tissues that resists deformation, it is responsive to stress and strain. An example of this is tooth movement, in which fibers embedded in the bone cause compression on one side of the tooth, resulting in

Fig. 2-8 Section of hyaline cartilage found in the adult in the thyroid or tracheal cartilages. The large cells (chondrocytes) are surrounded by a homogenous-appearing cartilage matrix. Only dark-stained nucleoli can be seen in the nucleus. Cells exist in lacunae, which are open spaces in the matrix. Some cells have divided, and two cells appear in the same lacunae.

Fig. 2-10 Fibrous cartilage with bundles of collagen fibers in the matrix. This cartilage is present in the vertebral and articular disks and contains type I collagen. The chondrocytes are arranged in parallel rows between collagen bundles.

Fig. 2-9 Elastic cartilage present in ear, epiglottis, auditory tube, and auditory canal. Elastic fibers are present in the matrix as well as type II collagen fibers, and a perichondrium is present.

| Haversian canals | Concentric lamellae | Lacunae |

Fig. 2-11 Cross section of compact bone. Tubular haversian canals are surrounded by concentric lamellae and lacunae appearing along the lamellae. This pattern indicates the deposition pattern of the bone. Between the haversian systems are some interstitial lamellae. In living bone, osteocytes would appear as live cells within the lacunae.

bone resorption and tension on the other, with subsequent bone formation. Bone is classified as **compact** (dense) or **cancellous** (spongy) (Figs. 2-11 and 2-12). Endochondral and membranous are terms describing their origin and are discussed in other chapters.

Blood

Blood conducts oxygen to the cells, returns carbon dioxide from the cells to the lungs, clots to prevent blood loss, and regulates pH through a buffer system (Fig. 2-13). It also regulates body temperature and provides protection from bacteria through its phagocytic and antigenic properties. Plasma is the fluid part of the blood in which the cells and particulate substances are suspended. Men have about 5 liters of blood, and women have about 4.5 liters, which is about 7% of body weight. The erythrocytes (red blood cells) are not true cells because they have no nucleus or other organelles. However, these cells do have the ability to take oxygen from the lungs, transport it to the tissues, and return carbon dioxide from these tissues to the lungs. Leukocytes (white blood cells) are

Fig. 2-12 Appearance of cancellous bone. Trabeculae of bone are seen with osteoblasts and osteoclasts appearing on their surface. In newly forming intramembranous bone, many osteoblasts would be on the surface of the trabeculae. A few elongated and flattened osteoblasts can be seen on the bone surface. Several thin-walled veins, which contain red blood cells, and scattered connective tissue cells can be seen in the field.

Bone matrix   Osteoblasts

Fig. 2-13 A, Polymorphonuclear leucocytes (white blood cells) are the most abundant of the WBCs. Neutrophils can squeeze through the capillary walls and into infected tissue where they kill invaders (e.g., bacteria) and engulf the remnants by phagocytosis. **B,** Monocytes leave the blood and become macrophages. A single macrophage surrounded by several lymphocytes and red blood cells can be seen. Macrophages are large, phagocytic cells that engulf foreign material (antigens) that enter the body. They are also responsible for phagocytosing dead or dying cells. **C,** Eosinophils are a type of white blood cell that contain granules and take up the red dye eosin. They accumulate wherever allergic reactions (e.g., asthma) take place. Their natural role is in the defense of parasites and other microorganisms. Allergies such as asthma are probably a malfunction of our protective mechanisms and are partially due to eosinophilic reactions. **D,** Basophils are a type of white blood cell that are filled with blue staining granules of chemicals including histamine, serotonin, bradykinin, heparin, and cytokines such as prostaglandins and leukotrienes. Basophils can also digest microorganisms and are responsible for allergy symptoms.

Table 2-2   Formed Elements of the Blood

Element		Number	Function
Erythrocytes		Male: 5.4 million/ml³ Female: 4.8 million/ml³	Oxygen and carbon dioxide pickup and transport
Leukocytes		5000-9000/ml³	
Granular	Neutrophils	55%-65%	Phagocytic to infectious agents
	Eosinophils	1%-3%	Helminthic parasitic diseases
	Basophils	0%-0.7%	Histamine, serotonin, heparin
Nongranular	Lymphocytes	20%-35%	Immunologic response, B, T, and NK cells
	Monocytes	3%-7%	Phagocytic, contribute osteoclasts
Platelets		5000-9000/ml³	Function in clot formation, stimulate cell division

of two types, granular and nongranular. Leukocyte cell types and function are shown in Table 2-2.

Details of cellular and other elements of blood are also noted in Table 2-2. Each type of connective tissue has specific associated cells and fibers with special functions and locations in the body (Table 2-3).

Lymphocytes

Lymphocytes arise and become functional in the bone marrow. They are responsible for the humorally activated immune system.

Lymphocytes circulate in the lymphatic vessels and in the bloodstream, functioning wherever they are called on by antigen actions. T cells have a number of different surface molecules that function into their being called into action. B memory cells also function as well as plasma cells.

Muscle Tissue

The reaction to stimulus is motion, and the basis of motion in a muscle cell is the change from chemical to mechanical energy by enzymatic cleavage of adenosine triphosphate (ATP). This is a result of the action of two proteins, **actin** and **myosin**, which are arranged in the direction of contraction. Muscle is located throughout the body and consists of three types: **skeletal** or **voluntary** (Fig. 2-14), **smooth** or **involuntary** (Fig. 2-15), and **cardiac** (Fig. 2-16). Skeletal muscle allows movement under voluntary control. The involuntary muscle

(smooth muscle) of the alimentary canal assists with digestion and movement of food through the alimentary tract. The involuntary (cardiac) muscle of the heart pumps blood through some 50,000 miles of blood vessels. Therefore, the three muscle types in the body have specific characteristics permitting individualized functions. However, some features of muscle are common to all types. For example, each entire muscle is covered with a **perimysium,** each muscle fascicle (a group of muscle fibers) is covered with an **epimysium,** and each muscle fiber with an **endomysium.** Each muscle type contains actin and myosin, which enables the contractions so vital to muscle function. Table 2-4 shows the muscles' locations and the cells that function within each.

 CLINICAL COMMENT

Muscle is one of the four tissue types found in the human. It is divided into three major types, each with its own unique characteristics. Cardiac and smooth muscle are considered to be involuntary, whereas striated muscle is voluntary. These muscles have their full complement of cells during development and increase in size only by increasing the volume of individual myocytes, rather than by increasing the number of cells.

TABLE 2-3 CLASSIFICATION OF CONNECTIVE TISSUE

Tissue type	Associated cells	Fibers		Location and function
I. Connective tissue proper A. Loose connective tissue	Fibroblasts, macro-phages, mast cells	Yellow elastic White collagen		Fascia, superficial and deep; organ framework support
B. Dense connective tissue 1. Dense regular	Fibroblasts, macrophages	White fibrou		Tendons, ligaments; muscle to bone attachment
2. Dense irregular	Fibroblasts, macrophages	Mostly white fibrous, elastic, and reticular fibers		Sheets, dermis, some sternum, capsules; support of organs
C. Loose connective tissue with special properties 1. Mucous connective tissue	Stellate fibroblasts	Collagenous		Umbilical and vocal cords; support
2. Elastic tissue	Fibroblasts	Yellow elastic		Ligamenta nuchae, vocal cords, support
3. Reticular tissue	Reticular cells	Fine reticular		Framework of lymph node and spleen
4. Adipose tissue	Fat cells	None		Scattered in all loose connective tissue and in deposits
5. Pigment tissue	Melanoblasts	None		Corium of dark skin Choroid and iris of eye
II. Cartilage A. Hyaline cartilage	Chondrocytes	Fine collagenous		Articular and nasal cartilages trachea, bronchi; support
B. Elastic cartilage	Chondrocytes	Elastic, collagenous		External; ear, Eustachian tube, epiglottis; support
C. Fibrous cartilage	Chondrocytes	Collagenous (dense)		Intervertebral disks; support
III. Bone A. Spongy or cancellous	Osteocytes, osteoblasts, osteoclasts	Collagenous		Center of long bones
B. Compact or dense	Osteocytes, osteoclasts, osteoblasts,	Collagenous		Outer shaft of bones
IV. Blood and lymph	Erythrocytes, leukocytes			Blood vascular and lymphatic systems

Striations   Nucleus

Fig. 2-14 Skeletal muscle fibers in longitudinal section. Cross striations are seen as alternating light and dark bands, indicating fiber contraction sites. Each large fiber contains a number of nuclei on the periphery. These are muscle fibers of the arms, legs, and body wall. They provide for body posture, locomotion, and arm movement and are controlled voluntarily.

Nucleus of smooth
muscle cell

Fig. 2-15 Smooth muscle fibers in longitudinal section. These can be compared with skeletal muscle. Smooth muscle fibers are spindle shaped with a large, longitudinal nucleus in the center of the fiber. Small amounts of connective tissue surround the fibers. This muscle surrounds the gastrointestinal tract and muscular blood vessels. It is controlled involuntarily.

TABLE 2-4 CLASSIFICATION OF MUSCLE

Type	Cell shape	Diagrams	Location
A. Skeletal wall, voluntary	Very long multinucleated fiber with cross-striations composed of actin (thin) and myosin (thick) components.		Bony skeleton or fascia, limbs and body, pharynx, upper esophagus
B. Smooth visceral, involuntary	Spindle-shaped fibers with a single elongated nucleus and myofilaments. Nuclei located in center of fiber.		Hollow organs, wall of intestines, ducts of glands, blood vessels
C. Cardiac muscle striated, involuntary	Long cross-striated fibers that branch and contain intercalated disks (junctional complexes). Some muscle fibers are specialized to conduct impulses: Purkinje's fibers. Nuclei in center of fiber.		Wall of heart, major veins opening into the heart

Fig. 2-16 Section of cardiac muscle found in the heart wall. Muscle fibers appear striated and are similar to skeletal muscle fibers, except that some of the fibers branch. The nuclei of these fibers are located centrally, as seen in smooth muscle, and the areas at the ends of the nuclei are pale staining.

 CLINICAL COMMENT

> The heart, which weighs less than a pound, is the size of a clenched fist, pumps 1899 gallons of blood a day (1.3 million gallons a year). This figure applies to a person who is resting; it increases significantly with exercise.

Consider the Patient...

> Osteoporosis is generally caused by a lack of sex hormones. Osteoporosis affects older men and women who lose calcium from their skeletons. Women lose calcium earlier (after age 40 to 45) than men (after age 60). Another possible cause of bone loss among older clients is a lack of protein (collagen) production, which results in brittle bones and loss of bone matrix.

ORGANS AND ORGAN SYSTEMS

Organ systems comprise the tissues in the body that are functionally integrated and specifically designed to perform designated functions. Cells, the basic structural and functional units of the body, may aggregate and form tissues or groups of tissues, which are organized together to form organs. These organs form for a specific function and relate to other organs to form organ systems. Figure 2-17 shows most of the body's organ systems, which are described as follows.

Integumentary or Skin System

The largest organ in the body is the skin, which has numerous functions (Fig. 2-18). One is the excretion of waste products, such as carbon dioxide, water, small amounts of salts, and urea. The skin also eliminates heat and serves as a protection against invasion of foreign materials, and the nerves of the skin receive stimuli from outside the body. The **epidermis** and **dermis** constitute the skin. The epidermis rests on a basement membrane that separates it from the dermis. The epithelial cells form membranes that are composed of closely associated cells with an intercellular substance between them. These varying functions are possible because of the skin's many layers of cells and the underlying layers of connective tissue that carry blood vessels, muscles, and nerves. Epithelium has five cell-type layers: a basal or germinating layer, a spinous layer called stratum spinosum, a layer of cells

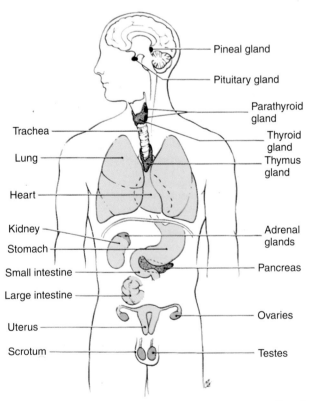

Fig. 2-17 Diagram of the human body, with glands listed on the right side and organs listed on the left.

with keratohyalin granules called the granular layer, a clear layer called the stratum lucidum, and the covering layer of keratinocytes that protects all the deeper layers.

The dermis has two layers: a superficial papillary layer and a deep reticular layer. The skin also has hair follicles (Fig. 2-19), sweat glands, and sebaceous glands, which assist in the multifunctional nature of the skin.

Neural System

The neural system is composed of the CNS and the peripheral nervous system. The CNS is the control center of the nervous system and is composed of the brain and spinal cord (Fig. 2-20). The brain is located in the cranium and is connected to the peripheral tissues by cranial nerves and to the spinal cord by spinal nerves. All sensation received anywhere in the body is relayed to the brain and spinal cord, which act on the sensation. The brain continues into the spinal cord, which is within the vertebral canal. This canal is a cylindrical space extending from the brain to the lumbar vertebrae. It is composed of 31 segments with spinal nerves coming from each. The spinal cord conveys impulses from the peripheral nervous system to the brain and from the brain to the peripheral tissues.

Nerve processes that carry information and convey it from the peripheral nervous system in muscles and

Fig. 2-18 Integumentary system. The skin is the largest organ in the body and serves to protect the body tissues from injury. The glands and nails arise from this layer of skin.

Fig. 2-19 Cross-section of a hair follicle. These epithelial structures arise from the basal cells of the skin.

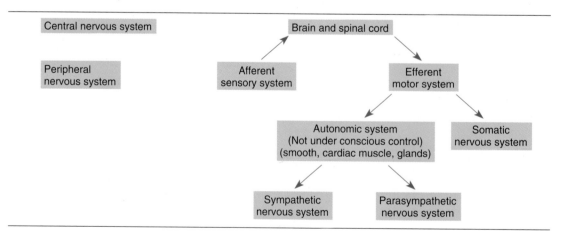

Fig. 2-20 Nervous system chart. This includes the brain, spinal cord, and all of the peripheral nervous system.

glands to the CNS are called the **afferent (sensory) system.** Other neurons that convey responses from the CNS to muscles and glands are located in the **efferent (motor) system.** These two systems are further divided into **somatic** and **autonomic nervous systems.** The nervous system is closely associated with the endocrine system, which is dependent on neural stimuli to function.

The somatic nervous system carries impulses to the voluntary muscles, such as the skeletal muscles, which are under conscious control. On the other hand, the efferent autonomic system carries impulses from the CNS to involuntary muscles, such as the smooth and cardiac muscles, and to all the glands. The viscera receive most of their impulses from this system.

The autonomic system produces responses involuntarily and is further divided into the **sympathetic** and **parasympathetic** divisions. In general, these two divisions modify each other: the sympathetic causes increased activity, and the parasympathetic modifies or decreases activity. Figure 2-21 outlines the nervous system.

Skeletal System

The skeletal system (Fig. 2-22) supplies the fundamental framework on which all the muscles and ligaments of the

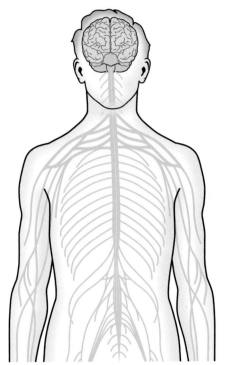

Fig. 2-21 Diagram of the nervous system. The brain, spinal cord, and peripheral nervous system function to regulate body activities.

Fig. 2-22 Skeletal system. A, Cartilage and bone. **B,** Skeletal system. The entire skeleton of the prenatal human is laid down in cartilage and gradually is transformed into bone. The last cartilage to change to bone is in the proximal and distal parts, as seen in this diagram. The adult skeleton, as seen in **B,** allows the body to stand erect and to move, providing attachment of the muscles, whereas the bone marrow provides origin of blood cells.

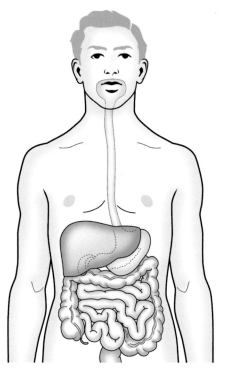

Fig. 2-23 The long tube of the digestive tract provides for physical and chemical breakdown of foods essential to bodily function. Many glands and organs are associated with and deliver their products into this tract.

Fig. 2-24 The liver is an important organ in the body. This organ filters the blood, removing all detrimental substances. The blood enters the liver peripherally and circulates through liver cords to the central vein. Note the large oval nuclei of the liver cells. This section of the liver tissue illustrates liver cell cords radiating from a central vein. Blood filters from the periphery of each liver (hepatic) lobule. This organ filters the blood and provides a storage area. Spaces between the cell cords are termed sinusoids.

Fig. 2-25 The pancreas is a second important organ associated with the digestive tract. This highly vascularized organ controls glucose production and elimination through the islets of Langerhans, rounded groups of cells found among the renal corpuscles. This organ's secretions enter the large intestine where it attaches to the stomach.

body are attached. Bone encloses the brain, spinal cord, and lungs and offers them protection. Bone marrow is also important in producing the hematopoietic system.

Digestive System

Functions of the digestive system's alimentary canal are to absorb, transform, and extract needed components from food ingested and to excrete all unused solid waste. In addition, carbon dioxide, water, and heat are lost. A long tube (approximately 26 feet) starts with the pharynx and esophagus, which conducts food to the stomach, a mixing and digestive chamber where food is reduced to liquid chyme (Fig. 2-23). Further digestion takes place in the small intestine, which adds glandular secretions from the liver, pancreas, and spleen. The large intestine, which absorbs nutrition, also dehydrates food and compresses it into solid waste. Digestion takes place throughout the tract through function of salivary glands in the oral cavity, gastric glands in the stomach, and liver, gallbladder, pancreas, spleen, and in the small intestine (Figs. 2-24 and 2-25). The walls of the tract are composed of functional layers: lining epithelium, connective tissue layers, and layers of muscle. Muscle aids in peristaltic movement of food through the tract.

Respiratory System

The function of the respiratory system is primarily to exchange gases in several phases. The process includes both inflow (inspiration) of oxygen and outflow (expiration) of carbon dioxide. The blood cells exchange oxygen and carbon dioxide with other cells in the body and with the pulmonary air sacs. The respiratory system includes the nasal chambers, in which the air is warmed by blood flowing close to the surface and which

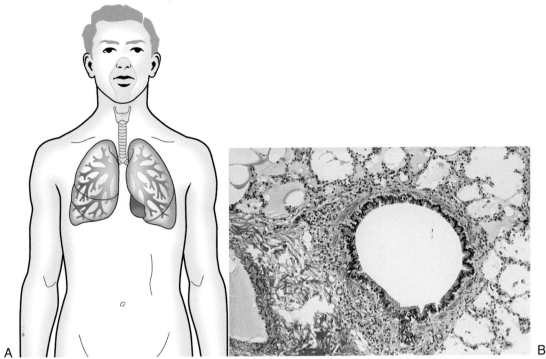

Fig. 2-26 A, Respiratory tract. Air enters the lung through the trachea, then enters the bronchi and the terminal bronchus to the air sacs seen on the *left.* **B,** A lung section showing a bronchiole in the left of the field and air sacs in the *upper right.* The bronchiole is lined with simple columnar ciliated epithelium, and signs of inflammation are seen in the cells surrounding the bronchiole.

becomes moist through the mucus secreted by goblet cells. These also trap dust particles. Cilia of the lining cells of the respiratory tract move these particulate substances to the pharynx and out of the respiratory system. In addition, the system includes the pharynx, trachea, and bronchi, which function as conduction chambers, and the lungs proper, which function in respiration (Fig. 2-26).

Vascular System

The vascular system includes the heart, large elastic arteries, smaller muscular arteries, and miles of capillaries, as well as veins that carry blood from the capillaries back to the heart. It is important to address the changes in the heart during pre- and post-natal life (Figure 2-27). The heart, which is the size of an adult's clenched fist, pumps an estimated 5 to 6 liters of blood approximately 60 times a minute. The function of the bloodstream is to carry oxygen to the cells in all areas of the body and to return carbon dioxide from these cells to the lungs. The blood vascular system provides nutrition from the walls of the alimentary canal and other organs. Blood also carries waste products to the kidneys, the gastrointestinal tract, and other organs of excretion, such as the skin.

Arteries function in conduction and distribution, capillaries in oxygen exchange and nutrition of the extracellular spaces, and veins in the return of blood to the heart. The blood vascular system additionally functions in blood clotting, and some white blood cells function in phagocytosis. Blood also conducts various hormones to their sites of action through the activities of the neuroendocrine system. Table 2-2 shows cellular and other elements of the blood.

Lymphatic System

The lymphoid organs are part of the immune system and consist of lymph nodes, thymus, and spleen (Figs. 2-28 and 2-29). Other aggregates of lymphatic tissue composed of lymphocytes are in the bone marrow, bloodstream, tonsils, Peyer's patches of the ileum in the small intestine, and other locations of the alimentary canal. A characteristic of the immune system is its ability to recognize and react specifically to macromolecules that are foreign to the body.

Muscular System

The striated muscles of the body represent the large muscles of the limbs, chest wall, and neck. They enable all of the actions of the body such as standing erect, walking, and other bodily movements. Striated muscle is made up of cylindrical fibers under voluntary control of the body. Striated muscle contraction functions on

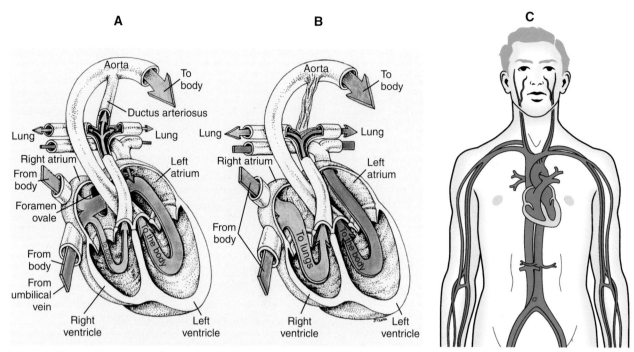

Fig. 2-27 The vascular system illustrating the heart. A, Before and 8 months after birth. Prenatally, oxygen comes from the placenta, and the oxygenated blood mixed with nonoxygenated blood enters the right side of the heart and is then sent to the left side of the heart, where it is pumped to the rest of the body. **B,** In the postnatal heart, the foramen ovale between the atria closes. **C,** Overview of the circulatory system, showing blood entering the right side of the heart.

Fig. 2-28 Lymphatic system. A, The lymphatic system of the human body. Lymph nodes, which are solid masses of lymphocytes and lymph channels, are located in all parts of the body. Note the system in the head and neck, thorax, abdomen, and limbs. **B,** The composition of a lymph node, with the dense composition of lymphocytes that serve as filters to remove bacteria from lymph vessels.

Fig. 2-29 The spleen is the largest lymphoid organ in the body. It is located in the upper left part of the abdomen. It serves as a filter for the blood and is active in destruction of old erythrocytes and in antibody production. It also produces both B and T cells.

Fig. 2-30 The thymus develops prenatally in the third pharyngeal arch and functions until puberty, when it then begins to atrophy. It primarily functions in T-cell production and in instructing these cells to become immunocompetent.

the all-or-none reaction. The myofibrils of muscle are arranged to permit contraction, which provides for movement of the body (see Fig. 2-14).

Endocrine System

The endocrine system includes the thyroid, parathyroid, and pituitary glands, ovaries, testes, pancreas, and adrenal medulla. A basic function of these glands is to secrete hormones into the vascular circulation, which then circulates and acts only on target cells through the second messenger, cyclic adenosine monophosphate (cAMP). Although 50 or more hormones traverse the bloodstream, each acts only on specific receptor cells. Hormones help regulate metabolism energy balance and

aid in regulation of involuntary smooth and cardiac muscle fibers. Hormones vary body activities, regulate centers of the immune system, play a role in growth and development, contribute to the process of reproduction, and regulate volume and composition of the extracellular environment. Some organs have endocrine function but also have other functions. Examples of these organs are the salivary glands, pancreas, testes, ovaries, thymus, hypothalamus, stomach, intestine, liver, kidneys, heart, and skin (Fig. 2-30). The hypothalamus is the major neural coordinating system between the nervous and endocrine systems.

Urinary System

The urinary system includes the kidneys, ureters, bladder, and urinary tract. The system filters toxic and unnecessary substances from the bloodstream and concentrates them before excretion. Kidneys excrete not only water, but also nitrogenous wastes and bacterial toxins (Fig. 2-31). The major function of the urinary system is to control blood volume and pressure and composition of the urine.

This system also restores water to the blood. In this manner, renin, atrial natiuretic factor, and vasopressin help to regulate blood pressure. Urine is stored in the urinary bladder until excreted.

Reproductive System

The male reproductive system includes the testes, prostate, and seminal vesicles, and the female system includes the ovaries, uterus, and vagina. The female produces eggs, and the male produces sperm along with secretions of the accessory glands that produce semen. The sperm and the egg each have half the chromosome complement that enables fertilization of the egg, which produces a zygote. The uterus then provides an environment in which the embryo can develop. The testes secrete the hormone testosterone, and the female system produces estrogen and progesterone to ensure development of the embryo.

Special Senses

The special senses system permits the detection of changes in the surrounding environment. This system includes vision, hearing, equilibrium, smell, and taste.

The eye focuses a distortion-free image on the retina. The retina responds to various colors and intensities and encodes spatial and temporal parameters for transmission to the brain.

The **ear** is composed of three parts: the external ear receives sound waves; the middle ear translates these waves into mechanical vibrations; and the internal ear receives the vibrations and changes them into specific impulses that are transmitted by the acoustic nerve to the brain.

Renal hilus

Renal artery & vein

Cortex

Medulla

Capsule

Ureter

Glomerulus

Cortex

Medulla

A

Urine

B

Fig. 2-31 Urinary system. A, The kidneys are filters, removing toxins but conserving water, proteins, glucose, salts, and other essential substances. The kidneys also help regulate blood pressure and acid-base balance. The kidneys then deliver the urine to the urinary bladder. **B,** Uriniferous tubules. All fluids pass through the tubule system as they carry fluid to the glomeruli and urine to the medullary area of the kidney. These highly cellular structures remove important elements and allow the urine to collect for passage to the urinary bladder. The glomeruli are important in recirculating and in toxin removal and retaining water, proteins, sugars, and other important elements.

Equilibrium is controlled by the vestibular organs, which are located in the internal ear.

The **olfactory organ** is located in the olfactory epithelium, which is a pseudostratified, ciliated columnar epithelium located in the roof of the nasal cavity. The olfactory cells are bipolar nerve cells, and their axons transmit to nerve trunks in the connective tissue underlying the olfactory epithelium. From there, olfactory impulses are transmitted to the brain.

The **taste modality** is located in cells of the taste buds, which are in the circumvallate papillae on the tongue's posterior dorsal surface. Taste is discussed in Chapter 14.

Consider the Patient...

A patient comes to the clinic with a puffy face and feels depressed. She describes her muscular weakness, inactivity, and need to spend much time in bed. She has a low heart rate. What do you suspect is causing her symptoms?

SELF-EVALUATION QUESTIONS

1. Describe four types of loose connective tissue that have special properties.
2. Describe two types of connective tissue proper.
3. Describe three types of cartilage and their locations in the body.
4. Describe cancellous and compact bone and the location of both types.
5. Describe two types of muscle that have involuntary movement and their functions.
6. What are the simple epithelial cell types, and where are they located in the body?
7. Describe the location of stratified squamous and columnar epithelium.
8. Discuss the function of the autonomic nervous system.
9. Describe how the sympathetic and parasympathetic nervous systems work together.
10. Name and briefly describe each of the nine organ systems.

Suggested Reading

Berman I: *Color atlas of basic histology,* ed 3, 2003, Appleton & Lange.
Fawcett D, Jensh R: *Bloom and Fawcett's concise histology,* London, 2002, Hodder Arnold.
Kerr J: *Atlas of functional histology,* St Louis, 1999, Mosby.
Le Douarin NM, Kalcherin C. *The neural crest,* ed 2, New York, 1999, Cambridge University Press.
Tortura GJ: *Principles of human anatomy,* ed 7, New York, 1995, Harper Collins College.
Weiss L: *Cell and tissue histology,* ed 5, New York, 1983, Elsevier.

3

DEVELOPMENT OF THE ORAL FACIAL REGION

CHAPTER OUTLINE

LEARNING OBJECTIVES

After reading this chapter the student will be able to:
- discuss the development of the oral pharynx, the pharyngeal arches including the pharyngeal pouches, the neural, vascular muscular components
- describe the skeletal components and the development of the tissues of the face

KEY TERMS

Alveolar process
Angular process
Aortic arch vessel
Auditory capsules
Basioccipital cartilages
Basion
Body
Common carotid arteries
Condylar
Coronoid process
Cranial base
Cranial base cartilages
Ethmoid
Ethmosphenoid and sphenoccipital articulations
Eustachian tube

External auditory canal
External carotid
Facial bones: zygomatic, maxillary, frontal, and temporal
Facial suture types: simple, serrated/interdigitating, squamosal
Facial sutures: zygomaticomaxillary, frontomaxillary, and zygomaticotemporal
Frontal, parietal, and squamous portions
Hyoid: superior hyoid, inferior hyoid
Incus
Inferior parathyroids
Internal carotid

Laryngeal cartilages
Malleus
Masseter, medial, and lateral pterygoid and temporalis muscles
Maxillary tissues
Meckel's cartilage bar, Meckel's cartilages
Middle ear
Nasion
Oropharyngeal membrane
Oropharynx
Palatine tonsils
Pharyngeal arch/mandibular arch
Pharyngeal pouches

KEY TERMS—cont'd

Premaxillary, maxillary, zygomatic,
  and petrous portions
Pulmonary circulation
Sella turcica
Sphenoid

Stapes
Superior parathyroids
Sutures
Synchondrosis
Syndesmosis

T cells
Temporal and interoccipital bones
Thymus
Tympanic membrane
Ultimobranchial body

OVERVIEW

This chapter concerns development and orientation of the tissues that form the human face and neck. During the fourth week of development, the human embryo consists of a flat disk that bends down at its anterior extremity as the overlying brain expands and enlarges. This action pushes the heart beneath the brain. A pit develops in the midline between the brain and the heart and becomes the oral cavity or stomodeum (see Fig. 3-2). Beneath this pit the first **pharyngeal arch,** termed the **mandibular arch,** forms. The **maxillary tissues** that form the cheeks grow from this first arch. Below the mandibular arch four other pharyngeal arches or bars appear during the fourth to seventh prenatal week. The second arch is called the **hyoid** (see Fig. 3-2). These parallel arches are important in the development of the face and neck, and each contains blood vessels, muscles, nerves, and skeletal elements. Aortic arch blood vessels, which course through each pharyngeal arch from the heart below to the brain above, are important to craniofacial development.

The first, second, and fifth of these vessels soon disappear. The third arch vessel quickly assumes the role of supplying nutrients to the tissues of the first and second arches. This third arch vessel also shifts the blood supply to the face from the internal carotid vessels to the external carotid. Muscles arise in each of the pharyngeal arches: the mandibular arch muscles become the masticatory muscles; the second arch muscles become the facial expression muscles; and the muscles of the third and fourth arches become the constrictor muscles of the throat. Cranial nerves enter each of these muscle masses as they arise. The fifth nerve enters the mandibular arch to innervate the muscles of mastication. The seventh innervates the second arch muscle mass, and other cranial nerves innervate the muscles of the neck. Cartilage also appears in each arch: **Meckel's cartilage bar** in the first, the **superior hyoid** in the second, the **inferior hyoid** in the third, and the **laryngeal cartilages** in the fourth. The **cranial base cartilages** arise to support the brain and from them come the auditory and olfactory sense capsules. All the creative events described in this chapter take place from the fourth to seventh prenatal weeks, the short time required for facial organization. Functions and tests for cranial nerves are discussed in Table 3-1.

DEVELOPMENT OF THE OROPHARYNX

The oropharynx is composed of the primitive oral cavity and the area of foregut called the pharynx. The oral pit first appears in the fourth week of development, when the neural plate bends ventrally as the neural folds develop to form the forebrain. This cephalocaudal bend pushes the heart ventrally, and the yolk sac becomes enclosed to form an elongating tube known as the foregut (Fig. 3-1).

The deepening oral pocket then appears between the forebrain and the heart and eventually becomes the oral cavity (Fig. 3-2). At its deepest extent is the **oropharyngeal membrane,** which ruptures in the fifth week, opens the oral cavity to the tubular foregut, and soon becomes the **oropharynx** (Figs. 3-3 and 3-4). The mandibular arch will grow laterally to the oral pit, developing the maxillary process, which forms the cheeks.

The enlarging heart now becomes positioned below the mandibular arch in the thorax and begins beating at the end of the fourth week (see Fig. 3-2). Blood is forced through the vessels in the pharyngeal arches supplying the face, neck, and brain. The forming face now grows away from the forebrain and presses against the chest and heart.

DEVELOPMENT OF THE PHARYNGEAL ARCHES

 CLINICAL COMMENT

From the initial development, each pharyngeal arch has a specific cranial nerve associated with it. The nerves and the musculature of each arch emerge together and follow defined pathways to their functional positions. These events are closely regulated genetically during development, and few errors occur.

Fig. 3-1 The embryo head bends anteriorly with the growth and expansion to the head. This pushes the heart ventrally and the oral pit (*stomodeum,* see Fig. 3-2) develops between the brain and the heart.

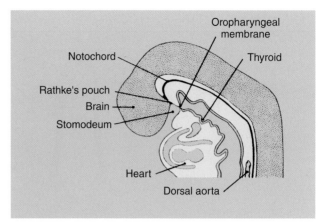

Fig. 3-3 Facial development in the fourth prenatal week. The oral pit is surrounded by the facial primordia, which are the frontonasal processes, the maxillary processes and the mandibular arch. The pharyngeal arches are defined by grooves between each arch. The heart develops in the thorax, which is in the pericardial cavity.

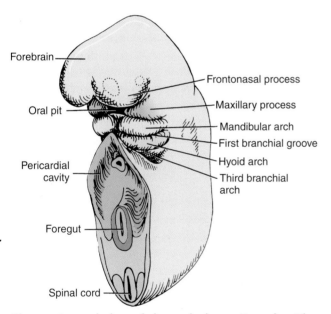

Fig. 3-2 Internal view of the oral pit at 3½ weeks. The oropharyngeal membrane separated the oral pit (*stomodeum*) and the pharyngeal cavities. The membranes will then rupture, allowing the two cavities to join.

Fig. 3-4 Sagittal view of pharyngeal arches with corresponding groove between each arch. The pharyngeal arches are seen in the wall of the pharynx. The aortic arch vasculature leads from the heart through these arches to the face.

The pharyngeal arches are so termed because they bend around the sides of the pharynx as bars of tissue. Each arch is separated by vertical grooves on the lateral sides of the neck at the fifth week. Within the pharynx, grooves called **pharyngeal pouches** separate each arch. These pouches match the pharyngeal clefts on the external aspects of the neck (see Fig. 3-4).

 Consider the Patient

A patient appears with a swelling in the lateral area of the neck and states that the swelling subsides from time to time but then resumes. He asks you what you think the cause may be.

TABLE 3-1 CRANIAL NERVES: FUNCTIONS AND TEST

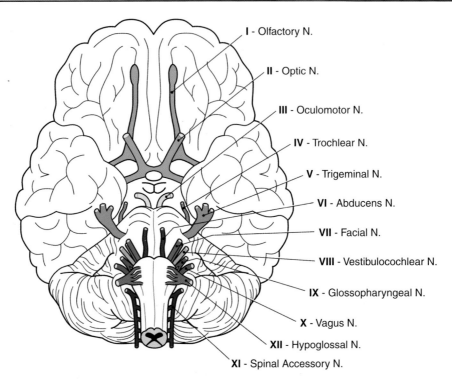

I - Olfactory N.
II - Optic N.
III - Oculomotor N.
IV - Trochlear N.
V - Trigeminal N.
VI - Abducens N.
VII - Facial N.
VIII - Vestibulocochlear N.
IX - Glossopharyngeal N.
X - Vagus N.
XII - Hypoglossal N.
XI - Spinal Accessory N.

Cranial nerve	Function	Test
I Olfactory	Smell	Odorous substance
II Optic	Vision	Vision chart
III Oculomotor	Eyelid and some eyeball	Coordinated following of an object
IV Trochlear	Superior oblique m.: eyeball	Look down at nose
V Trigeminal	Mastication, sensory for face and mouth	Bite down, touch face and gingiva
VI Abducens	Lateral rectus m.: eyeball	Gaze to the side
VII Facial	Muscles of facial expression, controls secretion of tears and saliva; taste (anterior 2/3 tongue)	Smile, frown, raise eyebrows, use a sweet or salty substance on anterior 2/3 of tongue
VIII Vestibulocochlear	Hearing and equilibrium	Tuning fork; equilibrium
IX Glossopharyngeal	Taste (posterior 1/3 tongue), salivary secretion, carotid blood pressure, and sensory posterior 1/3 of tongue, stylopharyngeus m.	Gag reflex, use a sweet or salty substance on posterior 1/3 of tongue
X Vagus	Motor to muscles of pharynx and larynx; parasympathetic to neck, thorax, and abdomen; sensory from pharynx, larynx, and gut; external ear; taste	Hoarseness, muscles responses after saying "Ah"
XI Spinal accessory	Motor to trapezius and sternocleidomastoid mm	Raise shoulders; turn head
XII Hypoglossal	Motor to tongue muscles except palatoglossal	Protrude tongue

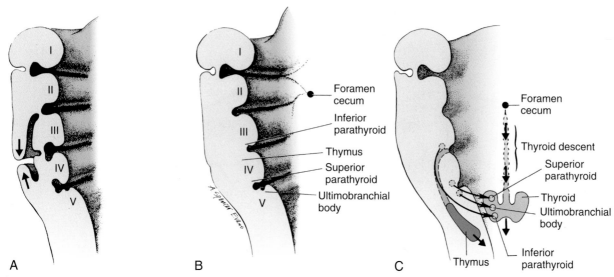

Fig. 3-5 Cross section of the pharyngeal arches. A, Tissues of pharyngeal arches 2 and 5 overgrow together, which results in disappearance of arches 2 to 5 and external smoothing of the neck. **B,** Resulting external appearance follows overgrowth. **C,** Contribution of the pharyngeal pouches.

The five arches with their clefts resemble the embryonic gill slits of fish and amphibians. This is one of many similarities between human embryos and other embryos during early development. The first arch is termed the mandibular arch because it will later form the bony mandible and the associated muscles of mastication, nerves, and blood supply. The second, or hyoid, arch forms the facial muscles, vessels, and hyoid bone. The third, fourth, and fifth arches consist of paired right and left bars that are divided before they reach the midline by the presence of the bulging heart (see Fig. 3-2). The arches become progressively smaller anterior to posterior. The outer surface of each arch is covered with ectoderm as are the inner surface of the first arch and the covering of the anterior surface of the second. This ectoderm is the epithelial lining of the oral cavity. The pharyngeal surface of the remaining four arches is, however, lined by endoderm, which is the same as the

lining of the gastrointestinal tract (see Fig. 3-4). The cores of the arches—the blood vessels, muscles, nerves, cartilages, and bones—will differentiate and are important in the development of the adult human face.

Pharyngeal Grooves and Pharyngeal Pouches

The first pharyngeal groove deepens to become the **external auditory canal** leading to the middle ear. The membrane at the depth of this tube becomes the **tympanic membrane.** The **middle ear** and **eustachian tube** develop from the corresponding first pharyngeal pouch. After the fifth week, no other pharyngeal grooves are seen externally as the tissues of the second and fifth arch grow over the other arches and grooves and make contact with each other (Fig. 3-5, *A*). This overgrowth obscures the tissue of both the arches and the grooves externally, although their internal structures are unaffected and provide an important role in facial and body development (Fig. 3-5, *A* and *B*).

The endodermal lining of the pharyngeal pouches differentiates into several important organs. The second pharyngeal pouch becomes the **palatine tonsils;** the third becomes the **inferior parathyroids** and **thymus;** the fourth becomes the **superior parathyroids;** and the fifth becomes the **ultimobranchial body** (Fig. 3-5, *C*).

The palatine tonsils function in the development of lymphocytes, which are important in the immunology of the body. The parathyroid glands regulate calcium balance throughout life. The thymus, located behind the sternum and between the lungs, is large at birth and

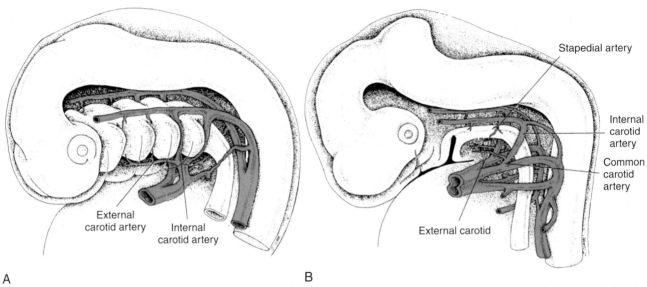

A   B

Fig. 3-6 Aortic arch development. A, At 4 weeks, the anterior aortic arch vessels have passed through the pharyngeal arch tissue and then disappear. The pharyngeal arch pouches project laterally between each arch. **B,** At 5 weeks, the third pharyngeal arch vessels become the right and left common carotid, which supplies the face by means of the internal carotid and stapedial arteries.

continues to grow until puberty, during which it begins to atrophy but continues to function. Although its full importance is unknown, the thymus produces **T cells** that destroy invading microbes and are therefore important to the body's immune system. The ultimobranchial body fuses with the thyroid and contributes parafollicular cells to the thyroid. The function of the ultimobranchial body remains unknown (Fig. 3-5, *B* and *C*).

Vascular Development

Each of the five pharyngeal arches contains a right and a left **aortic arch vessel** that leads from the heart through the arches to the face, brain, and posterior regions of the body (see Fig. 3-4). Not all of these paired aortic arches are present at the same time, however. The first and second begin to develop in the fourth week and disappear in the fifth week (Fig. 3-6). The third arch vessels then become prominent, taking over the facial area of the first two. As the fourth and fifth arch vessels arise, the fourth becomes prominent and the fifth disappears (Fig. 3-7). Next, the sixth arch vessels appear and become dominant along with those of the third and fourth.

The third arch vessels become the **common carotid arteries,** which supply the neck, face, and brain. The fourth arch vessels become the dorsal aorta, which supplies blood to the remainder of the body, and the vessels of the sixth arch supply the lungs with **pulmonary circulation** (Fig. 3-7).

An important feature of the common carotid arteries is the supply of blood to the face, neck, and brain from

Fig. 3-7 Details of aortic arch changes during early development of 3 to 5 prenatal weeks. Aortic arch vessels numbers 1, 2, and 5 disappear as the arches modify. Arch 3 becomes the common carotid and arch 4 becomes the dorsal aorta. The dorsal aorta then enlarges so that the common carotid arises from the dorsal aorta.

the **internal carotid** artery. However, after 7 weeks, the circulation to the face and neck shifts from the internal to the **external carotid** (Fig. 3-8). The internal carotid continues to supply the growing brain.

Muscular and Neural Development

Muscle cells in the first arch become apparent during the fifth week and begin to spread within the mandibular arch into each muscle site's origin in the sixth and seventh week (Fig. 3-9). By the tenth week, the muscles

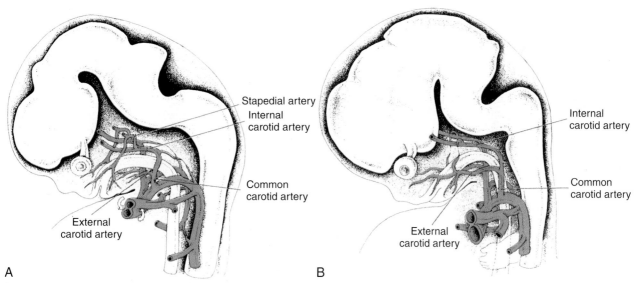

Fig. 3-8 **Shift in the vascular supply of the face. A,** The face and brain are first supplied by the internal carotid artery. **B,** The facial vessels at 7 weeks then detach from the internal carotid and attach to the external carotid.

of the second arch have formed a thin sheet that extends over the face and posterior to the ear (Fig. 3-10). As these muscles grow over the face, they develop into the various groups of muscles that attach to the newly ossifying bones of the facial skeleton. The muscle masses of the mandibular arch, on the other hand, remain in the first arch and become easily recognized muscles of mastication (Fig. 3-9, *A*). These are the **masseter, medial,** and **lateral pterygoid,** and **temporalis muscles.** They all relate to the developing mandible (Fig. 3-11).

The masseter and medial pterygoid form a vertical sling that inserts into the angle of the mandible. The temporalis muscle spreads into the infratemporal fossa that inserts into the developing coronoid process of the mandible. The lateral pterygoid extends horizontally from the neck of the condyle, and some fibers insert into the temporomandibular disk (see Chapter 13). The pharyngeal constrictor muscles in the fourth arch have differentiated in the neck and function to enclose the pharynx (see Fig. 3-11).

Nerves develop in conjunction with the developing muscle fibers. By the end of the seventh week, the fibers of the fifth nerve have entered the mandibular muscle mass, as has the seventh nerve in the facial muscle mass in the second arch (Fig. 3-12). As these muscle masses develop, the nerves are present and follow or lead them as they migrate to their position of differentiation, maturation, and function. The seventh nerve supplies the stylohyoid and stapedius muscles and the posterior belly of the digastric muscle. The ninth (glossopharyngeal) nerve enters the third arch and supplies the stylopharyngeal

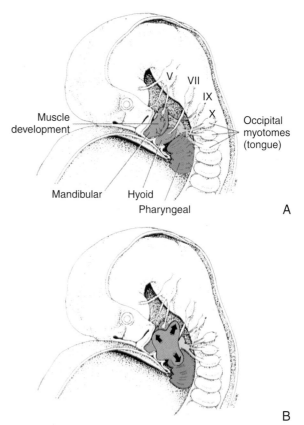

Fig. 3-9 **Development of the muscles and nerves of the pharyngeal arches. A,** Mandibular muscle mass expands to form the muscles of mastication. **B,** At 7 weeks, the muscles of the second arch grow upward to form the muscles of the face.

Frontalis muscle — Temporalis muscle — Occipitalis muscle

Medial pterygoid muscle — Masseter muscle

Fig. 3-10 The facial muscles grow from the second arch to cover the face, the scalp, and muscles posterior to the ear. These all become muscles of facial expression.

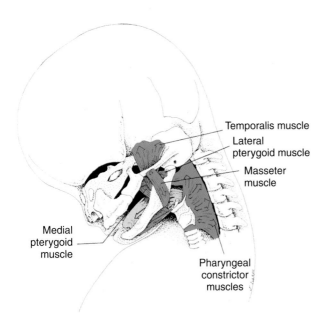

Temporalis muscle
Lateral pterygoid muscle
Masseter muscle

Medial pterygoid muscle

Pharyngeal constrictor muscles

Fig. 3-11 Masticatory muscles of the mandibular arch. The medial pterygoid and masseter muscles attach as a sling at the angle of the mandible. The temporalis muscle grows from the coronoid process into the temporal fossa, and the lateral pterygoid muscle extends from the condyle anteriorly to the sphenoid bone and the pterygoid bone in the temporal fossa.

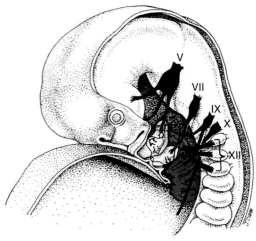

Fig. 3-12 Cranial nerves growing into the pharyngeal arches. Nerve V grows into the mandibular arch and nerve VII into the hyoid arch. Nerves V, IX, and X contribute to the tongue muscles, which are developing in the floor of the mouth.

and upper pharyngeal constrictor muscles. The tenth (vagus) nerve innervates muscles of the fourth arch, which are the inferior constrictors and laryngeal muscles. The tongue, which is primarily muscle, relates to the branches of the ninth nerve, which carries the sensory modality of taste from the taste buds located in the posterior one third of the tongue and to the seventh nerve, which carries the modality of taste from the taste buds on the anterior two thirds of the tongue. The fifth nerve is the sensory nerve to the same area of the anterior tongue (see Fig. 3-12). The tongue is a good example of muscle cell migration because it originates in the occipital myotome and migrates anteriorly into the floor of the mouth. During migration, the nerves mentioned enter the muscle mass and later carry out their functions (Fig. 3-13).

Cartilaginous Skeletal Development

The initial skeleton of the pharyngeal arches develops as cartilaginous bars. In the first arch, **Meckel's cartilages** appear bilaterally (see Fig. 3-13). The anterior aspects of these two cartilages approach each other near the midline but do not coalesce. Posteriorly, each terminates in an enlarged bulbous structure called the **malleus**. The malleus lies adjacent to a small cartilage called the **incus**. Farther posterior is a third body of cartilage, the **stapes** (see Fig. 3-13). These three bilateral cartilages later transform into bone and function in the middle ear as hearing bones.

Substantial evidence shows that the contact point of the malleus and incus is the articulation of the lower jaw for the first 20 weeks of prenatal life. Then the second temporomandibular joint, which is the articulation of the condyle and the temporal fossae, becomes

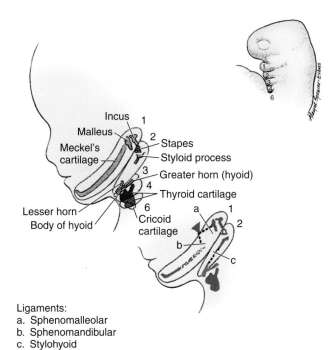

Ligaments:
a. Sphenomalleolar
b. Sphenomandibular
c. Stylohyoid

Fig. 3-13 Cartilages derived from the pharyngeal arches. Meckel's cartilage, malleus, and incus arise form arch 1. Stapes, styloid, and lesser horn of the hyoid form arch 2, the greater horn of hyoid forms arch 3, and thyroid and laryngeal cartilages form arches 4 and 5.

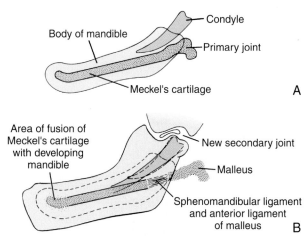

Fig. 3-14 Relationship between the primary and secondary temporomandibular joints. A, Meckel's cartilage with its posterior malleus-incus joint, which functions in jaw movements during the first 4 months of prenatal life. **B,** A shift to the condylar-temporal articulation that occurs after that time both prenatally and postnatally.

Fig. 3-15 The cartilages of the face and skull. Observe how the cranial base cartilage supports the maxillary and mandibular cartilages of the face. The locations of the nasal and auditory capsules and sphenoid are shown. All central skeletal elements arise in cartilage and later are transformed into bone.

functional (Fig. 3-14). Chapter 13 has further information about the temporomandibular joint.

The rod-shaped cartilage of the second or hyoid arch is known as Reichert's cartilage. The stapes, styloid process, lesser horn, and upper body of the hyoid arise from this arch (see Fig. 3-13). The third arch cartilage forms the greater horn and the lower part of the hyoid body. The fourth arch contributes to the hyoid cartilage, which then supports the gland. The fifth arch has no adult cartilage derivatives, and the sixth arch cartilage forms the laryngeal cartilage (see Fig. 3-13).

DEVELOPMENT OF THE CRANIOFACIAL SKELETON

Cartilages of the Face

The earliest formed skeletal elements in the craniofacial area are the cartilaginous nasal capsule **(ethmoid),** the **sphenoid,** the **auditory capsules,** and the **basioccipital cartilages.** All these cartilages initially arise as a single cartilaginous continuum in the midline underlying the brain (Fig. 3-15). Anteriorly, the nasal capsule contains the organ of smell. Laterally, the auditory capsules

protect the organs of hearing (see Fig. 3-15). The sphenoid cartilage is posterior to the ethmoid. It later forms wings of bone that spread out under the brain laterally (Fig. 3-16). Behind the sphenoid is the occipital cartilage. Although the ethmoid capsule, sphenoid, and basioccipital cartilages are formed as a single cartilaginous unit initially, they separate later to form individual bones. These cartilages underlie and support the brain and are known as the **cranial base.** The cranial base is determined by drawing a line from the nasal bone **(nasion)** to the **sella turcica** of the sphenoid to the **basion,** as seen in Figure 3-17. These cartilages are transformed into bone by endochondral bone formation.

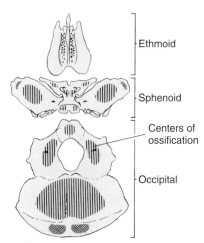

Fig. 3-16 A view of the base of the cranium showing the supporting structures of the brain. Cartilage centers *(lined areas)* initiate the formation of the cranial base bones with growth of these bones extending outward.

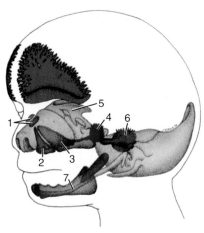

Fig. 3-18 Relationship of cranial cartilages to the membrane bones of the face at 8 weeks. The membrane bones are numbered: *1,* nasal; *2,* premaxillary; *3,* maxillary; *4,* zygomatic; *5,* sphenoid; *6,* temporal; *7,* mandible.

Fig. 3-17 Lateral view of the cranial base from which growth measurements are made. A line drawn from sella turcica to nasion to basion is a means of measuring facial growth.

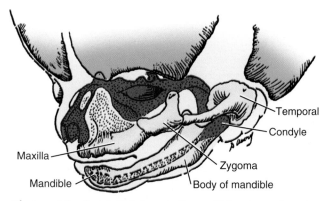

Fig. 3-19 The facial skeleton at the twelfth prenatal week. This figure illustrates the relationship of the maxillary, zygomatic, and temporal bones and their articulations. The membrane bone of the body and the cartilaginous condyle of the mandible are also shown.

Bones of the Face

The protective covering of the brain is formed by membrane bones. These bones are termed **frontal, parietal,** and **squamous portions** of the **temporal** and **interoccipital** bones (Fig. 3-18). Membrane bones form directly from connective tissue and do not initially form from cartilage.

CLINICAL COMMENT

Pharyngeal arch syndromes are seen clinically as combinations of such defects as underdevelopment of the mandible, retracted tongue, large tongue, small mouth, malformed ears, and cleft palate. A rare disorder, Treacher Collins syndrome, is directly attributable to pharyngeal arch deficiencies.

The **facial bones,** which also form in membrane bone, complete the facial skeleton. They develop overlying the nasal capsule and are called the **premaxillary, maxillary, zygomatic,** and **petrous portions** of the temporal bone (see Fig. 3-18). These bones initially appear as tiny ossification centers in the face and then increase in diameter, spreading anteriorly, posteriorly, and upward into the tissues surrounding the orbit (Fig. 3-19).

The maxillary bones also grow medially into the palate to support the palatine shelf tissue (Fig. 3-20). The bones of the maxilla grow as the facial tissues continue to develop. The height of the maxilla is due partially to the growth in length of the roots of the teeth.

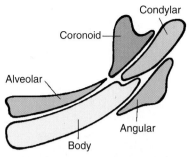

Fig. 3-21 Developing areas of the mandible and their responses to stimuli. The mandible develops from several parts, the condyle in cartilage is the articulation site, the coronoid develops in response to the temporalis muscle, the angular area is in response to the medial pterygoid and the masseter muscle, the mandible in membrane bone is the unifying structure fusing with all parts, and the alveolar process develops in response to the developing teeth.

Fig. 3-20 Cleared human palate at 8 months. Sutures are seen in the midline and between the premaxillary and maxillary bones and between the maxillary and the palatine bones in the posterior palate.

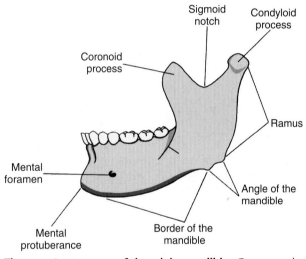

Fig. 3-22 Appearance of the adult mandible. Compare the difference of this adult mandible with the developing one in Figure 3-21. Observe in the adult mandible all parts have fused together to develop a strong, erect single bone.

The bony mandible grows laterally to the first arch cartilage as well as posteriorly to join the bony body with the cartilaginous condyle. Together, the body of the mandible and the cartilaginous condyle replace Meckel's cartilage (see Fig. 3-19).

The mandible develops as several units: a **condylar** unit forms the articulation, allowing movement of the mandible; the **body** is the center of all growth and function of the mandible; the **angular process** responds to the lateral pterygoid and masseter masticatory muscles; the **coronoid process** responds to the temporalis muscle development and attachment; the **alveolar process** responds to development of the teeth (Fig. 3-21). This development produces the mature mandible (Fig. 3-22).

CLINICAL COMMENT

Many facial defects result from a lack of transformation of the pharyngeal arches to their adult derivatives. Pharyngeal cysts and fistulas may appear along the sides of the neck because the epithelial-lined pockets remain as a result of the overgrowth of the arches. These defects may also open in the pharynx. Cysts and fistulas may result in swelling or draining of mucus from an opening on the side of the neck.

Sutures of the Face

A system of articulations develops between each of the major bones of the face to facilitate growth. These articulations are positioned in the direction of facial growth, which is forward, away from the brain, and downward to facilitate lengthening of the face. The articulations are termed **sutures** and are defined as fibrous joints in which the opposing surfaces are closely united. A suture develops between the **zygomatic, maxillary, frontal,** and **temporal facial bones.** Sutures are named for the two or more bones with which they articulate. Facial sutures are named **zygomaticomaxillary, frontomaxillary,** and **zygomaticotemporal** (see Fig. 3-22).

Fig. 3-23 Histology of a simple suture. Observe the opposing bony fronts with connective tissue and blood vessels between them. Osteoblasts appear along the opposing bony fronts and form bone to provide growth of this suture.

Interdigitating bone   Connective tissue of suture

Fig. 3-24 Histology of a serrated suture of the skull. Observe the interdigitating extensions of bone from both adjacent surfaces. Connective tissue appears between these bony fronts. This is a strong suture.

These articulations are growth sites that allow the associated bones to expand and to maintain orientation at their junctions by means of the fibrous attachment that controls their relationship with the adjacent bones. Such articulations may consist of a band of connective tissue termed **syndesmosis** (Fig. 3-23). In the center of this band are osteogenic cells, which along the periphery provide for new bone growth. The sutures of the face are

Bone   Connective tissue

Fig. 3-25 Histology of a developing squamous suture. These are overlapping sutures, and connective tissue and blood vessels appear between the bony fronts. For example, one squamous suture is between the parietal and temporal bones on the sides of the head.

of three types: **simple,** which is an uncomplicated band of tissue between bony fronts (see Fig. 3-23); **serrated,** which is an **interdigitating** type of suture (Fig. 3-24); and **squamosal,** which has a beveled or overlapping type junction (Fig. 3-25). Each connective tissue suture consists of a central zone of proliferating connective tissue cells with osteogenic cells along the peripheral bony fronts. Each suture is surrounded by a fibrous connective tissue (see Figs. 3-23 to 3-25). When the position of these sutures in the fetal skull is compared with the position of the sutures in the adult skull, the relationship of these articulations appears similar, although adult bones are larger (compare Figs. 3-26 and 3-27). When facial growth is complete, all of these sutures will become inactive, although the interface of the opposing bones remains and defines the boundary of the facial bones.

In contrast to the sutures of the external face, the articulations in the midline have interposing bands of cartilage. This type of articulation is termed **synchondrosis** and is located in the midline (Fig. 3-28). Synchondrosis articulations grow by forming new cartilage in the center of the suture as the cartilage is transformed into bone at the periphery of the cartilage. These cartilage articulations are of only one type and exist between the ethmoid and sphenoid and the occipital bones in the midline during the period of craniofacial growth. These are known as the **ethmosphenoid** and **sphenoccipital articulations.** Table 3-2 presents a summary of all structures that develop from the pharyngeal arches, pharyngeal grooves, and pharyngeal pouches.

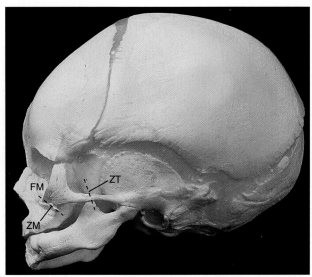

Fig. 3-26 Sutures of the developing skull of the newborn. *FM,* frontomaxillary; *ZM,* zygomaticomaxillary; *ZT,* zygomaticotemporal. The pterygopalatine suture is not present in the newborn but is present in the adult (see Fig. 3-27).

Resting zone   Proliferative zone   Ossification zone

Fig. 3-28 Histology of a cartilage suture located in the midline of the base of the skull. We can observe a band of cartilage with cartilage cells differentiating in the center of it. As they migrate peripherally, the cells become osteoblasts and form bone at the peripheral surfaces of the cartilage, as seen. Bony growth thus occurs in this suture. This suture is between the ethmoid and sphenoid bone.

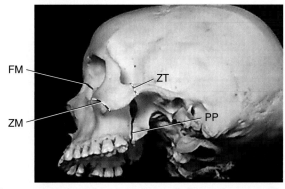

Fig. 3-27 Sutures of the adult human skull. *FM,* frontomaxillary; *ZM,* zygomaticomaxillary; *ZT,* zygomaticotemporal; and *PP,* pterygopalatine. Observe the difference in location of the sutures in the adult from those in the newborn.

6. Describe the origin and growth of the muscles of mastication.
7. Discuss the origin, descent, and function of the thyroid gland.
8. Discuss the origin and time of the shift in the facial blood supply.
9. Describe the cartilages of the early facial skeleton and the bones that replace them.
10. Name, locate, and describe the connective tissue sutures of the face.

SELF-EVALUATION QUESTIONS

1. What structures are derived from pharyngeal arch I?
2. What is the importance of Meckel's cartilage?
3. Identify the structures derived from pharyngeal arch II.
4. Rapid palatal expansion can be used by the orthodontist to increase the width of the hard palate. Why and when can the midpalatal suture be used to effect changes in the hard palate?
5. What are the contributions of pharyngeal pouches number 1, 2, 3, and 4?

Consider the Patient

> **Discussion:** The symptoms suggest a pharyngeal cleft and related cyst. Surgery would be recommended to correct this condition.

Suggested Reading

Avery JK: *Oral development and histology,* ed 3, Stuttgart, 2002, Thieme Medical.
Enlow DH: *Facial growth,* ed 3, Philadelphia, 1990, WB Saunders.
Sadler TW: *Langman's medical embryology,* ed 7, Baltimore, 1995, Williams & Wilkins.
Sperber GH: *Craniofacial embryology,* ed 5, Toronto, 2001, BC Decker.

TABLE 3-2 SUMMARY OF STRUCTURES THAT DEVELOP FROM PHARYNGEAL ARCHES, PHARYNGEAL GROOVES, AND PHARYNGEAL POUCHES

Branchial grooves	Branchial arch structures					Pharyngeal Pouches
Adult derivative	Arch no.	Cranial nerve	Branchiomeric muscles	Skeletal derivative	Aortic Arch	Adult derivative
External Auditory Meatus (1)	I Mandibular	V Trigeminal	Muscles of mastication, anterior belly of digastric, mylohyoid, tensor tympani, tensor palatini	Malleus, incus, sphenomandibular ligament, sphenomalleolar ligament (Meckel's cartilage)	I	1 Middle ear Eustachian tube
	II Hyoid	VII Facial	Muscles of facial expression, stapedius, stylohyoid, posterior belly of digastric	Stapes, styloid process, stylohyoid ligament, lesser cornu of hyoid, upper part of body of hyoid	II	2 Palatine tonsil
Cervical Fistula (2)	III	IX Glossopharyngeal	Stylopharyngeus	Greater cornu of hyoid, lower part of body of hyoid	III	3 Thymus, inferior parathyroid
(3, 4)	IV	X Vagus	Laryngeal musculature, pharyngeal constrictors	Laryngeal cartilages	IV	4 Superior parathyroid
	V	XI Spinal accessory	Sternocleidomastoid Trapezius		VI	5 Ultimobranchial body

4

DEVELOPMENT OF THE FACE AND PALATE

CHAPTER OUTLINE

Overview
Facial Development:
  Weeks 4 to 7
    Tissue Organization
     Fourth week
     Fifth week
     Sixth week
     Seventh week

Palatal Development: Weeks 7 to 9
  Medial and Lateral Palatal
    Processes
  Palatal Shelf Elevation and
    Closure
  Tongue Development
    Body and base
    Thyroid gland

Malformations
  Facial Clefts
  Palatal Clefts
  Other Defects
Self-Evaluation Questions
Consider the Patient Discussion
Suggested Reading

LEARNING OBJECTIVES

After reading this chapter the student will be able to:
- describe prenatal facial development during the fourth to seventh weeks of gestation
- describe palatal development during the seventh to ninth weeks of gestation
- explain how the tongue and thyroid develop
- discuss development of facial and palatal clefts and other facial defects

KEY TERMS

Auditory tube
Auricular hillocks
Cheeks
Cleft lip
Foramen cecum
Forehead
Frontal process
Frontonasal process
Hyoid
Internasal area
Lateral nasal process

Lateral palatine processes
Lingual tonsil
Lower jaw
Mandibular arch
Maxillary processes
Medial nasal process
Nasal fin
Nasolacrimal duct
Orbicularis oris
Oronasal optic groove
Palatal shelf elevation

Palatine and pharyngeal tonsils
Palatine shelf closure or fusion
Philtrum
Primary palate
Terminal sulcus
Thyroglossal cyst
Thyroglossal duct
Thyroglossal fistula
Tuberculum impar
Two lateral lingual swellings

OVERVIEW

This chapter describes the development of the human face and palate and defects that may occur during development. An understanding of this subject is important to the dental health professional for two reasons. First, the professional must understand the variability that can occur in facial form, and, second, he or she must be aware that the human face and palate are among the areas in the body most likely to develop malformations.

The human face develops early in gestation, during the fourth through seventh weeks, and the palatal processes begin to close during the eighth week. These two structures are closely related in time of development and sometimes have related malformations. The face develops from the tissues immediately surrounding the oral pit, but the forehead develops from the frontal area that lies above the pit (Fig. 4-1). The nose later develops from this area as well, so the name changes from *frontal area* to *frontonasal area* (Fig. 4-2). Below the oral pit is the mandibular arch, from which the mandible arises and articulates with the temporal bone. Lateral to the oral pit are the right and left maxillary processes, which develop from the mandibular arch. Cheek tissues come from these processes. Intraorally, the palate forms the mouth's roof, which separates the oral and nasal cavities.

First the medial palatal segment forms as part of the medial nasal segment. This segment provides the first separation of the oral and nasal cavities. Next, two lateral palatal shelves close anteriorly (not posteriorly) to the pharynx (see Fig. 4-12). At the same time, the tongue develops in the floor of the oral cavity but grows rapidly and expands into the nasal cavity. The tongue functions in palatine shelf closure because the shelves must override it before closure can be accomplished.

Many environmental factors can cause clefts of the face, palate, or both. These defects of the lip or palate may be unilateral or bilateral and also incomplete or complete.

FACIAL DEVELOPMENT: WEEKS 4 TO 7

Tissue Organization

The face develops primarily from tissues surrounding the oral pit. Above the oral pit is the covering of the brain termed the **frontal process,** from which develops the **forehead.** Lateral to the oral pit are the right and left **maxillary processes,** from which develop the **cheeks,** and below the oral pit is the **mandibular arch,** from which forms the **lower jaw.** In the fourth week, when the facial tissues have just begun to organize, they measure only a few millimeters in height and width and are

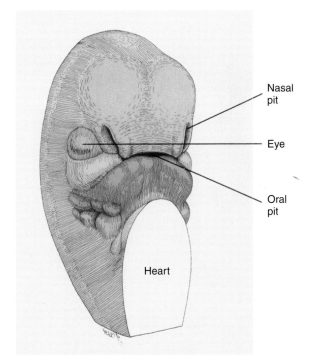

Fig. 4-1 Human face during the fourth prenatal week. Around the centrally located oral pit are grouped the frontal and maxillary processes and the mandibular arch. Although appearing unrelated at this time, these processes and the first arch form the human face.

Fig. 4-2 Human face during the fifth prenatal week. The nasal pits develop and appear on the sides of the face. The frontal process now becomes the frontonasal process.

only as thick as a sheet of paper. Further growth of the face from this minute assembly of tissue sites is anterior to the brain. Lying inferior to the mandibular arch is the second pharyngeal or **hyoid** arch, and its muscles expand into and contribute to the face. The hyoid arch also forms part of the external and middle ear.

Development of the human face is most easily described in terms of the changes that occur at weekly intervals from the fourth to the seventh prenatal weeks.

 CLINICAL COMMENT

> Syndromes associated with the pharyngeal arches are seen frequently as a group of defects. They can appear as a malformed mandible, defective ear, small mouth, enlarged tongue or unequal growth of the sides of the tongue, cleft lip or palate, and swelling or cysts or clefts of the front or sides of the neck. Usually, several or more defects appear simultaneously.

Fourth week

At 4 weeks' gestation, the oral pit is surrounded by several masses of tissue. Pharyngeal arches are also evident below the pit and on the sides of the neck. The frontal processes of the brain bulge forward and laterally to dominate the facial area. Below the frontal processes are two small wedge-shaped tissues termed the maxillary processes that lie lateral to the oral pit. Beneath the maxillary processes is the mandibular arch, which appears divided or constricted in the midline (see Fig. 4-1). The heart lies immediately below the face and is one of the fastest growing organs. During the fourth week, the heart begins to pump blood throughout the body.

 CLINICAL COMMENT

> Environmental factors play an important role in facial and palatal malformations. The period before the fifth week is the critical time during which these factors can affect facial development.

Fifth week

During the fifth week, the bilateral nasal placodes, or thickened areas of epithelium, appear in the upper border of the lip. They develop into nostrils as the tissues around these placodes grow, resulting in two slits opening into the oral pit. At this point, the frontal area becomes known as the **frontonasal process.** The nostrils deepen as the tissues around them continue to grow

anteriorly, and the **internasal area,** the distance between the nostrils, represents the width of the face. Gradually the frontal prominence diminishes and the face broadens. The eyes become prominent on the sides of the head. Throughout the fifth week, the mandibular arch loses its midline constriction (see Fig. 4-2).

Sixth week

At the beginning of the sixth week, the lateral parts of the face expand, broadening the face. This is also caused by lateral growth of the brain. The eyes and maxillary processes, which were located on the sides of the face in the fifth week, come to the front of the face. The mouth slit widens to the point at which the maxillary and mandibular tissues merge. The nasal processes are limited to the middle of the upper lip, which causes the face to appear more human. The upper lip is now composed of a medial nasal process and two lateral maxillary segments (Fig. 4-3). The medial nasal process is called the **philtrum.** A ridge of tissue surrounds each nasal pit. The tissue lateral to the pits is the **lateral nasal process,** and the tissue medial to the pits is the **medial nasal process.**

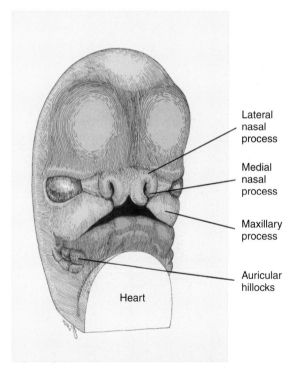

Lateral nasal process

Medial nasal process

Maxillary process

Auricular hillocks

Heart

Fig. 4-3 Human face during the sixth prenatal week. Nasal pits appear more centrally located in the medial nasal process. This is the result of growth of the lateral face, which also causes the eyes to approach the front of the face. The enlarged maxillary processes are near contact with the medial nasal process. Nasal pits may be sites of cleft lips. Auricular hillocks bordering the ear canal have merged.

The medial nasal process is in close contact with the medial aspect of the maxillary process, and the lateral nasal process is above the maxillary process. The border of the lip consists of two maxillary processes, and the medial third is the medial nasal. A lack of contact or fusion of the medial nasal and maxillary processes results in either a unilateral or bilateral **cleft lip.** The epithelial coverings of the medial nasal and maxillary processes normally contact and create a zone of fusion termed the **nasal fin** (Fig. 4-4). This epithelial fin is soon penetrated by connective tissue growth, which binds together the two maxillary and medial nasal parts of the lip. If this penetration were not to occur, the lip could pull apart. Soon the **orbicularis oris** muscle grows around the oral pit to provide support to the upper lip. The nasal pits continue behind the nasal fin to open into the roof of the mouth at 6 weeks (see Fig. 4-4). Extending from the nostrils to the eyes is an oblique groove, which is the **oronasal optic groove.** In the tissue beneath this groove, the **nasolacrimal duct** develops. A modification of the first pharyngeal groove into the ear canal or **auditory tube** also appears below the corners of the mouth. Six small hillocks of tissue, termed the **auricular hillocks,** are grouped around the external ear canal. Three of these come from the mandibular arch and three from the second or hyoid arch (see Fig. 4-3; Fig. 4-5).

Seventh week

By the seventh week, the face has a more human appearance (Fig. 4-6). The eyes approach the front of the face, and the nose represents less of the face than it did at the fourth week. The lateral growth of the brain, resulting in facial expansion, causes the eyes to appear on the front of the face, which makes it more recognizable as a human face. A third of the face has been added lateral to each nostril (see Fig. 4-6). The eyes are on the same horizontal plane as the nostrils, which will change after the bridge of the nose develops and lengthens. The upper lip has fused, producing a medially located philtrum. The mouth is limited in size with the change in facial proportions. The ear hillocks have fused and grown to form the ears (auricles). The ridges around the eyes will soon develop into eyelids (see Figs. 4-5 and 4-6). The danger of a cleft lip has passed. In just 3 prenatal weeks, separate tissue masses have enlarged, fused, and merged into a recognizable human face.

 CLINICAL COMMENT

> Because the face develops on the surface of the brain, defects of the anterior brain may result in developmental alteration of the facial form.

Fig. 4-5 Development of the external ear (auricles). A, The three auricular hillocks on the *left* are from the mandibular arch, and the three on the *right* are from the hyoid arch. **B,** Auricular hillocks begin to merge around the first pharyngeal groove. **C,** The hillocks merge. **D,** The ear is developed.

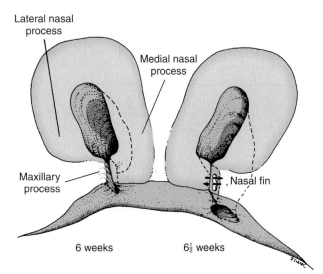

Fig. 4-4 Development of the floor of the nasal pit. On the *left,* the nares is in the process of closing. During this process, the medial nasal and maxillary process fuse as connective tissue grows through this area. On the *left,* there is space between the maxillary and medial nasal processes, and on the *right,* the two areas are in contact, and the resulting nasal fin is penetrated by the connective tissue of the developing lip.

PALATAL DEVELOPMENT: WEEKS 7 TO 9

Medial and Lateral Palatal Processes

The palate is the tissue that separates the oral and nasal cavities. This palate, although thin, is supported by bone, which provides rigidity. The palate develops from an anterior wedge-shaped medial part and two lateral palatine processes (Fig. 4-7, *A*). The medial part is also known as the **primary palate** because it develops first and is a floor to the nasal pits. Next, the **lateral palatine processes** develop from the maxillary tissues laterally and grow to the midline. This further limits the oral

cavity from the nasal cavity posteriorly to the nasopharynx (Fig. 4-7, *B*). As the palatine shelves grow medially, they contact the tongue, which grew upward into the nasal cavity during the seventh week. When the palatine shelves contact the tongue, they grow downward on either side of the tongue (Fig. 4-8).

Palatal Shelf Elevation and Closure

At its posterior limits, the tongue is below the palatine shelves. This is because posteriorly the tongue is attached to the floor of the mouth, and the posterior roof of the mouth is above the tongue. During the eighth prenatal week, the posterior shelves push together, forcing the tongue forward and down (Fig. 4-9). This action causes the palatal shelves to slide over the tongue (Fig. 4-10). The process is known as **palatal shelf elevation** and is presumed to take place rapidly, about as fast as the act of swallowing. For this reason, palatal shelf elevation has never been precisely recorded.

As soon as the palatine shelves reach the resulting horizontal position, the tongue broadens and pushes upward against the shelves, which helps mold them together (Fig. 4-11). The shelves have a final growth surge until they contact in the midline; this contact is known as **palatine shelf closure** or **fusion** (Fig. 4-12). The first site of contact is just posterior to the medial palatine process. From this point of initial contact, the shelves merge anteriorly and posteriorly. The final step in fusion is the removal of the midline epithelial

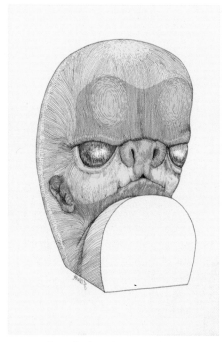

Fig. 4-6 Human face during the seventh prenatal week. The medial nasal and maxillary processes have merged. The eyes are closer to the front of face. The nose and eyes are on the same horizontal plane, which will change with vertical growth of face. The auricles of the ear have developed.

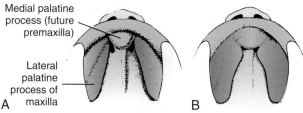

Medial palatine process (future premaxilla)

Lateral palatine process of maxilla

A   B

Fig. 4-7 The development of the palate. A, Medial and lateral palatine processes develop (enlarge). **B,** Lateral palatine processes move medially toward the midline and fuse with the medial palatine process.

Fig. 4-8 Coronal section of facial tissue showing tongue's growth upward into the nasal cavity during the seventh prenatal week. Palatine shelves (maxillary processes) contact the tongue during their medial growth. The tongue then grows down beside the palatal shelves. The tongue muscle begins to differentiate at this time.

barrier between the right and left shelves. This occurs by enzymatic action of epithelial cells, which results in self-destruction. As soon as the epithelial cells begin to break down and disappear, connective tissue grows through the midline and completes the fusion of the palate. This is the same process as the one that occurred in lip fusion and is illustrated in Figure 4-13. The fusion of the entire palate takes weeks while the palate grows in length. The palatal shelves also fuse with the overlying nasal septum in the midline of the face. This causes a complete separation of the oral and nasal cavities back to the nasopharynx. Then both the oral and nasal cavities open into the pharynx.

Tongue Development

Body and base

The tongue originates from the muscles of the occipital myotomes as described in Chapter 3 (see Figs. 3-9 to 3-11). From this posterior location the forming muscles migrate anteriorly into the floor of the mouth and are joined by other muscles of the first and second pharyngeal arches.

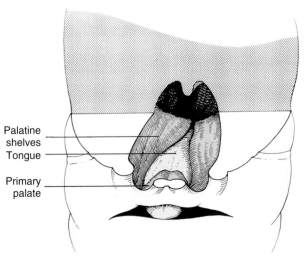

Palatine shelves
Tongue
Primary palate

Fig. 4-9 Palatine shelves position beside the tongue anteriorly and over the tongue posteriorly.

Fig. 4-11 Tongue with overlying palatal shelves at eighth week. The palatal shelves in a near-midline position underlying the nasal septum.

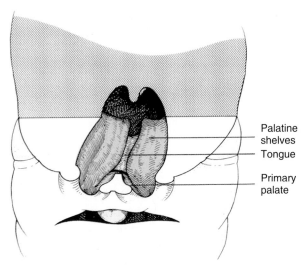

Palatine shelves
Tongue
Primary palate

Fig. 4-10 Elevation of palatine shelves over the tongue. The tongue's position over the palatine shelves during the elevation process early in the eighth week.

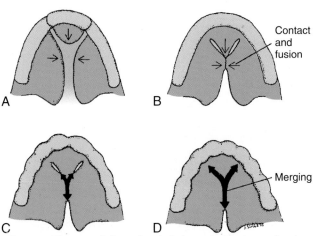

Contact and fusion

Merging

Fig. 4-12 Closure of the palatal shelves. A, Horizontal palatine shelf growth to attain contact in the midline. **B,** Initial contact behind the medial palatal segment. **C** and **D,** Tissues merge anteriorly and posteriorly from the point of initial contact.

The tongue is innervated by the fifth, seventh, ninth, and tenth cranial nerves. This extensive innervation is the result of the long distance the muscle cells migrate to reach the tongue and the varied functions the tongue performs. The muscles travel in the paths of these various nerves. The first pharyngeal arch tissue forms the anterior (movable) body of the tongue. The second and third arches form the posterior, immovable base of the tongue. Tissues of the tongue have three parts, the central **tuberculum impar** and the **two lateral lingual swellings** (Fig. 4-14). The lateral parts rapidly enlarge and merge, overgrowing the central tubercle. A U-shaped

sulcus develops around the anterior part of the tongue, separating it from the jaw tissues and allowing freedom of movement (Fig. 4-15). Gradually the three parts of the anterior tongue merge to form a unified structure. The surface of the body and base of the tongue are separated by a V-shaped groove called the **terminal sulcus.** Posterior to the terminal sulcus, the base of the tongue forms the **lingual tonsil** on the dorsal surface. The lingual tonsil forms part of the ring of tonsils (Waldeyer's ring) in the pharynx along with the **palatine** and **pharyngeal tonsils.** In later stages of development, several types of papillae differentiate on the oral mucosa of the tongue's dorsal body. The lingual tonsil differentiates on the surface of the tongue's base.

Thyroid gland

The thyroid gland develops as an epithelial proliferation from the **foramen cecum** on the surface of the tongue at the junction of the body and base. Cells arise and migrate ventrally in the throat, thus creating the thyroid gland (see Fig. 4-15; Fig. 4-16). Then the cells from the foramen cecum rim descend in the midline floor of the pharynx past the hyoid cartilages to the level of the laryngeal cartilage. Finally, by the seventh week, the thyroid descends to the front of the trachea. During this long migration, the thyroid gland remains attached to the tongue by an epithelial cord or duct termed the **thyroglossal duct,** which later becomes solid and eventually disappears (see Fig. 4-16). Chapter 3 presents further information about this process (see Fig. 3-5, *B*).

Cysts and fistulas are along the route of descent of the thyroid tissue. A **thyroglossal cyst** is a blind pocket lined with thyroid epithelium. This cyst appears as a swelling and is commonly found in the area of the hyoid bone. A **thyroglossal fistula** appears as a swelling that has an opening on the surface of the neck

Fig. 4-13 Coronal section of facial tissue showing palatal shelf fusion in the midline. After contact, the epithelial seam breaks down between the palatal shelves and the overlying nasal septum.

Nasal septum

Fused palatal shelves

Tongue

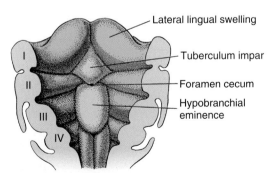

Fig. 4-14 Early tongue development. The body of the tongue develops from two lateral lingual swellings and a centrally located tuberculum impar. The base of the tongue develops from the second and third pharyngeal arches.

Lateral lingual swelling

Tuberculum impar

Foramen cecum

Hypobranchial eminence

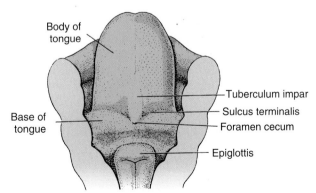

Fig. 4-15 Late tongue development illustrating body and base of the tongue. The foramen cecum is the initial site of the descent of the tubular downgrowth resulting in the thyroid gland.

Body of tongue

Base of tongue

Tuberculum impar

Sulcus terminalis

Foramen cecum

Epiglottis

Fig 4-16 Migratory path down front of neck of thyroid gland tissue. Epithelial cysts and fistulas may arise anteriorly in the midline along path of descent as well as remnants of thyroid tissue along path of descent. The site may be in the region of the thyrohyoid skeleton.

Fig 4-17 Clinical view of thyroglossal fistulas appearing in the anterior midline of the neck. These fistulas typically appear in the region of the thyrohyoid skeleton.

(Fig. 4-17). The gland finally acquires two lateral lobes joined by a thin central isthmus of cells. By the end of the third month of prenatal life, the gland becomes functional.

MALFORMATIONS

Facial and palatal clefts usually occur because of a combination of environmental and genetic factors. An individual's susceptibility to stress is one factor that can have adverse effects.

Cleft lip is the most common facial malformation. Genetic factors play a role, as shown by the differences between racial groups. In the white population of the

United States, the incidence of cleft lip is 1 in every 700 births. Proportionately, significantly fewer African-Americans have clefts, the incidence being only 1 in 2000 newborns. In the Asian population, the incidence is 3 in 2000 births. Asians with one child born with a cleft palate have a 1 in 25 chance of having a second child with the defect. The disparity is not surprising because congenital malformation affects races in different ratios. Evidence shows that a hereditary role exists along with various environmental susceptibility factors.

The incidence of clefts in male and female infants differs according to type of cleft. White boys have nearly twice the number of cleft lips or cleft lips and palates as girls. However, more white girls have cleft palates, which occur at the rate of about 1 in every 2000 births. Overall, cleft palate is less frequent than cleft lip or a combination of cleft lip and palate.

⧉ CLINICAL COMMENT

Clefts of the lips and palate usually occur early in development. These clefts vary in size and shape and usually occur along fusion lines. Most clefts today are corrected by surgical intervention in early life and give the patient an improved quality of life, thus allowing the baby to nurse and feed in an appropriate manner.

Facial Clefts

Facial clefts are classified according to position and extent. A cleft may affect one or both sides of the lip (unilateral or bilateral) and can be either incomplete or complete (Figs. 4-18 to 4-20). An incomplete cleft lip ranges in size from a notch to a deep groove in the upper lip but does not involve an opening of the nostril into the oral cavity (see Fig. 4-18). A true "harelip" is a midline cleft of the maxilla. The term *harelip* is used because a rabbit's upper lip develops with a midline cleft. The rabbit does not develop a medial nasal process, so the two maxillary processes meet in the midline. This condition, which is rare in humans, involves a notch in the medial nasal tissue that may be minute or may extend as a cleft into the nose (Fig. 4-21).

A cleft of the mandible may appear in the midline, although this also is rare (Fig. 4-22). A midline constriction in the mandible is observed during the fourth week. In this case, the early constriction did not disappear and later resulted in a separation of the mandible's halves. This condition is believed to occur because of pressure from the adjacent enlarged heart, which begins beating before the mandible's midline fusion.

Fig. 4-20 **Clinical view of bilateral complete cleft of the lip.** The medial labial process did not fuse on either side of the developing maxillary processes. This results in anterior extrusion of the medial labial process.

Fig. 4-18 **Clinical view of a unilateral cleft of the lip.** This partial cleft is located in the line of fusion of the medial nasal and maxillary processes.

Fig. 4-21 **Clinical view of a midline cleft of the lip.** This rare cleft occurs when the two parts of the medial nasal process fail to merge. The etiology of this condition can be seen in Figure 4-3.

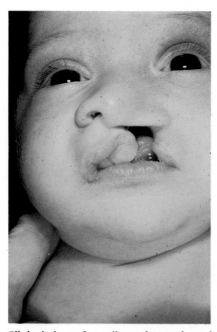

CLINICAL COMMENT

Cleft lip and cleft palate are among the most common congenital malformations. They appear in 1 of every 700 births in the white population and in 1 of 2000 births in the African-American population in the United States.

Fig. 4-19 **Clinical view of a unilateral complete cleft lip.** In this case, the maxillary and medial nasal processes did not fuse and then pulled apart during facial growth.

Palatal Clefts

All the preceding facial clefts involve the lip, but some may extend into the palate as unilateral and bilateral cleft lip and palate defects (Fig. 4-23). Because the palatine shelves meet in the midline, both unilateral and bilateral clefts of the palate are in the midline clefts. Clefts must, however, extend around the medial palatal segment before they proceed in the midline (see Fig. 4-23). Just as clefts of the lip can occur alone, clefts of the palate may occur as an isolated defect (Fig. 4-23, *B*). These palatal clefts can extend just a short distance into the posterior of the palate, can appear in the anterior, or can appear in both locations. However, most cleft palates occur in combination with cleft lips (Figs. 4-24 and 4-25).

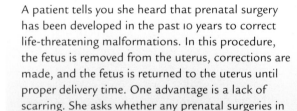

Consider the Patient

A patient tells you she heard that prenatal surgery has been developed in the past 10 years to correct life-threatening malformations. In this procedure, the fetus is removed from the uterus, corrections are made, and the fetus is returned to the uterus until proper delivery time. One advantage is a lack of scarring. She asks whether any prenatal surgeries in the area of dentistry may be of interest.

Fig. 4-24 Example of a unilateral complete cleft lip and palate. This ventral view of a cleft of the palate developed lateral to the medial palatal segment then posteriorly in the midline between the two palatal processes. This cleft occurs along the fusion lines of the palatal processes. The nasal tissue is also malformed.

Fig. 4-22 Clinical example of a midline cleft of the mandible. The two parts of the first pharyngeal arch, including the bony mandible, are separated at birth in this rare condition.

A   B

C   D

Fig. 4-23 Examples of cleft lip and palate. A, Cleft lip only. **B,** Cleft palate only. **C,** Unilateral complete cleft lip and palate. **D,** Bilateral complete cleft lip and palate.

Fig. 4-25 Example of a bilateral complete cleft lip and palate. This bilateral cleft extends lateral to the medial palatal process and then posteriorly in the midline.

Other Defects

Numerous other facial deformities appear clinically, some common and others rare. For example, Figure 4-3 shows the origin of an oronasal optic cleft extending from the mouth to the eye. The most common defects are various malocclusions of the teeth. Midfacial hypoplasia—such as Apert's and Crouzon's syndromes—is a less common abnormality. Chapter 3 describes the developmental aspects of the first and second pharyngeal arch syndromes.

SELF-EVALUATION QUESTIONS

1. From what four embryonic processes does the face arise?
2. During which 3 prenatal weeks does the face develop human characteristics?
3. When do the palatine shelves elevate and begin closure?
4. Name the upper lip's three segments. When do they begin to coalesce into one unit? → wk 8 .
5. From what structure does the nasal fin arise, and why is its disappearance important?
6. What is the origin of the auricles of the ear? From what pharyngeal arches do they arise?
7. Define the primary and secondary palates, explain when each appears, and discuss their relative importance.
8. Describe the process of palatal elevation and the tissues that are believed to contribute to this event.
9. Compare the ratios of facial and palatal defects in the Asian, white, and African-American populations.
10. From what three masses does the body of the tongue arise? What is the origin of the tongue base?

Consider the Patient

> **Discussion:** Prenatal surgery could correct defects such as cleft lip and cleft lip and palate without leaving scars.

Suggested Reading

Moore KL, Persaud TVN. *The developing human: clinically oriented embryology,* ed 7, St. Louis, 2003, Elsevier.

Sadler TW. *Langman's medical embryology,* ed 9, Baltimore, 2003, Lippincott Williams & Wilkins.

Sperber GH. Craniofacial embryology, ed 5, Toronto 2002, BC Decker.

5

DEVELOPMENT OF TEETH

LEARNING OBJECTIVES

After reading this chapter the student will be able to:

- describe the origin of the tooth formative cells and the role of induction in tooth formation
- describe the stages of tooth formation and the mineralization of enamel and dentin
- describe the development of the tissues that surround the developing teeth

KEY TERMS

Alveolar bone proper
Ameloblasts
Amelogenin
Bell stage
Bud stage
Cap stage
Cell signaling
Cementoid
Dental follicle
Dental lamina
Dental papilla
Dental pulp
Dentin

Desmosomes
Developmental or primary cuticle
Enamelin
Epithelial diaphragm
Epithelial rests
Epithelial root sheath/Hertwig's
  root sheath
Hemidesmosomes
Inner enamel epithelial cells
Intermediate cementum
Interradicular bone
Neural crest cells
Odontoblast process

Odontoblasts
Outer enamel epithelial cells
Predentin
Protective stage
Pulp proliferation zone
Reduced enamel epithelium
Stellate reticulum cells
Stratum intermedium cells
Successional lamina
Supporting bone
Terminal bar apparatus
Tomes' processes

OVERVIEW

In the human, 20 primary and 32 permanent teeth develop from the interaction of the oral epithelial cells and the underlying mesenchymal cells. Each developing tooth grows as an anatomically distinct unit, but the basic developmental process is similar for all teeth.

Each tooth develops through successive bud, cap, and bell stages (Fig. 5-1, *A* to *C*). During these early stages, the tooth germs grow and expand, and the cells that are to form the hard tissues of the teeth differentiate. Differentiation takes place in the bell stage, setting the stage for enamel and dentin formation (Fig. 5-1, *D* and *E*). As the crowns are formed and mineralized, the roots of the teeth begin to form. After the roots calcify, the supporting tissues of the teeth—the cementum, periodontal ligament, and alveolar bone—begin to develop (Fig. 5-1, *F* and *G*). This formation occurs whether the tooth is an incisor with a single root, a premolar with several roots, or a molar with multiple roots. Subsequently, the completed tooth crown erupts into the oral cavity (Fig. 5-1, *G*). Root formation and cementogenesis continue until a functional tooth and its supporting structures are fully developed (Fig. 5-1, *G* and *H*).

CLINICAL COMMENT

Developmentally missing permanent teeth can be a result of a genetic abnormality. When fewer than six teeth are missing, it is termed hypodontia, and when more than six teeth are missing, it is oligodontia.

INITIATION OF TOOTH DEVELOPMENT

Teeth develop from two types of cells: oral epithelial cells form the enamel organ and mesenchymal cells form the dental papilla. Enamel develops from the enamel organ, and dentin forms from the dental papilla. The interaction of these epithelial and mesenchymal cells is vital to the initiation and formation of the teeth. In addition to these cells, the **neural crest cells** contribute to tooth development. The neural crest cells arise from the neural tissue at an early stage of development and migrate into the jaws, intermingling with mesenchymal cells. They function by integrating with the dental papillae and epithelial cells of the early enamel organ, which aids in the development of the teeth. The cells also function in the development of the salivary glands, bone, cartilage, nerves, and muscles of the face. Chapter 1 discusses neural crest cells and explains the cell's migration (see Fig. 1-17).

The first sign of tooth formation is the development of **dental lamina** rising from the oral epithelium. Dental lamina develops into a sheet of epithelial cells that pushes into the underlying mesenchyme around the perimeter of both the maxillary and mandibular jaws (Fig. 5-2). At the leading edge of the lamina, 20 areas of enlargement appear, which form tooth buds for the

Fig. 5-1 Stages of tooth development. A, Bud. **B,** Cap. **C,** Bell. **D** and **E,** Dentinogenesis and amelogenesis. **F,** Crown formation. **G,** Root formation and eruption. **H,** Function.

Fig. 5-2 Development of tooth buds in the alveolar process. Anterior teeth are more advanced in development than posterior teeth. Anterior lamina has begun to degenerate as posterior lamina forms. When tooth buds have differentiated, lamina is no longer needed and degenerates.

20 primary teeth (see Fig. 5-2). At this early stage, the tooth buds have already determined their crown morphology of an incisor or molar. This is the result of gene expression. After primary teeth develop from the buds, the leading edge of the lamina continues to grow to develop the permanent teeth, which succeed the 20 primary teeth. This part of the lamina is thus called the **successional lamina** (Fig. 5-3). The lamina continues posteriorly into the elongating jaw and from it come the posterior teeth, which form behind the primary teeth. In this manner, 20 of the permanent teeth replace the 20 primary teeth, and 12 posterior permanent molars develop behind the primary dentition (see Fig. 5-3). The last teeth to develop are the third molars, which develop about 15 years after birth. Because the molars do not succeed the primary teeth, they do not form from the successional lamina but from the general lamina. The initiating dental lamina that forms both the successional and general lamina begins to function in the sixth

prenatal week and continues to function until the fifteenth year, producing all 52 teeth. In general, the teeth develop anteroposteriorly, which relates to the growing jaws. The posterior molars do not develop until space is available for them in the posterior jaw area. The second dentition does not develop until after the primary teeth are formed and functioning. Gradually the permanent teeth form under the primary crowns and later posteriorly to the primary molars.

STAGES OF TOOTH DEVELOPMENT

Although tooth formation is a continuous process, it is characterized by a series of easily distinguishable stages known as the bud, cap, and bell stages. Each stage is defined according to the shape of the epithelial enamel organ, which is a part of the developing tooth. The initial stage, the **bud stage,** is a rounded, localized growth of epithelial cells surrounded by proliferating mesenchymal cells (Fig. 5-4). Gradually, as the rounded epithelial bud enlarges, it gains a concave surface, which begins the **cap stage** (Fig. 5-5). The epithelial cells now become the enamel organ and remain attached to the lamina. The mesenchyme forms the **dental papilla,** which becomes the dental pulp. The tissue surrounding these two structures is the **dental follicle.**

After further growth of the papilla and the enamel organ, the tooth reaches the morphodifferentiation and histodifferentiation stage, also known as the **bell stage** (Fig. 5-6). At this stage, the inner enamel epithelial cells are characterized by the shape of the tooth they form (see Fig. 5-6). Also, the cells of the enamel organ have differentiated into the **outer enamel epithelial cells,** which cover the enamel organ, and **inner enamel epithelial cells,** which become the **ameloblasts** that form the enamel of the tooth crown. Between these two cell layers are the **stellate reticulum cells,** which are star shaped with processes attached to each other. A fourth

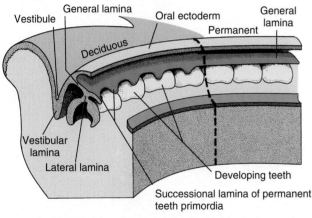

Fig. 5-3 Dental lamina formation is shown in relation to the general lamina. From the successional lamina come permanent teeth, which replace the primary teeth except for the permanent molars.

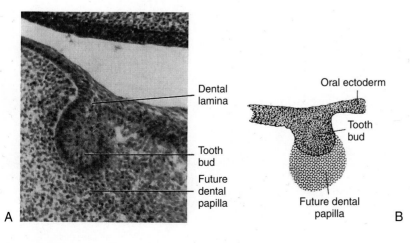

Fig. 5-4 Initiation of tooth development. A, Histology of the bud stage. **B,** Diagram of the bud stage.

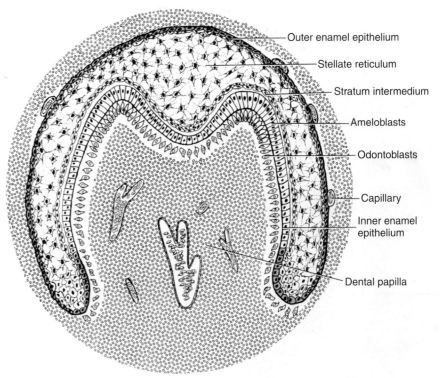

Fig. 5-5 Cap stage of tooth development. The enamel organ is outlined in *blue,* indicating that it is of ectodermal origin. The mesenchyme of the dental papilla surrounds the enamel organ.

Oral mucosa

Dental lamina

Enamel organ

Outer enamel epithelium

Inner enamel epithelium

Stellate reticulum

Dental follicle

Dental papilla

Fig. 5-6 Bell stage of tooth development. During this stage of tooth development, both odontoblasts and ameloblasts have fully differentiated in the cuspal region(s). Blood vessels develop in the dental papilla, whereas the only vascularized structure in the enamel organ is the outer enamel epithelium that contains a capillary plexus.

Outer enamel epithelium

Stellate reticulum

Stratum intermedium

Ameloblasts

Odontoblasts

Capillary

Inner enamel epithelium

Dental papilla

layer in the enamel organ is composed of **stratum intermedium cells.** These cells lie adjacent to the inner enamel epithelial cells. They assist the ameloblast in the formation of enamel. The function of the outer enamel epithelial cells is to organize a network of capillaries that will bring nutrition to the ameloblasts.

From the outer enamel epithelium, nutrients will percolate through the stellate reticulum to the ameloblasts. During the bell stage, cells in the periphery of the dental papilla become **odontoblasts.** These cells differentiate from mesenchymal cells. As the odontoblasts elongate and become columnar, they form a matrix of collagen fibers identified as **predentin.** After 24 hours, this increment of matrix calcifies and becomes **dentin.** When several increments of dentin have formed, the differentiated ameloblasts deposit an enamel matrix. Dentinogenesis always precedes amelogenesis. After the enamel organ is differentiated, the dental lamina begins to degenerate by undergoing lysis. The dental lamina disappears in the anterior part of the mouth, although it remains active in the posterior region for many years (see Figs. 5-2 and 5-3).

Cells interact through a system of effectors, modulators, and receptors called **cell signaling.** An example of such a system is epithelial-mesenchymal interaction in tooth development. The precursor cells, odontoblast and ameloblast, establish a positional relationship by means of effectors and receptors that are on the cell surface. The ameloblast differentiates first, causing the precursor odontoblast to locate itself adjacent. Then the odontoblast differentiates, establishing with the ameloblast a basement membrane that then forms a dentinal matrix. After this formation occurs, the ameloblast forms the enamel matrix. Thus it is not only cells, but also basal lamina and dentin matrix, that contain substances that cause cell changes and position.

DEVELOPMENT OF THE DENTAL PAPILLA

Densely packed cells characterize the dental papilla. This is evident even in the early bud stage, during which cells proliferate around the enlarging tooth buds at the leading edge of the dental lamina (Fig. 5-7). The papilla cells are believed to be significant in furthering enamel organ bud formation into the cap and bell stage. This cell density is maintained as the enamel organ grows. Cells of the dental papilla are found on close examination to be fibroblasts and appear to be in a delicate reticulum (Fig. 5-8). Blood vessels appear early in the dental papilla, initially in the central region along with nerve fibers associated with these vessels. The vessels bring nutrition to the rapidly growing organ. As the papilla grows, smaller vessels are also seen in the periphery of the area, bringing nutrition to the elongating odontoblasts (see Fig. 5-6). Cellular changes result in formation of a hard shell around the central papilla. As this occurs, the papilla becomes known as the **dental pulp.**

DENTINOGENESIS

As the odontoblasts elongate, they gain the appearance of a protein-producing cell. A process develops at the proximal end of the cell, adjacent to the dentinoenamel junction. Gradually the cell moves pulpward, and the cell process, known as the **odontoblast process,** elongates (Fig. 5-9). The odontoblast becomes active in dentinal matrix formation similar to an osteoblast when it moves away from a spicule of bone. Increments of dentin are formed along the dentinoenamel junction. The dentinal matrix is first a meshwork of collagen fibers, but within 24 hours it becomes calcified. It is called *predentin* before calcification and *dentin* after calcification. At that time, the dental papilla becomes the dental pulp as dentin begins to surround it. The odontoblasts maintain their elongating processes in dentinal tubules (see Fig. 5-9).

Dental papilla

Dental follicle

Degenerating lamina

Molar bud

Fig. 5-7 Histology of tooth development. Sagittal view of the human maxillary and mandibular molar tooth buds.

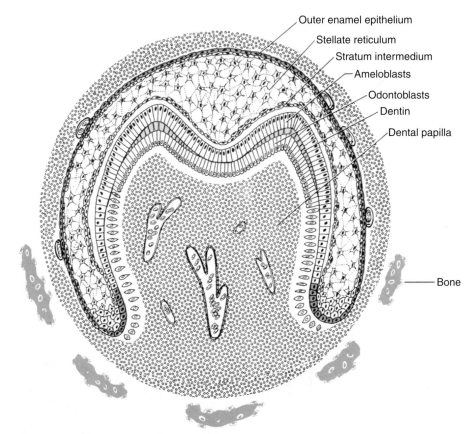

Outer enamel epithelium
Stellate reticulum
Stratum intermedium
Ameloblasts
Odontoblasts
Dentin
Dental papilla

Bone

Fig. 5-8 Dentinogenesis stage of tooth development. The initial formation of dentin *(yellow)* at the cuspal tips and the vascularized pulp organ are characteristic of the dentinogenesis stage. The dental follicular cells are differentiating around the enamel organ and alveolar bone proper is beginning to define the dental crypt.

When the odontoblasts are functioning, their nuclei occupy a more basal position in the cell, and the organelles become more evident in the cell cytoplasm. The appearance of granular endoplasmic reticulum, Golgi's complex, and mitochondria indicates the protein-producing nature of these cells (Fig. 5-10, *C* to *E*). The odontoblasts then secrete protein externally via vesicles at the apical part of the cell and along the cell processes (see Fig. 5-10). The collagenous dentinal matrix is laid down in increments like bone or enamel, which is indicative of a daily rhythm for hard tissue formation. The site of initial formation is at the cusp tips (see Fig. 5-8), and as further increments are formed, more odontoblasts are activated along the dentinoenamel junction (see Fig. 5-9). As the odontoblastic process elongates, a tubule is maintained in the dentin, and the matrix is formed around this tubule (Fig. 5-10, *C* and *D*).

Dentinogenesis takes place in two phases. First is the collagen matrix formation, followed by the deposition of calcium phosphate (hydroxyapatite) crystals in the matrix. The initial calcification appears as crystals that are in small vesicles on the surface and within the

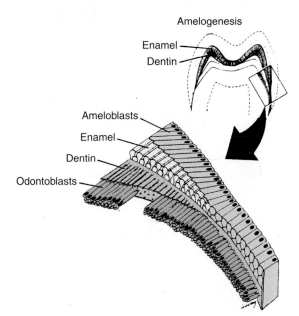

Amelogenesis
Enamel
Dentin
Ameloblasts
Enamel
Dentin
Odontoblasts

Fig. 5-9 Appositional stage of tooth development. During this stage of tooth development, both enamel and dentin are actively secreted until the crown is complete.

Fig. 5-10 Diagram of enamel and dentin formation. A, Initiation. **B,** Differentiation. **C,** Dentinogenesis. **D,** Apposition of enamel and dentin. **E** to **H,** Stages of enamel formation. **E,** Secretory stage of enamel formation. **F,** Early maturation. **G,** Late maturation. **H,** Protective stage in which the ameloblasts secrete the developmental cuticle. During maturation of enamel, an influx of mineral is accompanied by a loss of organic matter and water from the enamel matrix.

Fig. 5-11 Initiation of dentinogenesis. A transmission electron micrograph of a band of predentin, dentin, and enamel at the dentinoenamel junction. This initially secreted dentin is mantle dentin and is significantly different from the dentin that is formed by incremental deposition later in development. Calcification of the predentin will spread from nucleation sites within the matrix vesicles.

collagen fibers (Fig. 5-11). The crystals grow, spread, and coalesce until the matrix is completely calcified. Only the newly formed band of dentinal matrix along the pulpal border is uncalcified (Fig. 5-12). Matrix formation and mineralization therefore are closely related. Mineralization proceeds by an increase in mineral density of the dentin. As each daily increment of predentin forms along the pulpal boundary, the adjacent peripheral increment of predentin formed the previous day calcifies and becomes dentin (see Figs. 5-10 and 5-12; Fig. 5-13).

AMELOGENESIS

Ameloblasts begin enamel deposition after a few micrometers of dentin have been deposited at the dentinoenamel junction (Fig. 5-14). At the bell stage, cells of the inner enamel epithelium differentiate. They elongate and are ready to become active secretory ameloblasts. The ameloblasts then exhibit changes as they differentiate and pass through five functional stages: (1) morphogenesis, (2) organization and differentiation, (3) secretion, (4) maturation, and (5) protection (see Fig. 5-10). Golgi's apparatus appears centrally in the ameloblasts, and the amount of rough endoplasmic reticulum (RER) increases in the apical area (see Fig. 5-10, *D* and *E*). The row of ameloblasts maintains orientation by cell-to-cell attachments (desmosomes) at both the proximal and distal ends of the cell. This maintains the cells in a row as they move peripherally from the dentinoenamel junction depositing enamel matrix (see Fig. 5-9).

Short conical processes **(Tomes' processes)** develop at the apical end of the ameloblasts during the secretory stage (see Fig. 5-10, *E*; Fig. 5-15). Junctional complexes called the **terminal bar apparatus** appear at the junction of the cell bodies and Tomes' processes and maintain contact between adjacent cells (see Fig. 5-10, *E*).

Fig. 5-12 Calcification of dentin at the mineralization front.

As the ameloblast differentiates, the matrix is synthesized within the RER, which then migrates to Golgi's apparatus, where it is condensed and packaged in membrane-bound granules. Vesicles migrate to the apical end of the cell, where their contents are exteriorized and are deposited first along the junction of the enamel and dentin (Fig. 5-16). This first enamel deposited on the surface of the dentin establishes the dentinoenamel junction. Figure 5-17 is an electron micrograph of young enamel matrix formed along the dentinoenamel junction. The Tomes' process of the ameloblast indents the surface of the enamel (see Figs. 5-10, *E,* 5-15, and 5-16). This is because the center of the rod does not form at the same rate as the rod walls; this can best be seen in Figure 5-17. As the enamel matrix develops, it forms in continuous rods from the dentinoenamel junction to the surface of the enamel.

When ameloblasts begin secretion, the overlying cells of the stratum intermedium change in shape from

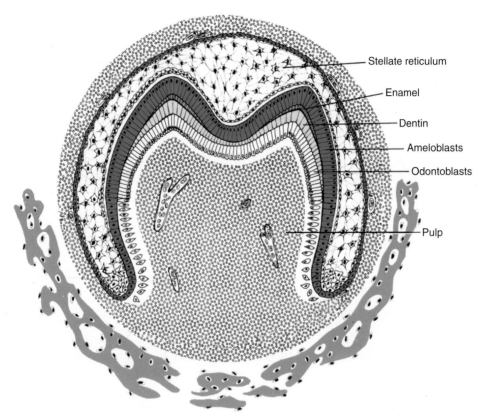

Fig. 5-13 Diagram of amelogenesis. Observe the thin layer of enamel secreted by the overlying ameloblasts at the cusp tips. Underlying the enamel is a layer of dentin formed by the odontoblasts. Observe the two layers of hard tissue that lie in apposition and form first at the cusp tips.

Fig. 5-14 Microradiograph of dentin illustrating incremental lines in dentin showing the deposition of dentin in increments.

Fig. 5-15 Diagram of Tome's process, the specialized secretory process of the ameloblast during enamel formation.

spindle to pyramidal (see Fig. 5-10, *B* to *F*). As amelogenesis proceeds, both of these cell layers, ameloblasts and stratum intermedium, are held together by cell junctional complexes termed **desmosomes,** with synthesis of enamel occurring in both cells. Substances needed for enamel production arrive via the blood vessels and pass through the stellate reticulum to the stratum intermedium and ameloblasts. In this manner, the protein **amelogenin** is produced. Only a few ameloblasts at the tip of the cusps begin to function initially (see Fig. 5-13). As the process proceeds, more ameloblasts become active, and the increments of enamel matrix become more prominent.

Growth of individual cusps by incremental deposition continues until tooth eruption. This occurs in posterior multicuspid teeth as the ameloblasts continue to differentiate from the inner enamel epithelium and form enamel. Cusps then coalesce in the intercuspal region of the crown (Fig. 5-18). In radiographs, cusps initially appear separated and are joined together as growth progresses. The inner enamel epithelium forms the blueprint for the shape of the developing crown.

Fig. 5-16 **Ultrastructure of the dentoenamel junction showing early enamel and dentin matrix formation.**

Labels in Fig. 5-16: Tome's process, Enamel, Dentinoenamel junction, Dentin, Predentin

CLINICAL COMMENT

Amelogenesis imperfecta is a genetic problem in which the enamel is poorly developed and mineralized. This can be the result of cellular malfunction resulting in defective enamel matrix formation.

CROWN MATURATION

As amelogenesis is completed and amelogenin is deposited, the matrix begins to mineralize (see Fig. 5-10, F to H). As soon as the small crystals of mineral are deposited, they begin to grow in length and diameter. The initial deposition of mineral amounts to approximately 25% of the total enamel. The other 70% of mineral in enamel is a result of growth of the crystals (5% of enamel is water). The time between enamel matrix deposition and its mineralization is short. Therefore the pattern of mineralization closely follows the pattern of matrix deposition. The first matrix deposited is the first enamel mineralized, occurring along the dentinoenamel junction. Matrix formation and mineralization continue peripherally to the tips of the cusps and then laterally on the sides of the crowns, following the enamel incremental deposition pattern (Fig. 5-19). Finally, the cervical region of the crown mineralizes. During this process, protein of the enamel changes or matures and is termed **enamelin.**

The mineral content of enamel is approximately 95% as it rapidly surpasses that of dentin (69%) to become the most highly calcified tissue in the human body. Because of the high mineral content of enamel, almost all water and organic material are lost from it during maturation (see Fig. 5-10, E to H).

As the ameloblast completes the matrix deposition phase, its terminal bar apparatus disappears, and the

Fig. 5-17 **Scanning electron micrograph showing interface between ameloblast and enamel matrix during amelogenesis.** Pits are result of presence of Tome's process.

Labels in Fig. 5-17: Human deciduous molar, Developing enamel surface, Height of field, 15–18 mm

Growth of cusps to predetermined point of completion

Fig. 5-18 **Diagram of growth areas of developing crown.** Growth occurs at cusp tips, then intercuspal zones and the cervical zone.

surface enamel becomes smooth (see Fig. 5-10, *F* and *G*). This phase is signaled by a change in the appearance of the cell as well as by a change in the function of the ameloblast. The apical end of this cell becomes ruffled along the enamel surface. The length of the ameloblast decreases, as does the number of organelles within it. The enamel has now reached the maturation phase, and the ameloblast becomes more active in absorption of the organic matrix and water from enamel, which allows mineralization to proceed (see Fig. 5-10, *F* to *H*).

The increased mineral content in enamel is dependent on the loss of fluid and protein. This process of exchange occurs throughout much of enamel maturation and is not limited to the final stage of mineralization. Even after the teeth erupt, mineralization of enamel continues.

Finally, after the ameloblasts have completed their contributions to the mineralization phase, they secrete an organic cuticle on the surface of the enamel, which is known as the **developmental** or **primary cuticle.** The ameloblasts then attach themselves to this organic covering of the enamel by **hemidesmosomes** (see Fig. 5-10, *H*). A hemidesmosome is half of a desmosome attachment plaque. Whereas a desmosome functions in attaching a cell to an adjacent cell, a hemidesmosome relates to the attachment of a cell to a surface membrane. The hemidesmosome attachment plaque is developed by the ameloblast, and this stage of plaque formation and attachment is known as the **protective stage** of ameloblast function. The ameloblasts shorten and contact the stratum intermedium and other enamel epithelium, which fuse together to form the **reduced enamel epithelium.** This cellular organic covering remains on the enamel surface until the tooth erupts into the oral cavity.

With mineralization of enamel complete and its thickness established, the crown of the tooth is formed (Fig. 5-20). The nearly completed crown with the reduced enamel epithelium is seen in Figure 5-21.

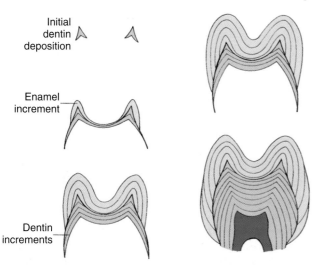

Fig. 5-19 Incremental pattern of enamel and dentin formation from initiation to completion. Development proceeds from upper left to lower right.

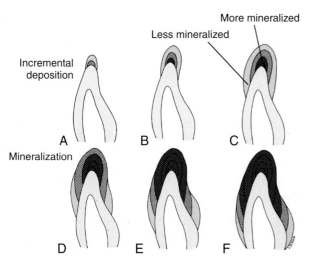

Fig. 5-20 Summary of enamel mineralization stages. A, Initial enamel is formed. **B,** Initial enamel is calcified as further enamel is formed. **C,** More increments are formed. **D,** Matrix deposition and mineralization proceeds. **E** and **F,** Matrix is formed on the sides and cervical areas of the crown.

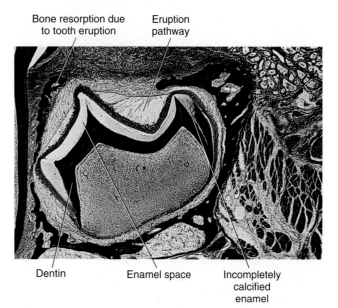

Fig. 5-21 Demineralized section of enamel of crown showing loss of mineralized enamel. Enamel matrix is present only at the cervical region where the matrix still contains developmental enamel proteins.

Meanwhile, dentin formation proceeds. The next stage of development will be root formation.

Consider the Patient

> A patient complains that white, chalky areas appear in the cervical enamel of some of his crowns. He asks what could cause this condition.

DEVELOPMENT OF THE TOOTH ROOT

Root Sheath

As the crown develops, cell proliferation continues at the cervical region or base of the enamel organ, where the inner and outer enamel epithelial cells join to form a root sheath (Fig. 5-22). When the crown is completed, the cells in this region of the enamel organ continue to grow, forming a double layer of cells termed the **epithelial root sheath** or **Hertwig's root sheath** (Fig. 5-22, *A*).

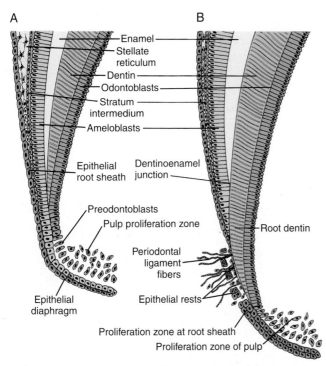

Fig. 5-22 Root formation, showing root sheath and epithelial diaphragm. A, Time of epithelial root sheath formation showing fusion of outer and inner enamel epithelium to form the epithelial root sheath, which includes the vertical epithelial root trunk and inward bending epithelial diaphragm. **B,** Later stage of root sheath development. Root dentin has formed below the cervical enamel on the surface of the pulp organ. Cementoblasts, periodontal ligament fibers, and epithelial rests are present in the ligament.

The inner cell layer of the root sheath forms from the inner enamel epithelium or ameloblasts in the crown, and enamel is produced. In the root, these cells induce odontoblasts of the dental papilla to differentiate and form dentin. The root sheath originates at the point that enamel deposits end. As the root sheath lengthens, it becomes the architect of the root. The length, curvature, thickness, and number of roots are all dependent on the inner root sheath cells. As the formation of the root dentin takes place, cells of the outer root sheath function in the deposition of **intermediate cementum,** a thin layer of acellular cementum that covers the ends of the dentinal tubule and seals the root surface. Then the outer root sheath cells disperse into small clusters and move away from the root surface as **epithelial rests** (Fig. 5-22, *B*). At the proliferating end, the root sheath bends at a near 45-degree angle. This area is termed the **epithelial diaphragm** (see Fig. 5-22). The epithelial diaphragm encircles the apical opening of the dental pulp during root development. It is the proliferation of these cells that causes root growth to occur.

As the odontoblasts differentiate along the pulpal boundary, root dentinogenesis proceeds and the root lengthens. Dentin formation continues from the crown into the root (Fig. 5-23). The dentin tapers from the crown into the root to the apical epithelial diaphragm. In the pulp adjacent to the epithelial diaphragm, cellular proliferation occurs. This is known as the **pulp proliferation zone** (see Fig. 5-22). It is believed that this area produces new cells needed for root lengthening. Dentinogenesis continues until the appropriate root length is developed. The root then thickens until the apical opening is restricted to approximately 1 to 3 mm, which is sufficient to allow neural and vascular communication between the pulp and the periodontium.

Fig. 5-23 Histology of root formation, showing root sheath and epithelial diaphragm. The highly cellular pulp proliferative zone is shown in the apical pulpal zone.

With the increase in root length, the tooth begins eruptive movements, which provide space for further lengthening of the root. The root lengthens at the same rate as the tooth eruptive movements occur (Fig. 5-24).

 CLINICAL COMMENT

> The presence of the epithelial root sheath determines whether a root will be curved or straight, short or long, or single or multiple.

Single Root

The root sheath of a single-rooted tooth is a tubelike growth of epithelial cells that originates from the enamel organ, enclosing a tube of dentin and the developing pulp (see Fig. 5-23). As soon as the root sheath cells deposit the intermediate cementum, the root sheath breaks up, forming epithelial rests (see Fig. 5-22, *B*; Fig. 5-25). The epithelial rests persist as they move away from the root surface into the follicular area. Mesenchymal cells from the tooth follicle move between the epithelial rests to contact the root surface. Here, they differentiate into cementoblasts and begin secretion of **cementoid** on the surface of the intermediate cementum. Cementoid is noncalcified cementum that soon calcifies into mature cementum (Fig. 5-26). The root sheath is never seen as a continuous structure because its cell layers break down rapidly once the root dentin forms. However, the area of the epithelial diaphragm is maintained until the root is complete; then it disappears.

Multiple Roots

The roots of multirooted teeth develop in a fashion similar to those of single-rooted teeth until the furcation zone begins to form (Fig. 5-27). Division of the

roots then takes place through differential growth of the root sheath. The cells of the epithelial diaphragm grow excessively in two or more areas until they contact the opposing epithelial extensions. These extensions fuse, and then the original single opening is divided into two or three openings. The epithelial diaphragm

Fig. 5-25 **Epithelial rests resulting from breakup of epithelial root sheath.**

Fig. 5-24 **Direction of root growth versus eruptive movements of the tooth.**

Fig. 5-26 **Cementum formation on the root surface after breakup of the epithelial root sheath.** Cementocytes can be seen on the surface as well as within the cementum.

surrounding the opening to each root continues to grow at an equal rate. When a developing molar is sectioned through the center of its root, it shows the root sheath as an island of cells (Fig. 5-28).

As the multiple roots form, each one develops by the same pattern as a single-rooted tooth. After the root is complete and the sheath breaks up, the epithelial cells migrate away from the root surface as they do in a single-rooted tooth. Cementum then forms on the surface of the intermediate cemental surface. The cementum usually appears cellular, although the cementum near the cementoenamel junction is less cellular than that at the apices of the root (Fig. 5-29). Because the apical cementum is thicker, it is said to require more cells to maintain vitality. The primary function of this cementum involves the attachment of the principal periodontal ligament fibers.

DEVELOPMENT OF PRIMARY AND PERMANENT TEETH

Primary and permanent teeth develop very similarly, although the time needed for development of primary teeth is much less than for the permanent teeth. Primary teeth begin development in utero, and the crown undergoes complete mineralization before birth, whereas the permanent teeth begin formation at or after birth. In Figures 6-1 and 6-2, the formation of the primary and permanent incisors is compared as is the first primary second molar and the permanent premolar. Any prenatal systemic disturbance will affect mineralization of the primary tooth crowns, whereas postnatal disturbances may affect the permanent tooth crowns.

Primary teeth function in the mouth approximately 8.5 years; this period of time may be divided into three periods: crown and root development, root maturation

and root resorption, and shedding of the teeth. The first period extends for about a year, the second for about 3.75 years, and the final stage of resorption and shedding lasts for about 3.5 years. In contrast, some of the permanent teeth may be in the mouth from the fifth year until death. One must also consider the permanent molars, which may be in the mouth only from the 25th year on until they are lost or death occurs. The permanent teeth may function seven or eight times as long as the primary teeth. This time of function of permanent teeth includes 12 years of development, 3 years longer than the primary teeth.

Many separate events occur within a few millimeters during development of the dentition. For a single primary tooth and its successor, an example of two possibly simultaneous events could be eruption with root formation of the primary tooth and mineralization of

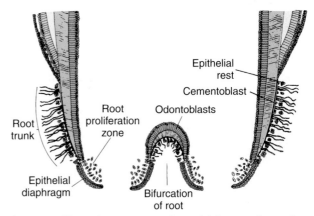

Fig. 5-28 Bifurcation root zone in multiple root formation. The root trunk is the junction area between the crown and the root bifurcation area.

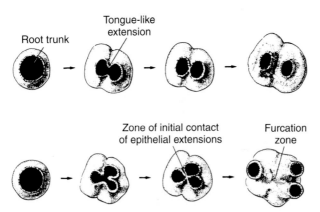

Fig. 5-27 Development of multirooted teeth. As the epithelial diaphragm grows, it may make contact and fuse to develop one-, two-, or three-rooted teeth.

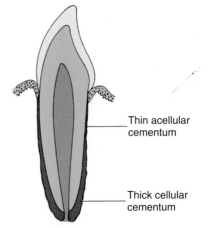

Fig. 5-29 Location of thin cementum on cervical area of root (younger individual) and additional apical cementum in an older individual.

the crown of the permanent tooth. Other examples of complex events during this mixed dentition stage are root resorption of the primary tooth and formation of the root of the permanent tooth. In a 6-year-old child one or more of these formative processes may be occurring in up to 28 of 32 permanent teeth, while some degree of resorption is occurring in the 20 primary teeth. Timing and coordination of myriad events allow continual function within the growing jaws.

In addition to the formative events, the primary teeth undergo root resorption and pulp degeneration.

DEVELOPMENT OF SUPPORTING STRUCTURES

The mesenchymal cells surrounding the teeth are known as the dental follicle (see Fig. 5-7). Some of these follicular cells, which lie immediately adjacent to the enamel organ, migrate during the cap and bell stages from the enamel organ peripherally into the follicle to develop the alveolar bone and the periodontal ligament (Fig. 5-30). These cells have been traced from this origin to the site where they differentiate into osteoblasts and form bone or fibroblasts, which form ligament fibers. After tooth eruption, these tissues serve to support the teeth during function.

Periodontal Ligament

Cells of the dental follicle differentiate into collagen-forming cells of the ligament and form cementoblasts, which lay cementum on tooth roots. Some cells of the ligament invade the root sheath as it breaks apart. Other cells of the ligament area form delicate fibers, which appear along the forming roots near the cervical region

of the crown. These are probably the stem cell fibroblasts that form more fiber groups, which appear as the roots elongate (Fig. 5-31). As these fibers become embedded in the cementum of the root surface, the other end attaches to the forming alveolar bone. Evidence suggests that these fibers turn over rapidly and are continually renewed as the location of origin is established. Collagen fiber turnover takes place throughout the ligament, although the highest turnover is in the apical area and the lowest is in the cervical region. Maturation of the ligament occurs when the teeth reach functional occlusion. At this time, the density of fiber bundles increases notably.

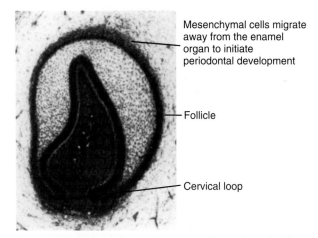

Mesenchymal cells migrate away from the enamel organ to initiate periodontal development

Follicle

Cervical loop

Fig. 5-30 Histology of enamel organ at time of cervical loop development. At this time, mesenchymal cells develop adjacent to the enamel organ on the external surface of the developing enamel organ and differentiate into follicular cells.

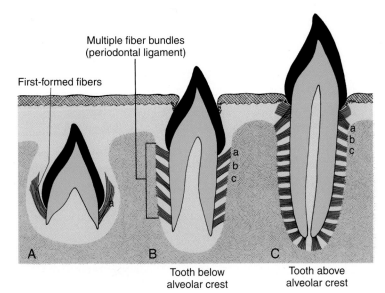

Multiple fiber bundles (periodontal ligament)

First-formed fibers

A

B

Tooth below alveolar crest

C

Tooth above alveolar crest

Fig. 5-31 Development of principal fibers of the periodontal ligament. A, Initial fiber development during preeruptive movements *(a)*. **B,** Secondary fiber development below alveolar crest as tooth moves into prefunctional occlusion *(b)*. **C,** Further fiber development and maturation of the principal fibers when the tooth reaches functional occlusion *(c)*.

Alveolar Process

As the teeth develop, so does the alveolar bone, which keeps pace with the lengthening roots. At first, the alveolar process forms labial and lingual plates between which a trench is formed where the tooth organs develop. As the walls lining this trench increase in height, bony septa appear between the teeth to complete the crypts (Fig. 5-32). When the teeth erupt, the alveolar process and intervening periodontal ligament mature to support the newly functioning teeth (Fig. 5-33). Bone that forms between the roots of the multirooted teeth is termed **interradicular bone.** In the mature form, alveolar bone is composed of **alveolar bone proper** and **supporting bone.** Alveolar bone proper lines the tooth socket, sustained by supporting bone, which is composed of both spongy and dense or compact bone. Supporting bone forms the cortical plate, which covers the mandible (Fig. 5-34).

In summary, tooth development involves the interactive events of two types of tissues: epithelial and mesenchymal. These tissues develop through the soft tissue stages of bud, cap, and bell. This level is followed by the hard tissue formative stages of dentinogenesis and amelogenesis. Root formation logically follows crown development. Each developmental progression includes morphologic changes in shape and size, which are coordinated with microscopic changes in cell shape and function. Most of these relationships are seen in Figure 5-35.

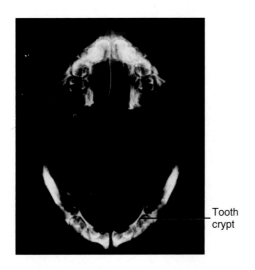

Tooth crypt

Fig. 5-32 Microradiograph of maxillary and mandibular arches showing alveolar bone and primary tooth crypts enclosing developing teeth.

Forming periodontal ligament fibers

Alveolar bone

Dentin

Cementum

Fig. 5-33 Developing periodontal ligament fibers. Density of fibers similar to **C** in Figure 5-31.

Fig. 5-34 Tooth in alveolar bone. Alveolar bone is composed of alveolar bone proper, which lines the socket, and supporting bone, which consists of spongy or cancellous bone and compact bone.

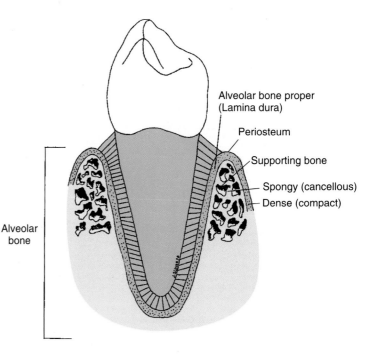

Alveolar bone proper (Lamina dura)

Periosteum

Supporting bone

Spongy (cancellous)

Dense (compact)

Alveolar bone

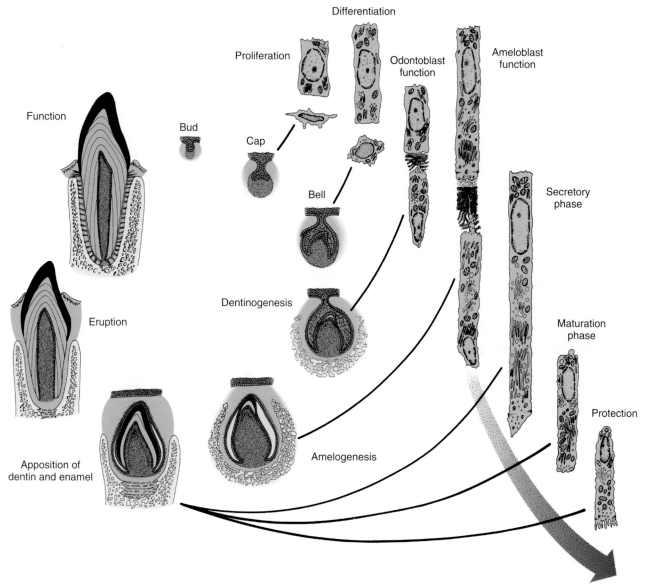

Fig. 5-35 Changes in formative cells of developing teeth shown on the *right* and correlated with morphologic changes of tooth organ on the *left*. Cell proliferation relates to the cap stage, whereas cell differentiation relates to the bell stage. Odontoblast function relates to dentinogenesis and ameloblast function to amelogenesis. The labels secretory phase, maturation phase, and protection phase relate to ameloblast function.

 CLINICAL COMMENT

Accessory root canals may connect the pulp with the periodontal ligament at any point along the root, although it usually appears near the root apex. Pulp or periodontal infection can spread by means of this route to the adjacent tissue. A periodontal pocket that is resistant to treatment could be caused by this defect.

SELF-EVALUATION QUESTIONS

1. What two cell types interact in tooth development?
2. Describe two characteristics of the bell stage of tooth development.
3. List and describe each stage of tooth development.
4. Describe the dental papilla. When does it become the dental pulp organ?
5. Describe the differentiation of the odontoblast and the initiation of dentin formation.
6. Why is dentinogenesis called the two-phases process?
7. What are the five phases of enamel production?

8. What structures enable the ameloblasts to move in a row rather than individually during enamel production?
9. What areas of enamel are first and last to calcify in the crown?
10. What two processes signal enamel completion?

 Consider the Patient

> **Discussion:** White, chalky areas in the cervical enamel of some crowns are caused by a lack of mineralization of the enamel. The chalkiness occurs in this location because this is the last area of the crown to calcify and sometimes the crown erupts before the cervical enamel has completely mineralized.

Acknowledgments

Dr. Nicholas P. Piesco and Dr. N.M. Elnesr contributed to the production of chapters in Avery JK: *Oral development and histology,* ed 3, Stuttgart, 2002, Thieme Medical. Some of the figures in that text have been used in preparation of this chapter.

Suggested Reading

Kallenbach E, Piesco NP: The changing morphology of the epithelium-mesenchyme interface in the differentiation of growing teeth of selected vertebrates and its relationship to possible mechanisms of differentiation, *J Biol Buccale* 6:229-240, 1978.

Marks SC et al: Tooth eruption, a synthesis of experimental observations. In Davidovich Z, editor: *The biological mechanisms of tooth eruption and root resorption,* Birmingham, AL, 1988, EBSCO Information Services, pp 161-169.

Robinson C, Kirkham J: Dynamics of amelogenesis as revealed by protein compositional studies. In *The chemistry and biology of mineralized tissues,* Birmingham, Alabama, 1985, EBSCO Media, pp 248-263.

Thesleff I, Vaahtokari A: The role of growth factors in the determination of odontoblastic cell lineage, *Proc Finn Dent Soc* 88(SI): 357-368, 1992.

Warshasky H et al: The development of enamel structure in the rat incisor as compared to the teeth of monkey and man, *Anat Rec* 299:371, 1981.

Wise GE, Marks SC Jr, Cahill DR: Ultrastructural features of the dental follicle associated with the eruption pathway in the dog, *J Oral Pathol* 14:15-26, 1985.

6

ERUPTION AND SHEDDING OF THE TEETH

CHAPTER OUTLINE

LEARNING OBJECTIVES

After reading this chapter the student will be able to:
- describe the three phases of tooth eruption: preeruption, prefunctional, and functional
- describe the initial growth of the tooth and the compensational changes that occur in the surrounding overlying and underlying tissues

KEY TERMS

Diphyodont
Eruption pathway
Extracellular phase
Fibroblast-fibroclast
Functional eruptive phase
Gubernaculum dentis or
  gubernacular cord

Intracellular phase
Intraoral occlusal/incisal movement
Mixed dentition period
Movement
Osteoblasts
Osteoclasts
Penetration

Preeruptive phase
Prefunctional eruptive phase
Root formation
Ruffled border
Shedding
Tissues: overlying, surrounding,
  underlying

OVERVIEW

Tooth eruption is the process by which developing teeth emerge through the soft tissue of the jaws and the overlying mucosa to enter the oral cavity, contact the teeth of the opposing arch, and function in mastication. The movements related to tooth eruption begin during crown formation and require adjustments relative to the forming bony crypt. This is the **preeruptive phase.** Tooth eruption is also involved in the initiation of root development and continues until the tooth's emergence into the oral cavity, which is the **prefunctional eruptive phase.** The teeth continue to erupt until they reach incisal or occlusal contact. Then they undergo functional eruptive movements, which include compensation for jaw growth and occlusal wear of the enamel. This stage is the **functional eruptive phase.** Eruption is actually a continuous process that ends only with the loss of the tooth. Each dentition, primary and permanent, has various problems during eruption and in the sequencing of eruption in the oral cavity. Teeth differ extensively in their eruptive schedules as well. This chapter describes these events. Finally, the process of tooth shedding or exfoliation of the primary dentition is discussed. Primary tooth loss results from three fundamental causes: root resorption, bone resorption, and size of crown too small to withstand mastication.

PREERUPTIVE PHASE

The preeruptive phase includes all movements of primary and permanent tooth crowns from the time of their early initiation and formation to the time of crown completion. Therefore this phase is finished with early initiation of root formation. The developing crowns move constantly in the jaws during the preeruptive phase. They respond to positional changes of the neighboring crowns and to changes in the mandible and maxilla as the face develops outward, forward, and downward away from the brain in its maturing growth path. During the lengthening of the jaws, primary and permanent teeth make mesial and distal movements. Eventually the permanent tooth crowns move within the jaws, adjusting their position to the resorptive roots of the primary dentition and the remodeling alveolar processes, especially during the mixed dentition period from 8 to 12 years of age.

Early in the preeruptive period, the permanent anterior teeth begin developing lingual to the incisal level of the primary teeth (Figs. 6-1 and 6-2). Later, however, as the primary teeth erupt, the permanent successors are positioned lingual to the apical third of their roots. The permanent premolars shift from a location near the occlusal area of the primary molars to a location

enclosed within the roots of the primary molars (see Fig. 6-2). This change in relative position is the result of the eruption of the primary teeth and an increase in height of the supporting structures. On the other hand, the permanent molars, which have no primary predecessors, develop without this type of relationship (Fig. 6-3). Maxillary molars develop within the tuberosities of the maxilla with their occlusal surfaces slanted distally. Mandibular molars develop in the mandibular rami with their occlusal surfaces slanting mesially (Fig. 6-3). This slant is the result of the angle of eruption as the molars arise from the curvature of the condyle of the posterior mandible. All movements in the preeruptive phase occur within the crypts of the developing and growing crown before root formation begins.

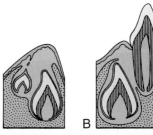

Fig. 6-1 Relative position of primary and permanent incisor teeth. A, Preeruptive period. **B,** Prefunctional eruptive period.

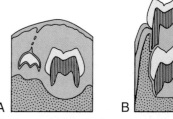

Fig. 6-2 Relative position of primary and permanent molar teeth. A, Preeruptive period. **B,** Prefunctional eruptive period.

Fig. 6-3 Human jaws at 8 to 9 years of age, during the mixed dentition period. Permanent teeth are replacing primary teeth, and positions of each are shown. The permanent mandibular molar has not emerged from the coronoid process.

PREFUNCTIONAL ERUPTIVE PHASE

The prefunctional eruptive phase starts with the initiation of root formation and ends when the teeth reach occlusal contact. Four major events occur during this phase:

1. **Root formation** requires space for the elongation of the roots. The first step in root formation is proliferation of the epithelial root sheath, which in time causes initiation of root dentin and formation of the pulp tissues of the forming root. Root formation also causes an increase in the fibrous tissue of the surrounding dental follicle (Fig. 6-4).

2. **Movement** occurs incisally or occlusally through the bony crypt of the jaws to reach the oral mucosa. The movement is the result of a need for space in which the enlarging roots can form. The reduced enamel epithelium next contacts and fuses with the oral epithelium (Fig. 6-5). Both these epithelial layers proliferate toward each other, their cells intermingle, and fusion occurs. A reduced epithelial layer overlying the erupting crown arises from the reduced enamel epithelium (Fig. 6-6).

3. **Penetration** of the tooth's crown tip through the fused epithelial layers allows entrance of the crown enamel into the oral cavity. Only the organic developmental cuticle (primary), secreted earlier by the ameloblasts, covers the enamel (Fig. 6-7).

4. **Intraoral occlusal** or **incisal movement** of the erupting tooth continues until clinical contact with the opposing crown occurs. The crown continues to move through the mucosa, causing gradual exposure of the crown surface, with an increasingly apical shift of the gingival attachment (see Fig. 6-7). The exposed crown is the clinical crown, extending from the cusp tip to the area of the gingival attachment. In contrast, the anatomic crown is the entire crown, extending from the cusp tip to the cementoenamel junction.

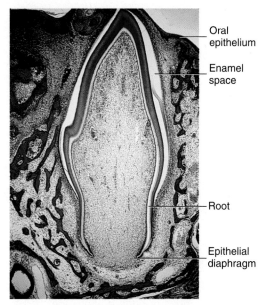

Oral epithelium

Enamel space

Root

Epithelial diaphragm

Fig. 6-5 Histology of an erupting cuspid tooth. The crown tip is in contact with oral epithelium.

Oral epithelium
Site of proliferation of reduced enamel epithelium

Enamel space

Epithelial diaphragm

Fig. 6-4 Histology of the prefunctional eruptive phase. The root develops, and reduced epithelium overlying crown approaches oral mucosa. Reduced enamel epithelium proliferates, anticipating fusion.

Fused oral and enamel epithelium

Reduced enamel epithelium

Enamel space

Oral epithelium

Fig. 6-6 Fused reduced enamel epithelium and oral epithelium overlie the enamel of crown. (Enamel space occurs as enamel is dissolved in preparation of slide.)

CLINICAL COMMENT

Hypereruption occurs with the loss of an opposing tooth. This condition allows the tooth or teeth to erupt farther than normal into the space provided.

Fig. 6-8 **Histology of a prefunctional erupting tooth.** Observe the appearance of the eruption pathway developed overlying the crown.

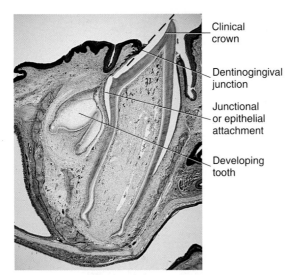

Fig. 6-7 **An erupting primary tooth appears in the oral cavity.** The permanent tooth's position is shown on the left. The *dotted line* indicates cuticle overlying the enamel surface of the erupting tooth.

Changes in Tissues

The prefunctional eruptive phase is characterized by significant changes in the **tissues overlying, surrounding,** and **underlying** the erupting teeth.

Overlying the teeth

The dental follicle changes and forms a pathway for the erupting teeth. A zone of degenerating connective tissue fibers and cells immediately overlying the teeth appears first (Figs. 6-8 and 6-9). During the process, the blood vessels decrease in number, and nerve fibers break up into pieces and degenerate. The altered tissue area overlying the teeth becomes visible as an inverted triangular area known as the **eruption pathway.** In the periphery of this zone, the follicular fibers, regarded as the **gubernaculum dentis** or **gubernacular cord** (Fig. 6-10), are directed toward the mucosa. Some scientists believe that these fibers guide the teeth in their movements to ensure complete tooth eruption.

Macrophages appear in the eruption pathway tissue. These cells cause the release of hydrolytic enzymes that

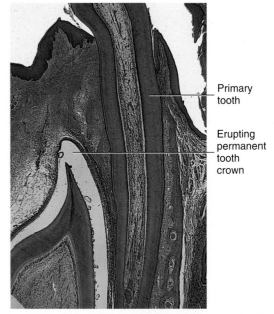

Fig. 6-9 **Observe the relation of the functional primary tooth root on the right to the permanent prefunctional erupting crown on the left.**

aid in the destruction of the cells and fibers in this area with the loss of blood vessels and nerves. Osteoclasts are found along the borders of the resorptive bone overlying the teeth. This bone loss adjacent to the teeth keeps pace with the eruptive movements of the teeth (see Fig. 6-9). **Osteoclasts** and **osteoblasts** constantly remodel the alveolar bone as the teeth enlarge and move forward in the direction of the growing face.

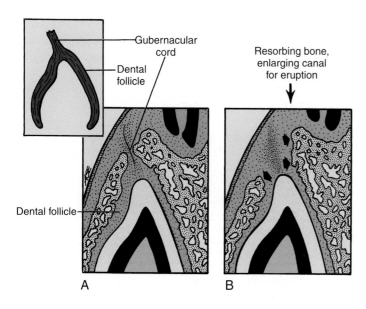

Fig. 6-10 Diagram of a developing eruption pathway.
A, Early developing eruption pathway **B,** Resorption of bone in eruption pathway.

Fig. 6-11 Foramina palatal to maxillary primary incisors. These are sites of eruption for permanent incisors.

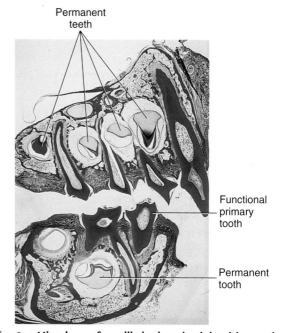

Fig. 6-12 Histology of maxilla in the mixed dentition period. Roots of erupted primary teeth are undergoing resorption. Crowns of developing permanent teeth appear below primary teeth.

Although the process of eruption for permanent teeth is similar to that of the primary teeth, the presence of primary teeth roots poses a problem. The resorption of their roots is similar to the process of bone resorption for the emergence of primary teeth. Permanent teeth establish an eruptive path lingual to the primary anterior teeth and the premolars under the primary molars. Permanent molars erupt into the alveolar free space behind primary teeth (see Fig. 6-9). Small foramina just posterior to the primary tooth row are evidence of the eruption sites of the anterior permanent teeth (Fig. 6-11). As the roots resorb, the primary crowns are lost or shed (Fig. 6-12). Dentin resorption is similar to bone resorption (see Fig. 6-10).

The resorptive process of primary and permanent teeth results from action of osteoclasts that arise from monocytes of the circulating bloodstream. These monocytes appear and fuse with others to form the multinucleated osteoclasts. Their function is to resorb the hard tissue. They do so by first separating the mineral from the collagen matrix through the action of the hydrolytic enzymes secreted by the osteoclasts. This enzymatic action is believed to occur within lacunae, which are developed by the osteoclasts. The osteoclast's cell membrane is in contact with the bone and becomes modified by an enfolding process termed the **ruffled border** (Figs. 6-13 and 6-14). This border greatly increases the surface area of the osteoclast and allows the cell to function maximally in bone resorption (Fig. 6-15).

Hard tissue resorption is believed to occur in two phases: the **extracellular phase,** in which the mineral is separated from the collagen and is broken into small fragments (see Fig. 6-15), and the **intracellular phase,** in which the osteoclast ingests these mineral fragments and continues the dissolution of this mineral. Crystals appear in cytoplasmic vacuoles of the osteoclast and are

Osteoclasts   Dentin
                                               of root

Fig. 6-13 **Histology of active resorption sites on primary tooth roots.** Osteoclasts appear in lacunae in root cementum and dentin.

Root resorption

Multinucleated osteoclast

Fig. 6-14 **Histology of osteoclasts in advancing resorption lacunae.** Observe the large multinucleated cells shown within the lacunae.

Fig. 6-15 **Osteoclast activity. A,** Osteoclasts in lacunae on bone surface. **B,** Large multinucleated osteoclasts with brush border in contact with bone spicule. **C,** High magnification of ruffled border of osteoclast showing mineral crystals passing into spaces between cell extensions. Unmasked collagen fibers are nearby. **D,** Clear zone on osteoclast surface. **E,** Ruffled border of osteoclast in constant motion or change.

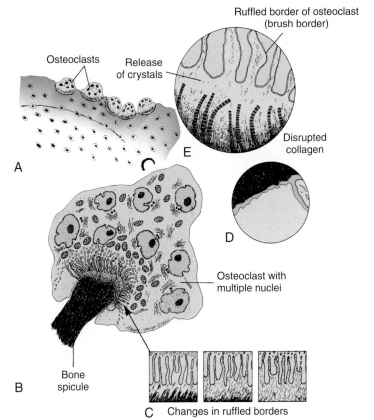

Osteoclasts   Release   Ruffled border of osteoclast
                   of crystals   (brush border)

Disrupted collagen

A   C   E

D

Osteoclast with multiple nuclei

Bone spicule

B

C   Changes in ruffled borders

gradually digested within them. Resorption of mineral occurs at the ruffled border interface outside the cell, and the mineral is then taken within the cell (Fig. 6-16). Special fibroblast **(fibroblast-fibroclast)** cells are believed to destroy the remaining collagen fibers secondarily by ingesting them in an intracellular phagolysosome system (Fig. 6-17). Amino acids resulting from this breakdown are used in the formation of collagen within this same cell and can be used in this same area for bone formation. Only the posterior permanent molars, which have no primary predeciduous teeth, erupt through alveolar bone (Fig. 6-18). Figure 6-19 summarizes what happens in the tissues overlying the teeth during their prefunctional eruptive phase. Bone loss has occurred as the tooth approaches the oral epithelium (Fig. 6-19, *A*). The tooth organ epithelium makes contact with the oral mucosa (Fig. 6-19, *B* and *C*). This contact causes stretching and thinning of the oral membrane and finally its rupture and penetration by the tooth (Fig. 6-19, *D* and *E*). Only a thin developmental cuticle then covers the tooth (Fig. 6-19, *E* and *F*). As the tooth emerges farther into the mouth, more crown is exposed, and as clinical contact with the opposing tooth is made, the epithelial attachment shifts to the cervical area (Fig. 6-19, *G*). Clinically, tooth eruption is seen as a blanching of the mucosa, and this condition may persist for several days because the eruptive process is neither rapid nor continuous. Each eruptive movement, however, results in greater exposure of the crown. With successive eruptive movements, the area of attached epithelium becomes lower on the clinical crown.

Surrounding the teeth

The tissues around the teeth change from delicately fine fibers lying parallel to the surface of the tooth to bundles of fibers attached to the tooth surface and

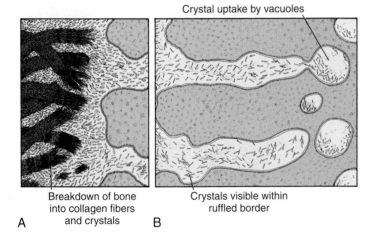

Crystal uptake by vacuoles

Breakdown of bone into collagen fibers and crystals

Crystals visible within ruffled border

A　　　B

Fig. 6-16 **Diagram of ruffled border of an osteoclast**. **A,** High magnification of unmasked collagen fibers. Mineral crystals are near the osteoclast surface. **B,** Diagram of uptake of crystals into osteoclast vacuoles.

Fig. 6-17 **Fibroblast (fibroblast-fibroclast) capable of synthesis of collagen as well as its breakdown.** Collagen fibers are phagocytosed into cells and are broken down to release amino acids. These amino acids are then used to form new collagen molecules.

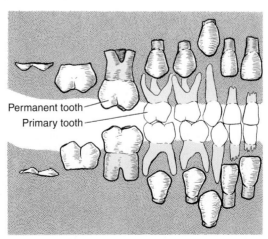

Permanent tooth
Primary tooth

Fig. 6-18 **The relationship between primary and permanent teeth during the mixed dentition period.**

extending toward the periodontium. The first fibers to appear are those in the cervical area as root formation begins (Fig. 6-20, *A*). As the root elongates, bundles of fibers appear on the root surface (Fig. 6-20, *B* and *C*). Fibroblasts are the active cells in both the formation and the degradation of the collagen fibers. With tooth eruption, the alveolar bone crypt increases in height to accommodate the forming root. After the teeth attain functional occlusion, the fibers gain their natural orientation (Fig. 6-20, *C*). Special fibroblasts have been found in the periodontium around the erupting teeth. These fibroblasts have contractile properties. During eruption, collagen fiber formation and fiber turnover are rapid, occurring within 24 hours. This mechanism enables fibers to attach and release and attach in rapid succession. Some fibers may detach and reattach later while

the tooth moves occlusally as new bone forms around it. Gradually the fibers organize and increase in number and density as the tooth erupts into the oral cavity. Blood vessels then become more dominant in the developing ligament and exert additional pressure on the erupting tooth (Fig. 6-21).

CLINICAL COMMENT

Teeth are considered submerged when eruption is prevented because of crowding or tipping of the adjacent teeth into the space created by the missing primary tooth. Retained primary teeth may be caused by the lack of development of the permanent successor.

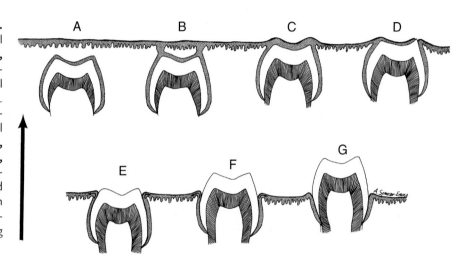

Fig. 6-19 Stages of tooth eruption. A, Tooth crown approaching oral epithelium in preeruptive stage. **B,** Contact of reduced enamel epithelium including the developmental cuticle fusing with oral epithelium. **C,** Fusion of reduced enamel epithelium including the developmental cuticle and oral epithelia. **D,** Thinning of fused epithelia. **E,** Rupture of oral epithelium, formation of the attached gingiva and emergence. **F,** Clinical crown appearance into the oral cavity (prefunctional stage). **G,** Tooth erupting into functional occlusion.

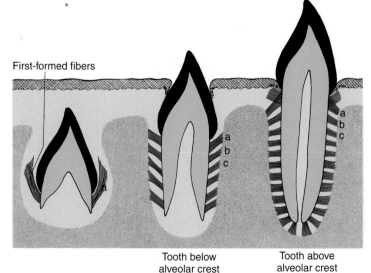

Fig. 6-20 Principal fiber development during tooth eruption. A, Origin of fibers at the cervical root area of crown. **B,** Fiber development with root growth. **C,** Change in orientation of the fibers with occlusal function. *a,* Initial fiber formation. *b,* Development of secondary fibers. *c,* Further fiber development. Initial fiber groups change direction with function.

Underlying the teeth

As the crown of a tooth begins to erupt, it gradually moves occlusally, providing space underlying the tooth for the root to lengthen (Fig. 6-22). In the fundic region these changes in the soft tissue and the bone surrounding the root apex are believed to be largely compensatory for the lengthening of the root. During root formation, the dentin of the root apex tapers to a fine edge that terminates in the epithelial diaphragm (Fig. 6-23). Fibroblasts form collagen around the root apex, and these fiber bundles become attached to the cementum as

it begins to form on the apical dentin. Fibroblasts appear in great numbers in the fundic area, and some of these fibers form strands that mature into calcified trabeculae. These trabeculae form a network, or bony ladder, at the tooth apex. This is believed to fill the space left behind as the tooth begins eruptive movement (see Fig. 6-23). Gradually this delicate bone ladder becomes denser as additional bony plates appear (Fig. 6-24). The bony plates remain until the teeth are in functional occlusion at the end of this phase. Dense bone then forms around the tooth's apex, and bundles of fibers attach to the apical cementum and extend to the adjacent alveolar bone to provide more support (Fig. 6-25).

CLINICAL COMMENT

Tooth eruption is a complex and multistep process, which includes different types of tooth growth and movements within the bony crypt in order for the tooth to erupt into the genetically designated area of the maxilla or mandible. To accomplish eruption, bone remodeling by osteoclasts (resorption of bone) and osteoblasts (bone deposition) must take place in a coordinated manner. Most important is the removal of bone overlying the crypt, which forms the eruption pathway. In experimental studies, it has been shown that without eruption pathway formation, the tooth will not erupt.

Fig. 6-21 Histology of erupting tooth with vascular injection. An outline of the blood vessels in the periodontium and tooth pulp is shown.

Labels: Pulp; Blood vessels in bone; Blood vessels in periodontal ligament

Fig. 6-22 Histology of erupting tooth with immature roots and open apex. As the tooth erupts, the roots will develop and fill in the wide pulpal tooth apex.

Labels: Pulp; Root tip; Zone of cell proliferation; Fundic region

Zone of
cell proliferation

Bone of
fundic region

Fig. 6-23 Histology of changes in fundic region during tooth eruption. Fine trabeculae of new bone appear near tooth apices that will aid in stabilizing the tooth during eruption.

Fig. 6-24 Diagram of a later stage of tooth eruption. The fundic region further develops a bony ladder.

Periodontal fiber bundles

Fig. 6-25 Histology of tooth in functional occlusion to show density of functioning periodontal fibers. Areas between fiber bundles are for blood vessels and nerves.

FUNCTIONAL ERUPTIVE PHASE

The final eruptive phase takes place after the teeth are functioning and continues as long as the teeth are present in the mouth. During this period of root completion, the height of the alveolar process undergoes a compensating increase. The fundic alveolar plates resorb to adjust for formation of the root tip apex. The root canal narrows as a result of root tip maturation, during which the apical fibers develop to help cushion the forces of occlusal impact. Root completion continues for a considerable length of time, even after the teeth begin to function. This process takes about 1 to 1.5 years for deciduous teeth and 2 to 3 years for permanent teeth.

The most marked changes occur as occlusion is established. At that time, the mineral density of the alveolar bone increases, and the principal fibers of the periodontal ligament increase in dimension and change orientation in their mature state. These fibers separate into groups oriented about the gingiva, the alveolar crest, and the alveolar surface around the root. Such fibers stabilize the tooth to a greater degree, and the blood vessels become more highly organized in the spaces between the bundles of fibers (see Fig. 6-25). Later in life, attrition and abrasion may wear down the occlusal or incisal surface of the teeth, causing the teeth to erupt slightly to compensate for this loss of tooth structure.

Posteruptive changes: attrition and formation of compensatory cementum

Thickened cementum

Fig. 6-26 Functional eruptive changes illustrating attrition of the incisal surface of enamel. Observe the compensatory deposition of cementum on the apical region of the root surface.

Any such change results in deposition of cementum on the root's apex (Fig. 6-26). Cementum is also deposited in the furcation area of a two- or three-rooted tooth.

CLINICAL COMMENT

Lack of eruption resulting from failure of root formation may be caused by crowding of teeth, crown-to-root fusion, and lack of development of the pulp proliferative zone.

POSSIBLE CAUSES OF TOOTH ERUPTION

Of the numerous causes of tooth eruption, the most frequently cited are root growth and pulpal pressure. Other important causes are cell proliferation, increased vascularity, and increased bone formation around the teeth. Additional possible causes that have been noted are endocrine influence, vascular changes, and enzymatic degradation. Probably all these factors have an influencing role, not necessarily independent of one another.

Although not all factors associated with tooth eruption are known, elongation of the root and modification of the alveolar bone and periodontal ligament are thought to be the most important ones. These events are coupled with changes overlying the tooth that produce the eruption pathway. Blood vessels in this area are compressed by the influence of the advancing crown and become nonfunctional. Connective tissue in the eruption pathway gradually disappears as the tooth epithelium and the oral epithelium fuse. In summary, the erupting tooth moves from an area of increased pressure to an area of decreased pressure.

CLINICAL COMMENT

The $^6/_4$ rule for primary tooth emergence means that from birth, 4 teeth emerge for each 6 months of age. Thus, 6 months, 4 teeth; 12 months, 8 teeth; 18 months, 12 teeth; 24 months, 16 teeth; and 30 months, 20 teeth.

SEQUENCE AND CHRONOLOGY OF TOOTH ERUPTION

The formula for the eruptive sequence of the primary and permanent dentition appears in Box 6-1. Table 6-1 shows the chronologic development and eruption of the primary dentition, and Table 6-2 shows the development and eruption of the permanent dentition.

6.1 | BOX | SEQUENCE OF TOOTH ERUPTION

PRIMARY

CI	LI	1M	Cu	2M
L	U	U	U	L
U	L	L	L	U

PERMANENT

UIM LCI UL LCU U1Pre U2Pre UCu L2M L3M
L1M UCI LL   L1Pre L2Pre   U2M U3M

TABLE 6-1   CHRONOLOGY OF DEVELOPMENT OF THE PRIMARY DENTITION*

Primary teeth listed in order of eruption (sequence)	Beginning calcification (Mo in utero)	Crown completed postnatally (Mo)	Appearance in the oral cavity (eruption time) (Mo)	Root completed (Yr)
Lower central incisor	3–4	2–3	6–8	1–2
Upper central incisor	3–4	2	7–10	1–2
Upper lateral incisor	4	2–3	8–11	2
Lower lateral incisor	4	3	8–13	1–2
Upper first molar	4	6	12–15	2–3
Lower first molar	4	6	12–16	2–3
Upper canine	4–5	9	16–19	3
Lower canine	4–5	9	17–20	3
Lower second molar	5	10	20–26	3
Upper second molar	5	11	25–28	3

The normal range of eruption times indicates a wide variation in eruption times. It is important to know that a difference of 1 or 2 months either side of the normal range does not necessarily indicate that a child's eruption time schedule is abnormal. Only deviations considerably out of this range should be considered abnormal.

TABLE 6-2   CHRONOLOGY OF DEVELOPMENT OF THE PERMANENT DENTITION

Permanent teeth listed in order of eruption (sequence)	Beginning calcification	Crown completed (Yr)	Appearance in the oral cavity (eruption time) (Yr)	Root completed (Yr)
Lower first molar	Birth	3–4	6–7	9–10
Upper first molar	Birth	4–5	6–7	9–10
Lower central incisor	3–4 mo	4	6–7	9
Upper central incisor	3–4 mo	4–5	7–8	10
Lower lateral incisor	3–4 mo	4–5	7–8	9–10
Upper lateral incisor	10–12 mo	4–5	8–9	10–11
Lower canine	4–5 mo	5–6	9–10	12–13
Upper first premolar	1–2 yr	6–7	10–11	12–14
Lower first premolar	1–2 yr	6–7	10–11	12–14
Upper second premolar	2–3 yr	7–8	10–12	13–14
Lower second premolar	2–3 yr	7	11–12	14–15
Upper canine	4–5 mo	6–7	11–12	14–15
Lower second molar	2–3 yr	7–8	11–12	14–15
Upper second molar	2–3 yr	7–8	12–13	15–16
Lower third molar	8–10 yr	12–16	17–20	18–25
Upper third molar	7–9 yr	12–16	18–20	18–25

 CLINICAL COMMENT

A lack of eruption may be related to fusion of tooth roots to the bony socket or to the crown of a permanent tooth. The condition is known as *ankylosis* because the tooth root fuses with underlying hard tissue.

 Consider the Patient

A patient complains about a retained primary tooth. She notes the absence of the permanent successor. How could you determine what has occurred?

SHEDDING OF PRIMARY TEETH

Humans are considered **diphyodont** because they possess two dentitions, primary and permanent. Teeth in the primary dentition are smaller and fewer in number than the permanent dentition to conform to the smaller jaws of the young person. Teeth in the permanent dentition are larger, longer, and more numerous, which the larger jaws of the adult can accommodate.

The primary dentition functions from about 2 to 8 years of age. Teeth from both dentitions are present in the **mixed dentition period,** which extends from about

8 to 12 years of age. This is an interesting period because only part of the primary teeth roots are present while they undergo resorption, and only part of the permanent roots are present while they are in the formative stage. In this way, nearly 50 teeth can be accommodated in the jaws during this 4-year span (see Fig. 6-12).

The period of tooth shedding follows the mixed dentition period. **Shedding** is the loss of the primary dentition caused by the physiologic resorption of the roots, the loss of the bony supporting structure, and therefore the inability of these teeth to withstand the masticatory forces.

The degeneration of primary pulp tissue is similar to that of the tissues in the eruption pathway with a loss of cells, nerves, and blood vessels. When a primary tooth is extracted, blood is still likely to be in the crown, although only the oral epithelium holds the tooth in the socket. Figure 6-27 shows the correlation between root growth and eruption. It illustrates changes that occur in the preeruptive *(A, B),* prefunctional *(C, D),* and functional eruptive *(E)* stages of the tissues overlying and around the root surface as the tooth develops functionally.

COMPARISONS OF THE PRIMARY AND PERMANENT DENTITIONS

This section will compare the morphology and histology of the primary and permanent dentition and describe some clinical problems in the developing jaw of the growing child as compared with the jaw in the adult and related characteristics of the developing primary and permanent teeth and their supporting structures (Table 6-3).

Tooth Number and Size

The main difference between the primary and permanent dentition is the number of teeth, which is 20 in the primary, and 32 in the permanent. The permanent teeth replacing the primary teeth are called *successional*. There are 12 permanent teeth, which have no predecessor. They are called *accessional*. As the permanent molars are added, arch length and occlusal surface are increased (see Fig. 6-18). Primary and permanent teeth differ in size and form. Several of these differences influence decisions about clinical treatment. Crowns of primary teeth are smaller than the crowns of their successors, with only a few key exceptions. Crowns of permanent incisors and canines are larger than their primary counterparts in all dimensions. (see Fig. 6-3). The difference between the cumulative mesiodistal diameters of the primary molars and canines and those of the permanent molars and canines is called the *leeway space*, which totals 1.3 mm in the maxillary arch and 3.1 mm in the mandibular arch.

Primary teeth resemble permanent teeth. Both permanent and primary incisors have single roots and incisal edges. Both primary and permanent canines also have single roots and a single cusp. Primary molars, however, bear no resemblance to the premolars that will succeed them. The crowns of the permanent molars are larger than crowns of primary molars; the latter have a larger mesiodistal diameter than crowns of the succeeding premolars. This difference has clinical significance in caries patterns on approximal surfaces and in cavity design for caries removal. Interproximal lesions will be cervical to the contact areas and of similar shape.

Roots

The roots of primary teeth are shorter than roots of permanent teeth and are more divergent. The flat curved roots of primary teeth permit development of the crown of the permanent successor (see Fig. 6-18). As the permanent teeth erupt, the roots of the primary teeth are resorbed. Root shape dictates the shape of the root pulp and is correlated with two important clinical considerations. First, curved roots with thin walls make mechanical access of root canals more difficult in primary molars than in permanent molars. Secondly, the flat ribbon-shaped root canals of the primary teeth are in sharp contrast to the tubelike canals of the permanent teeth. Significant developmental differences occur in the root canals of the primary molars; the root canal fills in unevenly with secondary dentin, which leaves calcified bridges, making endodontic instrumentation difficult.

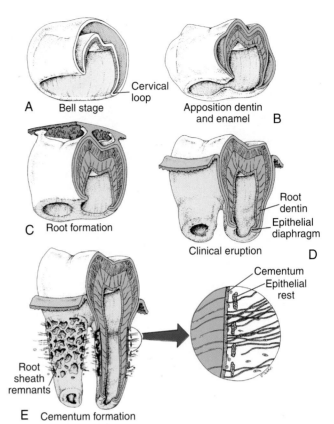

Fig. 6-27 Summary of tooth eruption. A, Early preeruptive changes in enamel organ at the bell stage. **B,** Late preeruptive changes as enamel and dentin form. **C,** Early prefunctional changes as the tooth moves to oral epithelium. **D,** Late prefunctional changes as the tooth emerges into the oral cavity. **E,** Functional eruptive phase with clinical contact. Root growth is shown with the root sheath detaching from the root surface. Epithelial rests and cementum formation by cementoblasts are now occurring.

Tooth Structure

Primary and permanent teeth have a similar enamel prism structure, except at the tooth surface. Primary teeth are more likely to have a prismless surface, and this reflects on the clinician's ability to etch the surface and provide an interface for attachment of sealants and other restorative procedures. Enamel is about twice as thick in permanent teeth as in primary teeth and is more highly pigmented. Primary tooth dentin is slightly softer than the permanent teeth.

Pulp Shape and Size

The coronal pulps of primary teeth are relatively larger than in permanent teeth. The largest pulp horn in primary molars is the mesiobuccal and the second largest is the mesiolingual. These differences are used in the

TABLE 6-3 BRIEF OUTLINE OF THE COMPARISON OF PRIMARY AND PERMANENT TEETH

	Primary	Permanent
Number of teeth	20	32
Enamel and dentin	Thinner	Thicker
Lifespan	Develop quicker: Span ~ 8 ½ yrs	Develop slower: Span ~ 6 yrs to ?
Size	Smaller except MD width of molars	Larger
Crown shape	Greater contour, especially at cervical area	Curved M/D/B/L
Contact areas	Flat	Point
Root shape	Curved molar roots	Straighter roots
Pulp chamber	Larger in relation to rest of tooth	Smaller
	Ribbon-like pulp in root	Oval shape in root
	MB pulp horn large in molars	
Accessory canals	More in bifurcation area than permanent teeth	More in apical area
MD width of incisors (difference is named incisor liability)	Smaller (incisors are more erect)	Larger (incisors have greater angulation)
MD width of primary molars and permanent premolars (difference is named leeway space)	Larger	Smaller (1.3 mm in maxillary, 3.1 mm in mandibular)
Root resorption	Normal	Pathological
Dentin hardness	Peripheral dentin ~Same	~Same
Central dentin	Softer	Harder
Pulpal dentin	Softer	Harder

design of dental restoration. Primary and permanent are similar in basic histological architecture and the vasculature, connective tissue and odontoblastic and subodontoblastic zones are similar in appearance. Permanent teeth have a larger number of nerves than primary teeth. The usual location of accessory canals in primary teeth is in the furcation zone and in permanent teeth at the apical one third of the completed root.

Arch Shape

Arch shape is similar in the anterior portion of the two dentitions but the permanent dentition extends further distally. Tooth-size differences are critical in assessment of potential space for permanent teeth to erupt into alignment.

The succession of smaller primary incisors with larger permanent incisors is called *incisor liability*, and the difference in the mesial distal dimension between the primary molars and permanent premolars is called the *leeway space*.

Root Resorption and Pulp Degeneration

The primary tooth roots have a higher susceptibility to resorption than permanent teeth. The process of

resorption is accompanied by gradual changes in the pulp. The first sign is a reduction in the number of cells in the pulp: nerve trunks degenerate and some fibrosis occurs. Blood vessels remain until the tooth is exfoliated.

During root formation, the primary tooth pulp is highly cellular. As the roots are completed, fewer cells and more fibers are evident. The proliferation of fibers continues during the root resorption phase with fiber bundles becoming more prominent.

Nerve fibers gradually organize in the pulp chamber of the primary tooth. As the tooth reaches functional occlusion, the nerve fibers form a parietal plexus. These nerve

Consider the Patient

Discussion: To answer this question, the dentist takes an x-ray film of the area to determine whether the permanent tooth is missing or displaced. In either case, the primary tooth is retained in position while the dentist determines the status of the permanent tooth and, if the tooth is present, aids its eruption into the proper place fibers are lost during resorption of the primary tooth roots, which makes teeth insensitive to pulpal pain at the time of exfoliation.

The periodontal support of primary and permanent teeth is similar in basic architecture.

SELF-EVALUATION QUESTIONS

1. Define tooth eruption and each of its phases.
2. Describe the changes overlying the tooth during eruption.
3. Describe the changes occurring around the tooth during eruption.
4. Describe the significant changes in the area underlying the teeth that relate to eruption.
5. What are the three fundamental causes of tooth shedding?
6. Give the sequence of eruption of the primary and permanent teeth.
7. What is the origin of osteoclasts?
8. Give the sequence of events that occur in hard tissue resorption.
9. Give the chronology of eruption for the primary teeth.
10. Give the chronology of eruption for the permanent teeth.

Acknowledgments

Dr. N.M. Elnesr contributed to the production of chapters in Avery JK: *Oral development and histology,* ed 3, Stuttgart, 2002, Thieme Medical. Some of the figures in that text have been used in preparation of this chapter.

Suggested Reading

Gorski JP, Marks SC Jr: Current concepts of the biology of tooth eruption, *Crit Rev Oral Biol Med* 3:185-206, 1992.

Marks S et al: Tooth eruption: a synthesis of experimental observations. In Davidovich Z, editor: *The biological mechanisms of tooth eruption and root resorption,* Birmingham, AL, 1988, EBSCO Media, pp 161-169.

Moxham BJ: The role of the periodontal ligament in tooth eruption. In Davidovich Z, editor: *The biological mechanism of tooth eruption and root resorption,* Birmingham, AL, 1988, EBSCO Media, pp 207-233.

Proffit WR: The effect of intermittent forces on eruption. In Davidovich Z, editor: *The biological mechanism of tooth eruption and root resorption,* Birmingham, AL, 1988, EBSCO Media, pp 187-191.

Wise GE, Marks SC, Cahill DR: Ultrastructural features of the dental follicle associated with the eruption pathway in the dog, *J Oral Pathol* 15:15-26, 1985.

7

ENAMEL

LEARNING OBJECTIVES

After reading this chapter the student will be able to:

- describe the physical features of enamel such as the structure of the enamel rods, incremental lines, lamellae, tufts, and spindles
- discuss how these affect the permeability of enamel
- discuss the surface characteristics and the etching of enamel

KEY TERMS

Enamelin
Gnarled enamel
Hunter-Schreger bands
Hydroxyapatite
Imbrication lines

Lines of Retzius
Microlamellae
Neonatal line
Perikymata
Prismless enamel

Spindles
Striae of Retzius
Tufts

OVERVIEW

Enamel, the hard protective substance that covers the crown of the tooth, is the hardest biologic tissue in the body. It consequently is able to resist fractures during the stress of mastication. Enamel provides shape and contour to the crowns of teeth and covers the part of the tooth that is exposed to the oral environment.

Enamel is composed of interlocking rods that resist masticatory forces. Enamel rods are deposited in a key-hole shape by the formative ameloblastic cells. Groups of ameloblasts migrate peripherally from the dentino-enamel junction as they form these rods. Ameloblasts take variable paths, which produces a bending of the rods. These cells maintain a relationship as they travel in different directions and produce adjacent rods. The enamel rod configuration viewed in incidental light appears as light and dark bands of rod groups termed **Hunter-Schreger bands.** Because these rods bend in an exaggerated, twisted manner at the cusp tips, they are called **gnarled enamel.**

All enamel rods are deposited at a daily appositional rate or increment of 4 μm. Such increments are noticeable, like rings in a cross section of a tree, and appear as dark lines known as **striae of Retzius** or **lines of Retzius.** The growth lines become apparent on the surface of enamel as ridges, known as **perikymata.** Two structures are noticeable at the dentinoenamel junction: **spindles,** the termination of the dentinal tubules in enamel, and **tufts,** hypocalcified zones caused by the bending of adjacent groups of rods.

Because enamel is composed of bending rods, which, in turn, are composed of crystals, minute spaces or gaps exist where crystals did not form between rods. This feature causes enamel to be variable in its density and hardness. Therefore, some areas of enamel may be more prone to penetration by small particles. This characteristic leads to tooth destruction by dental caries. After enamel is completely formed, no more enamel can be deposited.

 CLINICAL COMMENT

Perikymata are surface manifestations of the incremental lines usually found at the cervical of the crown. Some perikymata are more prominent and will present difficulties to the novice clinician, who may confuse them with calculus.

PHYSICAL PROPERTIES

Because enamel is very hard, it is also brittle and subject to fracture. Fracture is especially likely to occur if the underlying dentin is carious and has weakened the enamel's foundation.

Enamel is about 96% inorganic mineral in the form of **hydroxyapatite** and 4% water and organic matter. Hydroxyapatite is a crystalline calcium phosphate that is also found in bone, dentin, and cementum. The organic component of enamel is the protein **enamelin,** which is similar to the protein keratin that is found in the skin. The distribution of enamelin between and on the crystals aids enamel permeability. Enamel is grayish white but appears slightly yellow because it is translucent and the underlying dentin is yellowish. Enamel ranges in thickness from a knifelike edge at its cervical margin to about 2.5 mm maximum thickness over the occlusal incisal surface.

 CLINICAL COMMENT

Although enamel is the hardest tissue in the human body, it is permeable to some fluids, bacteria, and bacterial products of the oral cavity. Enamel exhibits cracks, checks, and microscopic spaces within and between rods and crystals, allowing penetration.

ROD STRUCTURE

Enamel is composed of rods that extend from their site of origin, at the dentinoenamel junction, to the enamel outer surface (Fig. 7-1). Each rod is formed by four ameloblasts. One ameloblast forms the rod head; a part of two ameloblasts forms the neck; and the tail is formed by a fourth ameloblast. Figure 7-2 shows the six-sided

Fig. 7-1 Enamel rods appear wavy in section of enamel as they extend from the dentinoenamel junction on the left to the enamel surface on the right. This figure is possible because the section is etched and viewed with a scanning electron microscope. (From Avery JK: *Oral development and histology,* ed 3, Stuttgart, 2002, Thieme Medical.)

design that is the shape of the ameloblast in contact with the forming keyhole- or racquet-shaped rod, which is columnar in its long axis. The head of the enamel rod is the broadest part at 5 *μ*m wide, and the elongated thinner portion, or tail, is about 1 *μ*m wide. The rod, including both head and tail, is 9 *μ*m long. The enamel rod is about the same size as a red blood cell (Fig. 7-3).

Each rod is filled with crystals. Those in the head follow the long axis of the rod, and those in the tail lie in the cross axis to the head (Figs. 7-4 and 7-5). The upper right rod head of Figure 7-4 indicates how the mineral is oriented during the rod's development, which forms the rod head and tail as seen on the left side of the figure.

The architecture of the mineral orientation is complex, especially when viewed in any direction other than cross section (see Fig. 7-5).

CLINICAL COMMENT

Enamel rods interlock to prevent fracture and splitting of the tooth. Enamel rod groups also intertwine, thereby preventing separation. The rod direction in the crown is normally perpendicular to the incisal surface, which provides additional support in preventing fracture.

Fig. 7-2 Diagram showing outline of six-sided ameloblasts overlying keyhole-shaped enamel rods. Parts of four cells form each enamel rod. Crystal orientation of three rods can be seen on the right side of the model. (From Avery JK: *Oral development and histology,* ed 3, Stuttgart, 2002, Thieme Medical.)

Fig. 7-4 The left side of diagram shows orientation of crystals in the forming rod head and tail. The right part shows how forming crystals pack in the rod from the cell complex *(arrows).*

Fig. 7-3 One rod is pulled out to illustrate how individual enamel rods interdigitate with neighboring rods. (From Avery JK: *Oral development and histology,* ed 3, Stuttgart, 2002, Thieme Medical.)

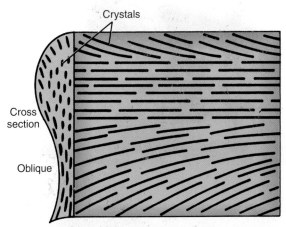

Fig. 7-5 Orientation of crystals in a mature enamel rod as indicated by cross section and side of a cut rod. (Modified from Avery JK: *Oral development and histology,* ed 3, Stuttgart, 2002, Thieme Medical.)

Rods form nearly perpendicular to the dentinoenamel junction and curve slightly toward the cusp tip. This unique rod arrangement also undulates throughout the enamel to the surface. Each rod interdigitates with its neighbor, the head of one rod nestling against the necks of the rods to its left and right (see Fig. 7-3). The rods run almost perpendicular to the enamel surface at the cervical region but are gnarled and intertwined near the cusp tips (Fig. 7-6). The surface of each rod is known as the rod sheath, and the center is the core. The rod sheath contains slightly more organic matter than the rod core (Fig. 7-7).

Consider the Patient

A patient has attrition of cusp tips in the enamel of the crowns. What do you expect when you look at the root length? Why would you see this?

Groups of rods bend to the right or left at a slightly different angle than do adjacent groups (see Fig. 7-6). It is believed that this feature provides the enamel with

strength for mastication and biting. When light is projected at the surface of a thin slab of enamel, light and dark bands appear. These bands are seen because the light transmits along the long axis of one group of rods but not along the adjacent rods, which lie at right angles. This is known as the Hunter-Schreger bands phenomenon (Fig. 7-8). These bands are named after the dental scientist who first noted the Schreger band effect microscopically. The repeating pattern from the cervical area to the incisal or occlusal areas can be seen along the long

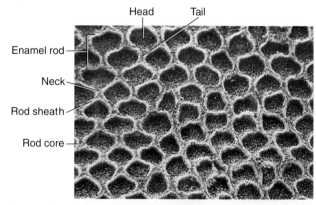

Fig. 7-7 Enamel rods in cross section. Each rod has a sheath and core. The rod sheath surrounds rod head and tail. This enamel sample has been etched to reveal organic matrix.

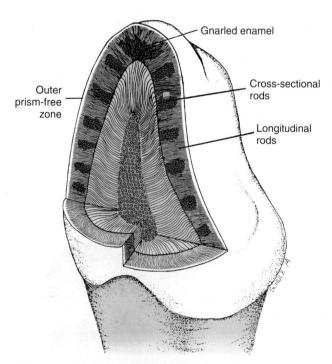

Fig. 7-6 Diagram of enamel rod orientation as shown in both longitudinal and cross section of the crown. Enamel rods are intertwined at the cusp tip; this is called gnarled enamel. Groups of outer enamel rods all run nearly perpendicular to the surface of the enamel, whereas inner groups of enamel rods alternate. Some appear in cross section while adjacent groups appear longitudinal. (Modified from Avery JK: *Oral development and histology,* ed 3, Stuttgart, 2002, Thieme Medical.)

Fig. 7-8 Photomicrograph of enamel taken by reflected light and illustrating phenomena of light and dark (Hunter-Schreger) bands.

axis of the tooth. Hunter-Schreger bands extend through one half to two thirds of the thickness of enamel as shown in a diagram (see Fig. 7-6) and a tooth section (see Fig. 7-8).

CLINICAL COMMENT

The rods that form enamel are woven during formation into a mass that resists average masticatory impact of 20 to 30 pounds per tooth. Enamel is thin in the cervical areas where masticatory impact is the least and thickest over the areas of crown cusps where impact is greatest.

INCREMENTAL LINES

The incremental lines in enamel are the result of the rhythmic recurrent deposition of the enamel. As the enamel matrix mineralizes, it follows the pattern of matrix deposition and provides the growth lines in enamel (Fig. 7-9). These lines may be accentuated because of a variation in the mineral deposited at the point of enamel hesitation in deposition. In some cases, the incremental lines are not visible. With enamel development, a row of ameloblasts covering the crown hesitates during deposition. These hesitation lines mark the path of amelogenesis. The spaces between the crystals entrap air molecules, accentuating these lines. Dr. Retzius, who first noted these "growth lines," termed them the striae of Retzius.

Part of the enamel of most deciduous teeth is formed before birth and part after birth. Because environment and nutrition change abruptly at the time of birth, a notable line of Retzius occurs at that time. This is known as the **neonatal line** (Fig. 7-10). Although the neonatal line is an accentuated incremental line, it can be seen microscopically that this line is prominent for another reason. The enamel internal to this line is of a different consistency from that external to it because it was formed before birth, and the external was formed after birth. The prenatal enamel has fewer defects than the postnatal. The staining of the postnatal enamel has numerous minute spaces that are stained with pigment.

CLINICAL COMMENT

Enamel is composed of mineral crystals that are the same as those found in dentin, cementum, and bone. Unlike bone and cementum, the mineral crystals in enamel are not replaced once deposited in enamel.

ENAMEL LAMELLAE

Enamel lamellae are cracks in the surface of enamel that are visible to the naked eye (see Figs. 7-9 and 7-11). Lamellae extend from the surface of enamel toward the dentinoenamel junction. Some lamellae form during enamel development, creating an organic pathway or tract. Spaces between groups of rods are another example of lamellae and may be caused by stress cracks that occur because of impact or temperature changes. Breathing cold air or drinking hot or cold beverages may cause small checks to occur in enamel, especially enamel weakened by underlying caries. Lamellae are not tubular defects but appear leaflike, extending around the crown (see Fig. 7-11). Lamellae are a possible avenue for dental caries.

Fig. 7-9 Photomicrograph of dentinoenamel junction showing dentin below and enamel above this junction. Enamel exhibits incremental lines, tufts, spindles, and lamella. Within dentin, a band of primary dentin is just below the dentinoenamel junction. At the lower border of this band of primary dentin is a row of interglobular spaces.

Enamel

Postnatal

Prenatal

Dentin

Fig. 7-10 Photomicrograph of section of enamel and dentin of primary tooth by transmitted light. The neonatal line is at the point of the *large arrow.* Enamel to the left of this line is a darker stain than enamel to the right of it. The enamel formed before birth is less pigmented and has fewer defects than postnatal enamel. Dentin exhibits numerous dead tracts as dark lines. Dead tracts are tubules filled with air; hence they appear black in transmitted light.

Fig. 7-11 Enamel lamellae. A, Diagram of possible location of leaflike enamel lamellae extending from the cervical to incisal enamel. **B,** Scanning electron micrograph of lamellae in enamel. (Enamel was decalcified away, and lamellar space was impregnated with resin for its maintenance.) (Modified from Avery JK: *Oral development and histology,* ed 3, Stuttgart, 2002, Thieme Medical.)

Lamella

Lamella

A

B

CLINICAL COMMENT

Temperature changes from breathing cold air or drinking hot or cold beverages may cause small checks or cracks to develop in enamel. This is especially evident in enamel weakened by underlying caries but can also appear in otherwise normal enamel.

ENAMEL TUFTS

Enamel tufts are another defect in enamel filled with organic material. They are located at the dentino-enamel junction and appear at right angles to it. They can extend one fifth to one tenth of the distance from the dentinoenamel junction to the outer surface of the tooth (Figs. 7-12 and 7-13). Tufts form between groups of enamel rods, which are oriented in slightly different directions at the dentinoenamel junction. These spaces are thus developed between adjacent groups of rods, which are filled with organic material termed enamelin. The interface of the junction of dentin and enamel is scalloped, and often tufts arise from these scalloped peaks (see Fig. 7-12).

ENAMEL SPINDLES

Spindles arise at the dentinoenamel junction and extend into enamel. These spindles are extensions of dentinal tubules that pass through the junction into enamel (see Fig. 7-13). Because dentin forms before enamel, the odontoblastic process occasionally penetrates the junction, and enamel forms around this process, forming a tubule. These small tubules may

— Enamel tufts

— Dentinoenamel
junction

— Dentin

Fig. 7-12 Transmitted light micrograph of the dentinoenamel junction area showing enamel tufts. In addition to tufts, scalloped dentinoenamel junction and fine enamel rod structure can be seen between tufts. Below the junction are dentinal tubules. (From Avery JK: *Oral development and histology,* ed 3, Stuttgart, 2002, Thieme Medical.)

Enamel
spindles

Dentinoenamel
junction

Fig. 7-13 Enamel spindles at the dentinoenamel junction are extensions of dentinal tubules that may contain odontoblastic processes in enamel. (From Avery JK: *Oral development and histology,* ed 3, Stuttgart, 2002, Thieme Medical.)

contain a living process of the odontoblast, possibly contributing to the vitality of the dentinoenamel junction. Tubules are found singularly or in groups and are shorter than tufts, only a few millimeters in length. The fingerlike spindles appear quite different than the broader and longer tufts.

SURFACE CHARACTERISTICS

The enamel surface may be smooth or have fine ridges. Such ridges result from the termination of the striae of Retzius on the surface of enamel (Fig. 7-14). These surface manifestations are ridges called perikymata or **imbrication lines.** Perikymata are produced by the ends of rod groups accentuated by hesitation of ameloblasts before the next group of rods contact the enamel surface (Fig. 7-15). This manifestation is more prominent on the facial surface of the tooth, near the cervical region (see Fig. 7-14). Another feature of outer enamel near its surface is the zone of **prismless enamel,** which is 20 to 40 μm thick. Throughout this zone, no Schreger band effect is noted. This zone is

Fig. 7-14 Fine ridges on the enamel surface of the crown are perikymata or imbrication lines. (From Avery JK: *Oral development and histology,* ed 3, Stuttgart, 2002, Thieme Medical.)

not accentuated except near the cervical region and in deciduous teeth. The prismless zone of enamel is important because it appears as a structureless microcrystalline environment of enamel rods oriented nearly perpendicular to the enamel surface. This enhances the

Fig. 7-15 **Scanning electron micrograph of perikymata in Figure 7-14 at a much higher magnification, which shows alternating ridges and valleys.** (From Avery JK: *Oral development and histology,* ed 3, Stuttgart, 2002, Thieme Medical.)

Fig. 7-16 **Transmission electron micrograph of a cross section of enamel rods that shows differences in rod sheath and rod core crystal orientation.** (From Avery JK: *Oral development and histology,* ed 3, Stuttgart, 2002, Thieme Medical.)

integrity of the enamel surface and should be recognized when a bevel for restorations is prepared.

 CLINICAL COMMENT

> When caries has spread from the tooth's surface to near the dentinoenamel junction, the hypocalcified tufts allow a lateral spread along this junction. Other hypocalcified structures in enamel such as lamellae and incremental lines can also modify the spread of caries.

PERMEABILITY

 CLINICAL COMMENT

> Decalcifying agents such as lemon juice and sodas can remove the mineral from the surface of the enamel crystals. However, the various constituents of saliva, including calcium and phosphate, help to maintain the integrity of the enamel surface.

Enamel permeability is a feature of clinical importance. The passage of fluid, bacteria, and bacterial products through enamel is an important consideration in clinical therapy. Permeability of enamel is caused by several factors, some of which are evident as they relate to leakage around faulty restorations and decomposition of the tooth by dental caries. These latter examples need no further explanation, but fluid and fine particles can also pass through unbroken enamel by

way of pathways described previously in this chapter, such as lamellae, cracks, tufts, and spindles. These all contribute to the microporosity of enamel. The minute spaces between or around enamel rods and through crystal spaces within rods are also important and are called **microlamellae.** Differences in crystal orientation can cause enamel to have minute spaces, which can be seen at high magnification (Fig. 7-16). Also, surface irregularities, such as those found in central fissures and near the cervical region, are important in influencing permeability.

Enamel and dentin are both composed of hydroxyapatite crystals, although the crystals in enamel are about 30 times larger than those in dentin (Fig. 7-17). Crystal size is a factor in the extreme hardness of enamel in contrast to dentin.

 CLINICAL COMMENT

> Some etched areas of enamel can be remineralized by solutions of sodium fluoride or stannous fluoride. Tests show that the fluoride ion penetrates the porous etched surface enamel. Low levels of fluoride stimulate remineralization.

ETCHING

Etching with dilute acids, such as citric acid, may alter the surface of enamel. This dilute acid selectively etches

Enamel

Dentin

Fig. 7-17 Dentinoenamel junction. Enamel is above and dentin below. Crystallites of enamel and dentin are different in size and orientation. Whereas crystals of human enamel may be 90 nm (900 Å) in width and 0.5 μm in length, those of dentin are only 3 nm (30 Å) in width and 100 nm (1,000 Å) in length. Crystals of dentin are similar in size to bone. (Electron micrograph × 35,000.)

Rod sheath

Rod core

Fig. 7-18 Acid-etched enamel rod core dissolved to greater extent than rod sheath, which provides for attachment of sealant.

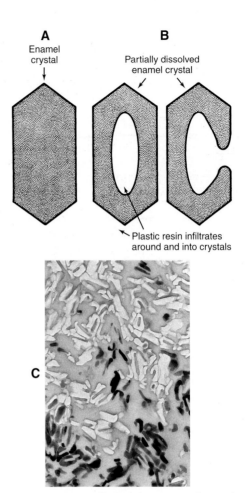

A Enamel crystal

B Partially dissolved enamel crystal

Plastic resin infiltrates around and into crystals

C

Fig. 7-19 A, Intact enamel crystal. **B,** Loss of crystal core in acid-etched enamel. **C,** Demineralized enamel crystals. Medium-toned areas show plastic replacing enamel, lightest areas are dissolved crystals, and the darkest areas are intact enamel crystals.

the ends of the enamel rods and provides adherence of a plastic sealant to the surface of enamel rods (Fig. 7-18). The rod sheath resists demineralization to a greater extent than the rod core. The core of the crystal is rich in coronated apatite and is more sensitive to demineralization than the peripheral hydroxyapatite (Fig. 7-19). The purpose of this procedure is to produce an intact surface and thus prevent caries.

 CLINICAL COMMENT

The use of sealants, especially in children, can help prevent caries in susceptible areas of the teeth. In order for the sealant to be effective, the surface enamel must be etched to improve adhesion.

Consider the Patient

Discussion: A radiograph would reveal a lengthened root with excessive cemental deposition that is due to hypereruption of the tooth. Because of the hypereruption, space is provided for compensating cemental deposition.

SELF-EVALUATION QUESTIONS

1. Describe the shape and size of the enamel rods.
2. Define Hunter-Schreger bands.
3. Define striae of Retzius. What is a synonym?
4. Describe gnarled enamel. Where is it located?
5. What are perikymata and imbrication lines?
6. What are the location and importance of tufts?
7. Define and give the cause of neonatal lines.
8. What is prismless enamel?
9. What is the inorganic component of enamel, dentin, and bone?
10. What is the organic component of enamel?

Suggested Reading

Bhaskar SN, editor: *Orban's oral histology and embryology,* ed 11, St Louis, 1991, Mosby.

Boyd A, Lester KS, Martin LB: Basis of the structure and development of mammalian enamel as seen by electron microscopy, *Scanning Microsc* 2:1479-1490, 1988.

Diekwisch T, et al: Membranes, minerals, and proteins of developing vertebrae enamel, *Micros Res Tech* 59(5):373-395, 2002.

Fernhead RW: *Tooth enamel V,* Yokohama, 1989, Florence.

Kodaka T, Natajima F, Higashi S: Structure of the so-called "prismless" enamel in human deciduous teeth, *Caries Res* 23: 290-296, 1989.

Satchell PG, et al: Conservation and variation in enamel protein distribution during vertebrate tooth development, *J Exper Zoology* 294(2):91-106, 2002.

Zeichner-David M, et al: Control of ameloblast differentiation. In Ruch JV, editor: Odontogenesis: embryonic dentition as a tool for developmental biology, *Int J Dev Biol* 39:69-92, 1995.

Zeichner-David M, et al: Timing of the expression of enamel gene products during mouse tooth development, *Int J Dev Biol* 41: 27-38, 1997.

8

DENTIN

CHAPTER OUTLINE

Overview
Physical Properties
Dentin Classification
   Primary Dentin
   Secondary Dentin
   Reparative or Tertiary Dentin
Predentin
Tubular and Intertubular
   Relations

Primary and Secondary Tubules
Intratubular or Peritubular
   Dentin
   Intertubular Dentin
Incremental Lines
Granular Layer
Odontoblastic Cell Processes
Dentinoenamel Junction
Permeability

Repair Process
Self-Evaluation Questions
Consider the Patient Discussion
Suggested Reading

LEARNING OBJECTIVES

After reading this chapter the student will be able to:
• describe the various types of dentin and the structures they contain
• describe the dental process that lies in the dental tubules
• discuss the relationship of the enamel to the dentin at their junction

KEY TERMS

Dead tracts
Dentin: circumpulpal, globular,
   granular, interglobular,
   intratubular, mantle, peritubular,
   primary, reparative, response,
   sclerotic, secondary, tertiary,
   transparent

Granular layer of Tomes
Imbrication lines
Incremental lines
Interglobular spaces
Lines of von Ebner
Neonatal line
Osteodentin

Predentin
S curve
Smear layer

OVERVIEW

This chapter focuses on dentin, the hard tissue that constitutes the body of the tooth. Dentin is a living tissue not normally exposed to the oral environment. Root dentin is covered by cementum, and crown dentin is covered by enamel. Dentin, like bone, is composed primarily of an organic matrix of collagen fibers and the mineral hydroxyapatite. It is classified as **primary, secondary,** or **tertiary** on the basis of the time of its development and the histologic characteristics of the tissue. Primary dentin is the major component of the crown and root and consists of both **mantle** dentin and **circumpulpal** dentin. Mantle dentin is deposited first, along the dentinoenamel junction, in a band about 150 *µm* wide. The collagen fibers of this dentin are larger than those of the circumpulpal dentin, which forms later. Mantle dentin is separated from the circumpulpal dentin by a zone of disturbed dentin formation called **globular dentin,** which is noted because of the spaces between the globules, termed **interglobular spaces.** Globular dentin is believed to be a result of deficient mineralization. Dentin continues to form, although the collagen fibers are smaller, until the teeth erupt and reach occlusion. As the teeth begin to function, the dentin is termed secondary dentin. Dentin is responsive to the environment. When caries or mechanical trauma affects the pulp, dentin is deposited underlying that area and is termed **response, reparative,** or tertiary dentin. This dentin is deposited to protect the pulp. Bordering the pulp is **predentin,** which is newly formed dentin before calcification and maturation. Predentin is composed of collagen fibers, which calcify within 24 hours as the odontoblasts deposit a new band of collagen fibers.

In addition to classifying dentin, this chapter describes properties and characteristics of dentin. Like osteoblasts that form bone, the odontoblasts that form dentin lie on the surface of the forming hard tissue. Unlike bone, the odontoblastic processes exist in tubules and penetrate the dentin from the pulp to the dentinoenamel junction. Dentin, like bone, is deposited by appositional growth and produces **incremental lines.** In addition, a **granular dentin** anomaly appears along the root surface. This anomaly may also be caused by the cementum that forms adjacent to the root dentin during development. The odontoblasts may die because of trauma or old age, and **dead tracts** then develop in dentin. The tubules may later calcify as they fill with mineral. When this occurs, the dentin is termed **sclerotic** or **transparent dentin.**

PHYSICAL PROPERTIES

Dentin, which forms the bulk of the tooth, is yellowish in contrast to the whiter enamel. It appears darker if a root canal procedure has been performed. Dentin is composed of 70% inorganic hydroxyapatite crystals, 20% organic collagen fibers with small amounts of other proteins, and 10% water by weight. With 20% less mineral than enamel, dentin is softer, although it is slightly harder than bone or cementum. Therefore, it is more radiolucent than enamel but much more dense or radiopaque than pulp. Dentin is resilient or slightly elastic, and this allows the impact of mastication to occur without fracturing the brittle overlying enamel. This resilience is partly the result of the presence throughout the matrix of tubules, which extend from the dentinoenamel junction to the pulp.

CLINICAL COMMENT

Metallic restorations, such as gold inlay, crown, or silver amalgam, are excellent thermal conductors. Therefore, it is appropriate to place a cement base under these restorations to protect the pulp by minimizing pain conduction.

DENTIN CLASSIFICATION

Dentin includes primary, secondary, and tertiary dentin. Based on structure, primary dentin is composed of mantle and circumpulpal dentin. Examples of these classifications are given in Figure 8-1, *A*. Figure 8-1, *B*, shows the **S curve** of the dentinal tubules through primary and secondary dentin. Primary dentin forms the body of the tooth; secondary dentin forms only after tooth eruption and is a narrow band that borders the pulp. Tertiary or reparative dentin is formed only in response to trauma to the pulp.

Primary Dentin

Mantle dentin is the first primary dentin formed. It is deposited first at the dentinoenamel junction (Fig. 8-2) and extends approximately 150 *µm* from the junction pulpward to the zone of **interglobular** or globular dentin. Mantle dentin is so named because it serves as a covering or mantle over the rest of the dentin. Circumpulpal dentin directly underlies mantle dentin and comprises the bulk of the tooth's primary dentin. Circumpulpal dentin may be 6 to 8 mm thick in the crown and a little thinner in the roots.

Zones of dentin have structural differences. Mantle dentin is composed of large collagen fibers, some of which are 0.1 to 0.2 *µm* in diameter, in contrast to the circumpulpal dentinal matrix, which is 50 to 200 nanometers (nm). Thus, the fibers in circumpulpal dentin are ten times smaller than those in mantle dentin. Mantle dentin is also slightly less mineralized and contains fewer defects than circumpulpal dentin.

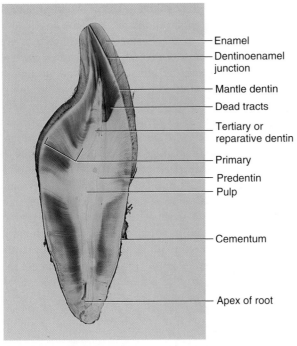

- Enamel
- Dentinoenamel junction
- Mantle dentin
- Dead tracts
- Tertiary or reparative dentin
- Primary
- Predentin
- Pulp
- Cementum
- Apex of root

A

B

Fig. 8-1 **Tooth section of enamel dentin and diagram of tooth. A,** Incisor tooth section illustrating structures in enamel, dentin, and cementum. **B,** Diagram of dentin showing S curvature of the dentinal tubules, especially at the *arrow*. (Modified from Avery JK: *Oral development and histology,* ed 3, Stuttgart, 2002, Thieme Medical.)

- Enamel
- Dentinoenamel junction
- Mantle dentin
- Interglobular dentin

Fig. 8-2 **Histologic section of mantle dentin.** Area bounded by dentinoenamel junction above and interglobular dentin below.

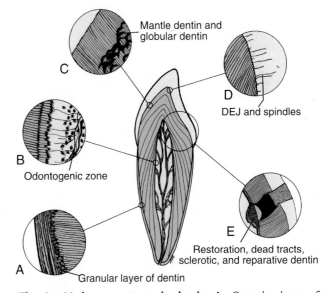

Mantle dentin and globular dentin

C

D

DEJ and spindles

B

Odontogenic zone

A

Granular layer of dentin

E

Restoration, dead tracts, sclerotic, and reparative dentin

Fig. 8-3 **Various structures in dentin. A,** Granular layer of dentin and adjacent cementum. **B,** Odontogenic zone and predentin. **C,** Mantle dentin and interglobular or globular dentin. **D,** Dentinoenamel junction *(DEJ)* and spindles. **E,** Restoration, dead tracts, sclerotic dentin, and reparative dentin.

Mantle dentin is nearly free of developmental defects. It interdigitates with enamel at the scalloped dentinoenamel junction peripherally and in the zone of globular dentin centrally. The area of globular dentin usually exists only in the crown but may extend into the root. Such a zone of dentinal matrix is not completely mineralized, and the area of globular calcospherites has not fused correctly (see Figs. 8-2 and 8-3, *C*).

Globular dentin contains hypomineralized areas between the globules, termed *interglobular spaces.* Figure 8-3 shows examples of various structures in dentin. Interglobular spaces are not true spaces but are less mineralized areas between the calcified globules. The dentinal tubules run without interruption through

this zone, indicating a defect in mineralization, not a defect in matrix formation (see Fig. 8-2). Interglobular dentin is especially noticeable with vitamin D deficiency, which affects mineralization of teeth and bones. Primary dentin constitutes the bulk of dentin in crowns and roots of teeth. It is characterized by the continuity of tubules from pulp to dentinoenamel junction and by incremental lines that indicate a daily rhythmic deposition pattern of approximately 4 μm of dentin.

 CLINICAL COMMENT

The sensitivity of dentin is an important clinical consideration after placement of a restoration that conducts heat or cold. Dentin responds to such stimuli by deposition of reparative dentin and by changes in the dentin tubules underlying the restoration. The sensitivity of the tooth will diminish after a few weeks because of these changes.

Secondary Dentin

Secondary dentin forms internally to primary dentin of the crown and root. It develops after the crown has come into clinical occlusal function and the roots are nearly completed (Fig. 8-4). This dentin is deposited more slowly than primary dentin, and its incremental lines are only about 1.0 to 1.5 μm apart. Dental scientists theorize that after the crown begins clinical function, the brain signals the dentin to slow the rate of production. This keeps the pulp from being obliterated by the previous rapid rate of dentin formation. The tubules of primary and secondary dentin are generally continuous unless the deposition of secondary dentin is uneven. In molar teeth, for example, more secondary dentin is deposited on the roof and floor of the coronal pulp chamber than on the lateral walls. This leads to protection of the pulpal horns as occlusal function occurs.

Reparative or Tertiary Dentin

Reparative or tertiary dentin results from pulpal stimulation and forms only at the site of odontoblastic activation.

Whether the formation is the result of attrition, abrasion, caries, or restorative procedures, this dentin is deposited underlying only those stimulated areas (Figs. 8-5 and 8-6). It may be deposited rapidly, in which case the resulting dentin appears irregular with sparse and twisted tubules and possible cell inclusions (Fig. 8-6, *B* to *E*). Odontoblasts, fibroblasts, and blood cells have been found in this type of dentin. In contrast, if it is formed slowly because of fewer stimuli, the dentin appears more regular, much like primary or secondary dentin (Figs. 8-5 and 8-6, *A*). Reparative dentin at times resembles bone more than dentin and is then termed **osteodentin** (Fig. 8-6, *C*). It can also appear as a combination of several types (Fig. 8-6, *E*). Recent terminology suggests that the term *reparative dentin* be used when the original odontoblasts function in deposition and that *response dentin* be used when newly recruited odontoblasts begin depositing dentin. The latter case occurs with a more severe injury to the tooth.

Consider the Patient

Case 1: A patient complains of pain in a tooth after placement of a large gold crown. The tooth is very sensitive to hot or cold fluids or foods. Why?

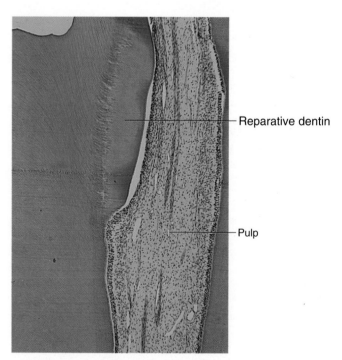

Fig. 8-5 Reparative dentin. Reparative dentin formed in localized area under cavity preparation. Open tubules underlying the cavity floor caused the response of reparative dentin.

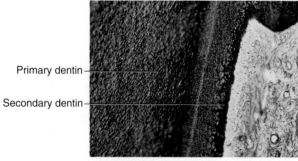

Fig. 8-4 Primary dentin *(left)* and secondary dentin *(right).* Note the demarcation between the two. (From Bhaskar SN, editor: *Orban's oral histology and embryology,* ed 11, St. Louis, 1991, Mosby.)

PREDENTIN

Predentin is a band of newly formed, unmineralized matrix of dentin at the pulpal border of the dentin (Fig. 8-7). Predentin is evidence that dentin forms in two stages: first, the organic matrix is deposited, and second, an inorganic mineral substance is added. Mineralization occurs at the predentin-dentin junction, and predentin becomes a new layer of dentin. During primary dentin formation, 4 μm of predentin is deposited and calcified each day. After occlusion and function, this activity decreases to 1.0 to 1.5 μm per day.

TUBULAR AND INTERTUBULAR RELATIONS

Primary and Secondary Tubules

As dentin is formed by odontoblasts, space is provided for the lengthening process of the odontoblast that moves pulpward from the amelodentinal junction. The tubules normally begin at this junction but may extend into the forming enamel matrix. The process begins forming before either enamel or dentin matrix begins forming. Thus, the spindles that are extensions of the odontoblastic process extend a short distance into

Fig. 8-6 **Normal and reparative dentin. A,** Normal dentin. **B to E,** Reparative dentin: **B,** decrease in number of tubules; **C,** cell inclusions; **D,** irregular and twisted tubules; **E,** combination of types.

Fig. 8-7 **Photomicrograph of predentin zone that borders pulp with mature dentin above.** Odontogenic zone is below predentin and comprises odontoblasts and cell-free and cell-rich zones.

enamel. The odontoblastic process then forms an S curve, which extends to the pulp. As the process elongates, it branches, and its secondary processes appear at nearly right angles to the main process (Fig. 8-8). These cells and their processes give the dentin vitality. The surface area ratio of the dentinoenamel junction to the pulpal surface is about 1:5. Therefore, the tubules are farther apart at the dentinoenamel junction than at the pulpal surface (see Figs. 8-1 and 8-8). In addition, the tubules are smaller in diameter in the outer dentin (1 μm) than

at the pulpal border (3 to 4 μm). The ratio of the number of tubules at the dentinoenamel junction to the number at the pulpal border is about 4:1. This relates to the odontoblast's gradual increase in size as its process grows in length. Also, more tubules are in the crown than in the root. Approximately 30,000 to 50,000 tubules per square millimeter exist in the dentin near the pulp. The lateral branches of the odontoblastic processes are seen throughout dentin, crown, and root. These lateral branches are termed canaliculi, secondary branches, or microtubules (see Fig. 8-8) and are less than 1 μm in diameter. Some of these lateral branches lead to an adjacent dentinal tubule, and some appear to terminate in the intertubular matrix. Each of these secondary tubules contains branches of the odontoblastic process.

Intratubular or Peritubular Dentin

The dentinal matrix that immediately surrounds the dentinal tubule is termed **intratubular** or **peritubular** dentin (Fig. 8-9). Peritubular dentin is present in tubules throughout dentin except near the pulp. It is called peritubular because it is a hypermineralized collar surrounding the tubules. However, because it is formed within and at the expense of the tubules, *intratubular dentin* is a more accurate term. Intratubular dentin is missing from the dentinal tubules in interglobular dentin. This is an area of deficient mineralization like the area of predentin, which is also not calcified. In some areas, the hypermineralized intratubular dentin completely fills the tubules, as in the area near the dentinoenamel junction overlying the pulp horns. This condition is also found in the peripheral tubules of the root near

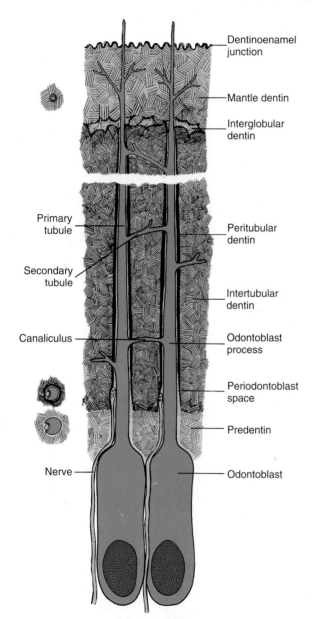

Fig. 8-8 Odontoblast process in the dentinal tubule and extending from the dentinoenamel junction above to the pulp below. Side branches of odontoblast processes in tubules are in inner dentin called secondary tubules and in outer dentin termed canaliculi. (Modified from Bhaskar SN, editor: *Orban's oral histology and embryology,* ed 11, St. Louis, 1991, Mosby.)

Labels for Fig. 8-8:
Dentinoenamel junction
Mantle dentin
Interglobular dentin
Primary tubule
Peritubular dentin
Secondary tubule
Intertubular dentin
Canaliculus
Odontoblast process
Periodontoblast space
Predentin
Nerve
Odontoblast

Fig. 8-9 Diagram of dentinal tubules showing peritubular and intertubular dentin. Note that side branches of dentinal tubules are in the intertubular dentin. (Modified from Bhaskar SN, editor: *Orban's oral histology and embryology,* ed 11, St. Louis, 1991, Mosby.)

Labels for Fig. 8-9:
Peritubular dentin
Intertubular dentin

Intertubular
dentin

Occluded
tubules

Near-
occluded
tubule

Fig. 8-10 Scanning electron micrograph of sclerotic dentinal tubules. The micrograph shows the minute size of nearly occluded dentinal tubules and some completely occluded tubules. Tubule occlusion is a mechanism to protect the pulp. (From Avery JK: *Oral development and histology,* ed 3, Stuttgart, 2002, Thieme Medical.)

the cementum. These are areas of very small tubules and areas where external stimulation may play a role. *Sclerotic dentin or transparent dentin* (Fig. 8-10) is the term for dentin with tubules that are completely obliterated. The name is derived from the transparent nature of dentin, which manifests itself when the tubules are no longer present. Sclerotic dentin increases in amount with age and is believed to be another mechanism to protect the pulp, like reparative dentin. Permeability to the pulp is eliminated in these areas, and sclerotic dentin is found in areas of attrition, abrasion, fracture, and caries of the enamel.

 CLINICAL COMMENT

Dentinal tubules increase in size by the loss of intratubular or peritubular dentin. This dentin is subject to decalcification by caries or acid cleansing of the cavity, which removes the smear layer. This dentin is about 40% more highly calcified than the remainder of the dentin.

Intertubular Dentin

The main body of dentin is located between or around the dentinal tubules. Intertubular dentin is the body of dentin, which comprises the crown and root. This dentin consists of the same type of organic matrix fibers (type I collagen fibers and inorganic crystals of

hydroxyapatite) as that of intratubular dentin. Intertubular dentin, however, is less highly calcified and changes little throughout life. The collagen fibers of the matrix form a meshwork oriented nearly perpendicular to the intratubular dentin. They exhibit a typical 640-Angstrom (Å) cross banding similar to those of bone or cementum.

 CLINICAL COMMENT

Dentin is a permeable hard tissue with tubules leading from the dentinoenamel junction to the pulp. Therefore, in cavity preparation, sealing of dentinal tubules is a requisite of effective restorative clinicianry.

INCREMENTAL LINES

All dentin is deposited incrementally, which means that as a certain amount of matrix is deposited daily, a hesitation in activity follows. This hesitation in formation results in an alteration of the matrix known as incremental lines, **imbrication lines,** or **lines of von Ebner.** Although daily lines are difficult to distinguish, lines formed by increments over several days (possibly every 5 days), resulting in 20-μm lines, are believed to be the ones von Ebner described (Fig. 8-11). Analysis of soft x-ray films has shown these lines to represent hypocalcified bands, at least in the primary teeth and the permanent first molars, indicating that dentin is formed before birth. Prenatal dentin and postnatal dentin are separated by an accentuated contour line known as the **neonatal line** (Fig. 8-12). This line reflects the abrupt change in environment that occurs at or near birth.

GRANULAR LAYER

When a thin, calcified section of root is studied under transmitted light, a granular-appearing layer of dentin is seen underlying the cementum that covers the root. This layer is known as the **granular layer** or **granular layer of Tomes** (Fig. 8-13). This zone increases slightly in width, proceeding from the cementoenamel junction to the root apex. The zone is believed to be the result of a coalescing and looping of the terminal portions of the dentinal tubules. It is possible that the odontoblast is initially disoriented as it begins dentin formation. The odontoblast turns at right angles to the root surface and proceeds pulpward, causing the dentinal matrix in this area to be defective (Fig. 8-14).

ODONTOBLASTIC CELL PROCESSES

Odontoblastic cell processes are cytoplasmic extensions of the cell body that are positioned at the pulp-dentin border. Opinions vary about whether these processes extend through the entire thickness of dentin. This difference in opinion is caused in part by the difficulty in preserving and visualizing these processes. Recently, improved techniques of immunofluorescence labeling, freeze fracture, and polymer replacement have revealed that these processes extend to the dentinoenamel junction (Fig. 8-15). In some instances, they also extend

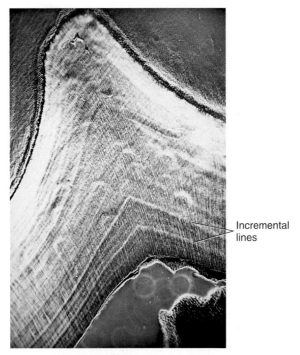

Incremental
lines

Fig. 8-11 Microradiograph of 20-μm incremental lines (lines of von Ebner) in dentin. Fine daily incremental lines can be seen microscopically between the 20-μm lines.

Prenatal
enamel

Neonatal
lines

Dentinoenamel
junction

Neonatal line
in dentin

Fig. 8-12 Neonatal line is seen at birth in both enamel and dentin because the prenatal has fewer defects than postnatal. The neonatal line is more easily seen in enamel because of the color change between prenatal and postnatal. Dentin has a neonatal line that is difficult to see at this magnification, but is located midway through dentin.

into the enamel for a short distance as enamel spindles (Fig. 8-16). The odontoblastic processes are largest in diameter near the pulp (3 to 4 μm) and taper to 1 μm near the dentinoenamel junction. These processes divide near the dentinoenamel junction to end in several branched processes (Fig. 8-17).

Periodically along the odontoblastic process, lateral branches arise at nearly right angles to the main odontoblastic process, extend into the intertubular dentin, and sometimes extend into adjacent dentinal tubules (Fig. 8-18). Within the odontoblastic process are microtubules, small filaments, occasional mitochondria,

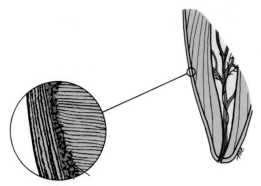

Fig. 8-13 Diagram of the appearance and location of the granular layer of dentin along the cementodentinal junction of the root.

Fig. 8-15 Photomicrograph of odontoblasts *(bottom)* **with their processes intact and extending upward to dentinoenamel junction** *(top).* Peritubular and intertubular dentinal matrix has been removed, exposing odontoblastic processes.

Fig. 8-14 Histologic appearance of the granular layer of dentin *(center)* **and cementum** *(right),* **with periodontal ligament remnants** *(far right).*

Fig. 8-16 Spindles, which are extensions of dentinal tubules, pass across the dentinoenamel junction into inner enamel.

Dentinoenamel junction

Branching dentinal tubule

Dentin

Fig. 8-17 Scanning electron micrograph of dentinal tubules branching near the dentinoenamel junction.

Fig. 8-18 Scanning electron micrograph of dentin near the dentinoenamel junction, illustrating the odontoblastic processes. Side branches of odontoblastic process extend into intertubular dentin.

Consider the Patient

Case 2: A patient asks why carious dentin does not elicit pain during its removal.

CLINICAL COMMENT

A carious attack can sometimes result in the death of the odontoblast underlying the surface lesion. The dentinal tubules normally contain a living odontoblast process, dentinal fluid, and sometimes a nerve terminal. After the odontoblast dies, the dentinal fluid will crystallize and fill the dentinal tubule with sclerotic dentin (transparent dentin), thus preventing further insult to the pulp.

DENTINOENAMEL JUNCTION

The junction between dentin and enamel, termed dentinoenamel junction, is scalloped, which enhances contact and adherence of the two structurally different tissues. This can be seen microscopically in Figures 8-13 and 8-16. Scalloping has been found to be accentuated in the cusps where the incisal or occlusal contact is greatest. Features in addition to scalloping that characterize the dentinoenamel junction are enamel spindles and fine branching of the terminal dentinal tubules in the dentin (see Figs. 8-16 and 8-17). The odontoblastic processes extend to the dentinoenamel junction unless stimulation has caused a change in the tubule and its contents. Figure 8-18 shows the processes with their side branches, and Figure 8-19 gives an example of changes in dentin underlying a restoration. Loss of tubular contents results in dead tracts (black streaks), which indicate air

and microvesicles. All these structures are indicative of the protein-synthesizing character of the odontoblast. Collagen is deposited along the predentin border and to a lesser extent along the tubule wall. Nerve terminals can be seen close to the odontoblastic cell body and within the dentinal tubule in the region of the predentin. These are described in Chapter 9. Loss of the odontoblastic process usually results in the appearance of dead tracts in dentin. In the dentin underlying an area of attrition or a carious lesion, odontoblasts may die and processes disintegrate, producing a group of open tubules that contain debris and spaces. If these tubules are open to overlying caries, bacteria may enter them and migrate to the pulp, causing inflammation. The areas of dead tracts may appear black when the teeth are sectioned and viewed by transmitted light because air may penetrate these tubules and create this appearance (Fig. 8-19).

Fig. 8-19 Black dead tracts *(open tubules)* **underlie a black (dense) restoration that appears associated with sclerosed dentinal tubules.** Tubules lie adjacent to the reparative dentin, which is seen on the roof of the pulp chamber. Each of these tubules probably resulted from stimulation from the overlying restoration.

in the tubules. Below the dead tract area in Figure 8-19 is sclerosed dentin, which protects the pulp from bacteria or bacterial products in the tubules underlying the restoration.

 CLINICAL COMMENT

Dentin is a vital tissue that contains living cell processes. Because these branching processes permeate the dentin so completely, it is not possible to touch a cavity preparation in dentin with an explorer without inflicting pain.

PERMEABILITY

The outer surface of dentin is approximately five times larger in surface area than the inner surface. Because the tubule diameter is only 1 µm near the dentinoenamel junction, the tubules are farthest apart at this junction. They are, however, much closer together at the pulpal surface because the tubules are larger (3 to 4 µm) and the dentinal surface is five times smaller (Fig. 8-20). The tubules are consequently cone shaped and permit increased permeability from the cavity wall or floor to the pulp. The system of branching tubules increases

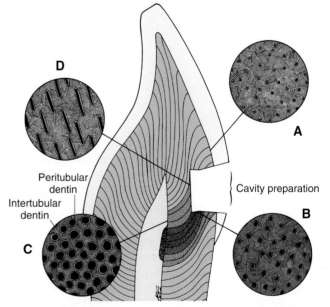

Fig. 8-20 Location and differences in size of dentinal tubules at the dentinoenamel junction *(A)* and at pulp *(C)* and relationship between tubules in cavity floor *(B and D)* and the pathway of caries through dentin. Size of tubules at the pulp border *(C)* can be compared with those in the floor of the cavity *(B and D)* and at the dentinoenamel junction *(A)*. Deposition of reparative dentin underlies invading caries. (Modified from Avery JK: *Oral development and histology,* ed 3, Stuttgart, 2002, Thieme Medical.)

the permeability. Also, because the peritubular dentin is more highly calcified than is the intertubular, the etching of a cavity causes an increase in the diameter of the tubule. The only feature that protects the pulp is that it has higher osmotic pressure than the area of the dentinoenamel junction. Fluid is constantly being forced outward by this increased pressure of the pulp. Therefore, when some dentinal tubules are cut, a small vesicle of fluid appears on the cut surface of the cavity preparation. Against the direction of this flow, minute particles such as bacteria or bacterial products percolate down the dentinal tubules to the pulp. Again, loss of the odontoblastic process, which produces a dead tract, results in increased permeability. For these reasons, the permeability factor is a major consideration in cleansing of the cavity preparation and the placement of a cavity liner to prevent microleakage. In Figure 8-20, the shaded area indicating caries signifies that bacteria find the shortest distance to the pulp along the dentinal tubules. The figure also shows the deposition of reparative or response dentin to the cavity preparation.

The tubules of dentin are effectively blocked by the production of a **smear layer** on the floor or walls of the cavity during preparation. The smear layer is composed of the fine particles of cut dentinal debris that are produced by cavity preparation. These particles enter the tubules as smear plugs at the cut surface of the cavity preparation. The effectiveness of the plug is dependent on the size of the tubules and the size of the cut particles of dentin.

REPAIR PROCESS

Dentin is laid down throughout life. Pathologic effects of dental caries, attrition, abrasion, and cavity preparation cause changes in dentin. The changes are described as odontoblastic degeneration, formation of dead tracts, calcification of tubules leading to sclerosis, and tertiary or reparative dentin formation. Stimulation of the odontoblasts leads to increased dentinogenesis underlying an area of pathologic change. If the stimulation is mild enough for the odontoblast to survive, new or reparative dentin will be formed. This is believed to be a protective mechanism of the pulp to maintain its vitality. A second situation arises after death and degeneration of the odontoblast. When dead tracts appear, sclerosis of the dentin may occur, and further reparative dentin in the pulp forms. In this instance, the pulp is again protected by this walling off action, which blocks the tubules underlying the area of trauma (see Figs. 8-19 and 8-20). With appropriate coverage, pulps can maintain their vitality. Dead tracts and sclerosis of dentin do not occur if leakage is

Fig. 8-21 Thin section of two human mandibular molar teeth in situ with gold crowns. The pulp of the first molar appears normal with no sign of sclerotic dentin or dead tracts.

prevented. An example of this is shown in Figure 8-21, in which the pulp is viable in the first molar under a full crown. The pulp in the second molar is not visible because the crown was not cut through its center. This unusual section shows teeth and the surrounding supporting bone.

 CLINICAL COMMENT

The pulp is covered by smear layer dentinal particles, which block the tubules and aid in walling off the pulp, and by the formation of reparative dentin.

 Consider the Patient

Discussion 1: Metals are good conductors of heat and cold. (Similar complaints may result after placement of an amalgam or an inlay.) However, the clinician can offer the patient assurance that the tooth will respond to the pain with internal healing. The clinician knows that reparative dentin forms slowly and eventually will insulate the pulp nerves from the metal restoration. Within 6 months or a year following such a restoration, the patient may note that the pain no longer exists. This indicates that the reparative dentin has formed.

Discussion 2: The odontoblastic process is believed to function in pain conduction in dentin and is nonliving in carious dentin. During cavity preparation, pain arises only from the adjacent living dentin.

SELF-EVALUATION QUESTIONS

1. Name the type of dentin that comprises the greater part of the crown and root.
2. Name the newly formed area of collagen matrix that borders the pulp.
3. Describe the location and composition of the granular layer of dentin.
4. Name several factors that affect the permeability of the dentin.
5. What are the location and composition of mantle dentin?
6. What is the smear layer and what is its importance to permeability of dentin?
7. Why is dentin considered a vital tissue?
8. What is sclerotic dentin and where is it most likely to be seen?
9. What is secondary dentin and when does it form?
10. What is interglobular dentin and how does it form?

Suggested Reading

Bleicher F, et al: New genes involved in odontoblast differentiation, *Adv Dent Res* 15:30-33, 2001.

Boskey A: The role of extracellular matrix in dentin mineralization, *Crit Rev Oral Biol Med* 2:369-388, 1991.

Holland GR: The odontoblast process: form and function, *J Dent Res* 64:499-514, 1984.

Linde A: Structure and calcification of dentin. In Bonucci E, editor: *Calcification in biological systems,* Boca Raton, FL, 1992, CRC Press, pp 269-311.

Pashley DH: Dentin permeability and dentin sensitivity, *Proc Finn Dent Soc* 88(S1):31-38, 1992.

Pashley DH: Smear layer: overview of structure and function, *Proc Finn Dent Soc* 88(S1):225-242, 1992.

Priam F, et al: New cellular models for tracking the odontoblast phenotype, *Arch Oral Biol* 50(2):271-277, 2005.

Szabo J, Trombitas K, Szabo I: The odontoblast processes branches, *Arch Oral Biol* 26:331, 1984.

Trowbridge HO, et al: Response to thermal stimulation in human teeth, *J Endocrinol* 66:40, 1980.

Yamamoto T, et al: The structure of the cemento-dentinal junction in rat molars, *Ann Anatomy* 182(2):185-190, 2000.

9

DENTAL PULP

CHAPTER OUTLINE

Overview
Anatomy of the Pulp
  Coronal Pulp
  Radicular Pulp
  Apical Foramina and Accessory
    Canals
Histology of Pulp
  Odontoblasts

Fibroblasts
Other Pulpal Cells
Fibers and Ground Substance
Vascularity
Nerves
Nerve Endings
Pain and the Pulp-Dentin
  Complex

Functions of the Pulp
Regressive Changes
  Fibrous Changes
  Pulp Stones
  Diffuse Calcifications
Self-Evaluation Questions
Consider the Patient Discussion
Suggested Reading

LEARNING OBJECTIVES

After reading this chapter the student will be able to:

- describe the anatomy of the pulp and the histology of the odontoblasts, fibroblasts, Schwann cells, the endothelial cells of the arteries, veins and capillaries, pericytes and perivascular cells, and undifferentiated cells within the pulp proper and macrophages
- describe the structure of the blood vessels
- discuss the extracellular matrix of the pulp, predentin and dentin, pulp stones, and diffuse calcifications and changes that take place during the aging process

KEY TERMS

Adventitia
Apical foramen
Basophils
Capillaries
Cell-free zone
Cell-rich zone
Coronal pulp
Denticles
Direct innervation theory
Endothelial cells
Eosinophils
Erythrocytes
False denticles
Formative

Free, attached, or embedded
  denticles
Gap junction
Hydrodynamic theory
Inductive
Intermediate junction
Intima
Leukocytes
Lymphocytes
Macrophages
Media
Nutritive
Odontogenic zone
Parietal layer of nerves

Pericytes
Plexus of Raschkow
Precapillaries
Protective
Radicular pulp
Reparative
Schwann's cells
Terminal arterioles
Tight (zonula occludens) junction
Transduction theory
True denticles
Undifferentiated cells
Zone of Weil/Weil's basal layer

OVERVIEW

Dental pulp is the soft connective tissue located in the central portion of each tooth. It has a crown (coronal part) and a root (radicular part). Pulp is a delicate, specialized connective tissue containing thin-walled blood vessels, nerves, and nerve endings enclosed within dentin. Each pulp opens into the tissue surrounding the tooth, the periodontium, through the apex of the root canal. Accessory canals may be present at the apex of the tooth.

Pulp has a central zone and a peripheral zone, which are observed in both the coronal and radicular pulp. The central zone contains large arteries, veins, and nerve trunks that enter the pulp from the apical canal and proceed to the coronal pulp chamber. Fibroblasts are the preponderant cell, existing in an intercellular substance of glycosaminoglycans and collagen fibers. Odontoblasts are the second most prevalent cell. The odontogenic zone in the periphery consists of odontoblasts and cell-free and cell-rich zones. Adjacent to the cell-rich zone is a parietal layer of nerves.

Odontoblasts form dentin throughout life, which causes the pulp to grow smaller with time. The terminal blood cells in the periphery are in thin-walled capillaries situated among the odontoblasts. Larger vessels with muscle cell support in their walls exist centrally and are under sympathetic control. Several theories exist concerning pain conduction through dentin. The hydrodynamic theory is the most popular. It defines the movement of the odontoblast into contact with pulpal and intratubular nerve endings. Recent findings indicate, however, that odontoblasts are capable of receiving, conducting, and transmitting impulses to nerve endings in close proximity.

Pulp has several functions, such as initiative, formative, protective, nutritive, and reparative activities. All these clinical features are important to the production and maintenance of teeth.

Pulp may regress after trauma or with age and may contain diffuse areas of collagen fiber bundles and pulp stones. These pulp stones may be attached, embedded, or free in the pulp tissue. Pulp may also contain diffuse calcifications.

ANATOMY OF THE PULP

Human beings have 52 pulps in their teeth, 20 in the primary dentition and 32 in the permanent (Fig. 9-1). All pulps have similar morphologic characteristics, such as a soft, gelatinous consistency in a chamber surrounded by dentin, which contains the peripheral extensions of the pulpal odontoblasts. The total volume of the pulps of the permanent dentition is approximately 0.38 ml, and the mean volume of a single human tooth is 0.2 ml. The pulps of molar teeth are approximately four times larger than those of the incisors (see Fig. 9-1).

Coronal Pulp

The two forms of pulpal tissue are coronal and radicular (Figs. 9-2 and 9-3). **Coronal pulp** occupies the crown of the tooth. It is much larger than root pulp and has a structure different from the root tissue. In general, the coronal pulp follows the contour of the outer surface of the crown. Coronal pulp has six surfaces: mesial, distal, buccal, lingual, occlusal, and the floor. Coronal pulp has pulp horns, which are protrusions of pulp that extend into the cusps of the teeth. The number of pulp horns depends on the number of cusps (see Fig. 9-1). At the

Fig. 9-1 Three-dimensional diagram of pulp organs of permanent human teeth. *Upper row,* Maxillary arch; left central incisor through third molar; *lower row,* mandibular arch; left central incisor through third molar. (Modified from Bhaskar SN, editor: *Orban's oral histology and embryology,* ed 11, St. Louis, 1991, Mosby.)

A   B   C   D

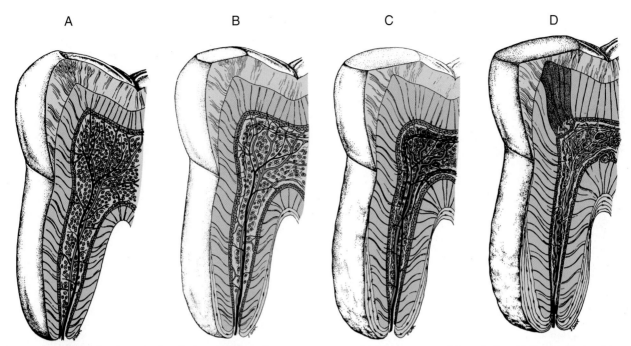

Fig. 9-2 Diagram of series of pulps during the life cycle. A, Young stage. **B,** After some attrition. **C,** At middle age. **D,** In old age. Pulp size and number of cells decrease, and fibrous tissue increases. Attrition also affects pulp horn with appearance of dead tracts and sclerotic dentin. (Modified from Bhaskar SN, editor: *Orban's oral histology and embryology,* ed 11, St. Louis, 1991, Mosby.)

cervical region, the coronal pulp joins the root pulp. With age, the coronal pulp decreases in size because of continued dentin formation (see Fig. 9-2).

Radicular Pulp

Pulpal root canals extend from the cervical region to the apex of the root. **Radicular pulp** of the anterior teeth is

Coronal pulp

Radicular pulp

Cementum around apical canal

Fig. 9-3 Calcified section of older tooth showing decreased size of coronal and root pulp.

singular, whereas the posterior teeth have multiple root pulps. Radicular pulp is tapered or conical and, like coronal pulp, becomes smaller with age because of continued dentinogenesis (see Figs. 9-2 and 9-3). The apical canal may become narrowed by cementum deposition.

 Consider the Patient

> A patient calls a pink incisor to the dentist's attention. He wants to know what causes this symptom.

 CLINICAL COMMENT

> Radiographic knowledge of the pulp chamber's shape and the extension of pulp horns into the overlying cusps is important in providing safe restorative dentistry. Pulp horns present a potential problem for pulp exposure.

Apical Foramina and Accessory Canals

The **apical foramen** is the opening of root pulp into the periodontium. This opening varies from 0.3 to 0.6 mm, being slightly larger in the maxillary teeth than in the mandibular teeth. The apical foramen generally is centrally located in the newly formed root apex but becomes more eccentrically located with age (see Figs. 9-3

Fig. 9-4 Section of tooth apex illustrating an accessory canal *(upper arrow)* and main apical canal *(lower arrow).*

and 9-4). If several apical canals exist, the larger is designated the apical foramen, and the more lateral ones are called the accessory canals (see Fig. 9-4). Accessory canals may result from the presence of blood vessels obstructing dentin formation or from a break in the epithelial root sheath to induce initial root formation. The incidence of accessory canals is about 33% in permanent teeth. Accessory canals are located on the lateral sides of the apical region and may be found in the bifurcation area of multirooted teeth. Clinically, accessory canals are important because they represent contact of the pulp with the periodontal tissues. If inflammation of the pulp is present, it can spread to the periodontium or vice versa.

CLINICAL COMMENT

The presence of accessory pulp canals in an area where periodontal pathologic conditions exist may allow bacteria to spread into the pulp. If a pathologic condition exists in the pulp, on the other hand, it could be disseminated to the periodontium through such an accessory canal.

HISTOLOGY OF PULP

The pulp consists of coronal and root pulp. Coronal pulp is larger and contains many more elements than root pulp. Root pulp acts as a conducting tube to carry blood to and from the coronal area to the apical canal. Both pulp areas contain the same elements, although the cells, fibers, blood vessels, and nerves are more numerous in coronal pulp. Centrally, the pulp is composed of large veins, arteries, and nerve trunks surrounded by fibroblasts and collagen fibers embedded in an intercellular matrix (Fig. 9-5, *A*). Peripherally along the dentin in both coronal and radicular pulp are the formative cells of dentin, odontoblasts. The **odontogenic zone** includes these odontoblasts, the **cell-free zone,** and the cell-rich zone (Fig. 9-5, *B*). The cell-free zone is known as the **zone of Weil** or **Weil's basal layer.** Adjacent to this zone is a zone of high cell density called the **cell-rich zone,** and pulpal to this zone is the **parietal layer of nerves** (Fig. 9-5, *B*). Thus, the peripheral area of pulp is highly organized. The odontogenic zone appears most notably in coronal pulp and relates to the process of dentin formation, although the function of the cell-rich and cell-free zones in this process is still uncertain. In addition to the regions of the central and peripheral pulp is the area of the pulp horns. Here the odontoblasts are crowded and appear palisaded in contrast to their appearance in the remainder of the coronal area (Fig. 9-6). In the middle area, root pulp odontoblasts are short and cuboidal.

Odontoblasts

Odontoblasts line the perimeter of the pulp from the time they begin organizing to form dentin to the time they are in quiescence and no longer producing dentin. Odontoblasts are small and oval when they first differentiate but soon become columnar (Fig. 9-7). These cells then develop processes or extensions around which dentin forms. As the process lengthens, the amount of dentin thickens. Then the odontoblastic process develops many side branches. When these branches develop, space is provided in the dentin for them (Fig. 9-8). Odontoblasts are larger in coronal pulp than in the root and appear columnar in pulp horns (see Fig. 9-6). These tall, columnar cells are about 35 μm long in the pulp horns, whereas in radicular pulp they are more cuboidal, and cells of the apical region appear flat. The process of the odontoblast is the largest part of the cell, extending from the pulp to the dentinoenamel junction. In the crown, the process could be several millimeters long, but it is shorter in the root.

The active cell has a large nucleus in its basal part and a Golgi's apparatus in its apical part. Abundant rough-surface endoplasmic reticulum and numerous mitochondria are scattered through the cell body (Fig. 9-9). The process arises from the odontoblast at the predentinal border, where the cell constricts as the process enters the dentinal tubule (see Fig. 9-8). The process passes through the predentin, where a few mitochondria are located. As it continues into the mineralized dentin, the process is devoid of major organelles but contains filaments and microtubules throughout its length to

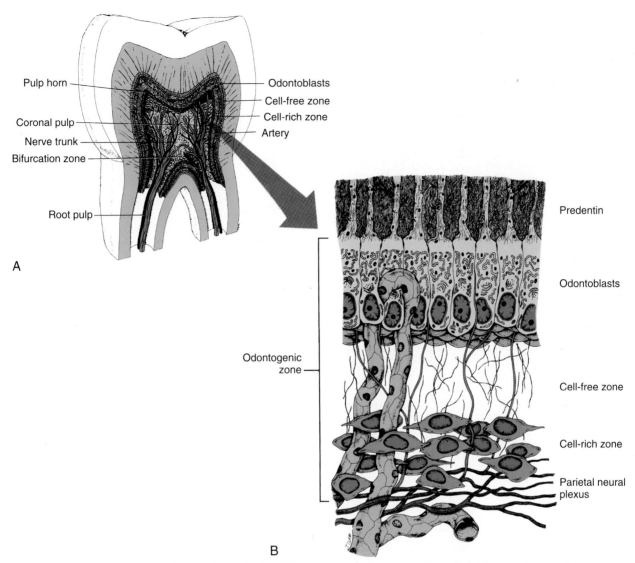

Fig. 9-5 Diagram of pulp organ illustrating pulpal architecture. A, There appears high organization of the peripheral pulp and the appearance of centrally located nerve trunks *(dark)* and blood vessels *(light)*. **B,** Odontogenic zone of pulp. *Top to bottom:* Predentin, odontoblasts, cell-free and cell-rich zones, and parietal layer of nerves. (Modified from Bhaskar SN, editor: *Orban's oral histology and embryology,* ed II, St. Louis, 1991, Mosby.)

Fig. 9-6 Photomicrograph of odontoblasts in the coronal area of the pulp organ. Pulpal capillaries are shown among these cells.

the dentinoenamel junction. How far the process extends into the dentin has been the subject of much discussion. Recent evidence indicates that it extends all the way to, and in some instances through, the dentinoenamel junction and into the enamel as spindles (see Fig. 9-8).

Three types of junctional complexes are found between adjacent odontoblasts: **tight (zonula occludens), gap,** and **intermediate junctions** (Fig. 9-10). Each junction has a different function. Adhering junctions or desmosomes are beltlike areas around these cells that possibly function in maintaining positional relationship between cells. This also prevents substances in the pulp from passing into the dentin. Gap junctions are openings between odontoblasts for communication of cell electrical impulses and passage of small molecules

D
Apposition

A
Morphogenic

B
Organization differentiation

C
Formation

Enamel
organ

Dental
pulp

Initiation

Differentiation

Dentinogenesis

Dentin
matrix
mineralization

Fig. 9-7 Changes in an odontoblast during its differentiation from a preodontoblast (A) to beginning function (D). In the enamel organ, an ameloblast differentiates first and an odontoblast second, but an odontoblast then forms dentin before an ameloblast forms enamel.

(see Figs. 9-10 and 9-11). In this manner, the odontoblasts can have synchronous activity. If stimuli reach the odontoblasts, this information spreads throughout the cell layer by gap junctions. Although odontoblasts are generally believed to live as long as the tooth is viable, inactivity and aging of the odontoblasts result in loss of organelles and a reduction of cell size.

 CLINICAL COMMENT

The pulp horns recede with age. This is a protective measure performed by the pulp cells. Also, reparative dentin forms under cavity preparations or other areas of trauma. Cells in the pulp can be called on to become new odontoblasts and to form dentin at required sites.

Fibroblasts

Fibroblasts are the most numerous cells in pulp because they are located throughout pulp. These cells are characterized by their functional state. In young pulp, fibroblasts produce collagen fibers and ground substance. At that time, they have a large oval nucleus that is centrally located and has multiple processes (Fig. 9-12). Higher magnification of a fibroblast (Fig. 9-13) illustrates Golgi's apparatus, adjacent abundant rough-surface endoplasmic reticulum, and mitochondria. This fibroblast is a protein-producing cell. In aging, these cells appear smaller and shaped like a spindle, with few organelles.

Other Pulpal Cells

Nerve cells in the pulp include **Schwann's cells** (Fig. 9-14). These cells form the myelin sheath of nerves and are associated with all pulp nerves. In addition, **endothelial cells** lining the capillaries, veins, and arteries of the pulp can be visualized (Fig. 9-15). Accompanying most blood vessels are **pericytes** and numerous **undifferentiated cells** found in normal pulp. They function as a cell pool and are called into action when new odontoblasts or fibroblasts are needed. For example, this may happen when reparative dentin is needed for pulp exposure. **Macrophages,** normal constituents of the pulp, function in pulp maintenance because of the turnover of

Fig. 9-9 Electron micrograph of tight, intermediate, and gap junctions, which are located between odontoblasts. Cell organelles may also be seen above the region of nuclei. (From Avery JK: *Oral development and histology,* ed 3, Stuttgart, 2002, Thieme Medical.)

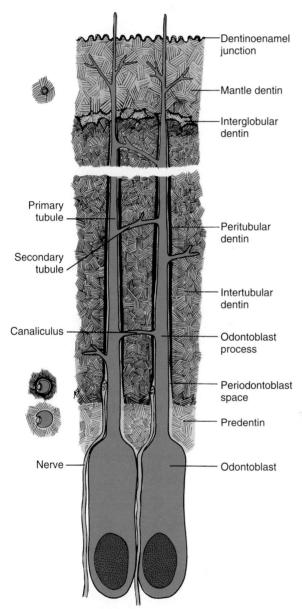

Fig. 9-8 Odontoblast and process extend through the entire thickness of dentin into the inner enamel, as noted at the top of the picture. Side branches of odontoblastic process are shown, and cross section of tubules is at the left. (Modified from Bhaskar SN, editor: *Orban's oral histology and embryology,* ed 11, St. Louis, 1991, Mosby.)

Fig. 9-10 Diagram of the three types of junctional complexes found between adjacent odontoblasts. Their locations can be noted in central diagram, and an illustration of a unit membrane is at upper right. (Modified from Bhaskar SN, editor: *Orban's oral histology and embryology,* ed 11, St. Louis, 1991, Mosby.)

Fig. 9-11 Electron micrograph of junctions between four odontoblasts in the region of cell nuclei. Cell membranes meet at thickened dense-staining zones where junctions are formed, as indicated by *arrows*. These dark zones are gap junctions that allow passage of small molecules between odontoblasts.

Fig. 9-12 Pulp fibroblasts, collagen fibers, and blood vessels in young pulp. (From Avery JK: *Oral development and histology,* ed 3, Stuttgart, 2002, Thieme Medical.)

Fig. 9-13 Electron micrograph of pulp fibroblasts showing rough-surface endoplasmic reticulum and mitochondria. (From Bhaskar SN, editor: *Orban's oral histology and embryology,* ed 11, St. Louis, 1991, Mosby.)

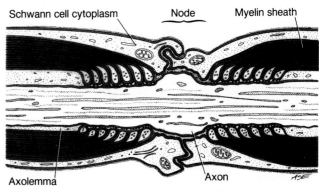

Fig. 9-14 Pulpal nerve axon surrounded by Schwann's cell cytoplasm.

cells in pulp (Fig. 9-16). **Lymphocytes** are also found in pulp-free spaces and probably function in an immune system of pulp. **Erythrocytes,** lymphocytes, **leukocytes, eosinophils,** and **basophils** are found in pulp blood vessels.

Fibers and Ground Substance

Collagen fibers exist in the extracellular matrix, which surrounds the cells. Collagen originates from the pulpal fibroblasts throughout pulp. Both type I and type III collagen have been found in pulp. Type I is probably produced by odontoblasts because this is the type of collagen found in dentin, the tissue that the odontoblasts produce. Type III is probably produced by pulp fibroblasts. In young pulp, fibers are relatively sparse and the tissue appears delicate (see Fig. 9-12). Around the fibers is the ground substance of pulp. This substance is the environment that provides life for cells in pulp and

throughout the body. If pulp is irritated, fibers may accumulate rapidly. However, older pulp contains more collagen of both bundle and diffuse types (Fig. 9-17).

Vascularity

The pulp organ is highly vascularized, with vessels arising from the external carotid arteries to the superior and inferior alveolar arteries. It drains by the same veins. Although the periodontal and pulpal vessels both originate from these vessels, their walls are different. The walls of the periodontal and pulpal vessels become quite

Myelinated nerve

Nonmyelinated nerve

Red blood cell

Endothelial cell

Schwann cell nucleus

Fig. 9-15 Electron micrograph of an arteriole in the central pulp. The lumen is surrounded by endothelial cells forming the intimal layer and of muscle cells forming the media. At right are myelinated nerves; large nuclei belong to accompanying Schwann's cells. (From Avery JK: *Oral development and histology,* ed 3, Stuttgart, 2002, Thieme Medical.)

Dentin

Odontoblast process

Zone of inflammation in pulp

Fig. 9-16 Area underlying dentin with leukocytes, lymphocytes, and macrophages apparently responding to an irritant that resulted in inflammation. The odontoblastic processes in dentinal tubules are degenerating.

thin as they enter the pulp because the pulp is protected within a hard, unyielding container of dentin. These thin-walled arteries and arterioles enter the apical canal and pursue a direct route up the root pulp to the coronal area (Fig. 9-18). Along the way, vessels produce branches that pass peripherally to a plexus that lies in and adjacent to the odontogenic zone of the root (Fig. 9-19). Blood flow is more rapid in the pulp than in most areas of the body, and the blood pressure is quite high. The diameter of the arteries varies from 50 to 100 μm, which equals the size of arterioles in other areas of the body. These vessels have three layers: the inner lining, or **intima,** which consists of oval or squamous-shaped endothelial cells surrounded by a closely associated fibrillar basal lamina; a middle layer or **media,** which consists of muscle cells from one to three cell layers thick (Fig. 9-20); and an outer layer, or **adventitia,** which consists of a sparse layer of collagen fibers forming a loose network around the larger arteries. Smaller arterioles with a single layer of muscle cells range from 20 to 30 μm, and **terminal arterioles** of 10 to 15 μm are

also present. **Precapillaries** measuring 8 to 12 μm and **capillaries** measuring 8 to 10 μm in diameter are present in the peripheral pulp. Capillaries are endothelial-lined tubes that form a network among the odontoblasts (see Fig. 9-19). Numerous investigators have shown that lymphatic vessels are present in pulp. These vessels are thin walled, irregularly shaped, and larger than capillaries and have an incomplete lamina supporting the intima and media.

CLINICAL COMMENT

The vitality of pulp results in part from the apical canal's ability to remain open. This opening can become blocked, however, as the tooth ages and cementum becomes deposited around the apical canal. Thin walls of veins are the first structure affected by cemental constriction of the apices; vascular congestion can occur, leading to pulpal necrosis.

Fig. 9-17 Collagen bundles in an older pulp organ. Trauma may also have contributed to collagen in this pulp.

Diffuse collagen fibers

Collagen bundles

Collagen bundles

Fig. 9-18 Vascular injection to illustrate blood vessel organization in pulp and periodontium. Larger vessels conduct blood in the central pulp, and smaller capillaries are in the peripheral pulp.

Coronal pulp

Periodontium

Root pulp

Fig. 9-19 Vascular injection into blood vessels to illustrate the network of capillaries among odontoblasts in the odontogenic zone. Dentin, which protects pulp, is seen at the top of the picture. The central pulp is in the lower part of the micrograph. (From Avery JK: *Oral development and histology,* ed 3, Stuttgart, 2002, Thieme Medical.)

Dentin

Capillaries

Odontogenic zone (odontoblasts)

Central pulp

Lumen of
vessel

External
adventitial
fibers

Endothelial
cell

Muscle
cells

Fig. 9-20 Ultrastructure of a pulp arteriole in the central pulp area. The lumen is surrounded by endothelial cells; a nucleus is seen below. These cells compose the intima layer. Surrounding the intima is a layer of muscle cells that form the media. External adventitial fibers are also present. (From Avery JK: *Oral development and histology,* ed 3, Stuttgart, 2002, Thieme Medical.)

Nerves

Several large nerves enter the apical canal of each molar and premolar, and single nerves enter the anterior teeth. These nerve trunks traverse the radicular pulp, proceed to the coronal area, and branch as they extend peripherally (Fig. 9-21). Nonmyelinated axons also enter with the myelinated axons, but they are smaller. A young molar may have as many as 350 to 700 myelinated axons and 1,000 to 2,000 nonmyelinated axons entering the apex.

The large nerve trunks are invested with Schwann's cells (see Figs. 9-14 and 9-15). Later, as the pulp organ matures, the subodontoblastic plexus is apparent in the roof and lateral walls of the coronal pulp and, to a lesser extent, the root canals. This network, comprising both myelinated and nonmyelinated axons, is known as the parietal layer of nerves or nerve **plexus of Raschkow** (see Figs. 9-21 and 9-22). From the parietal layer, the nerves pass into the odontogenic zone and then terminate among the odontoblasts or extend into the dentinal tubules with the odontoblastic process.

Nerve Endings

Most pulpal nerve endings are in the odontogenic region of the pulp horns. Some terminate on or in association with the odontoblasts (Figs. 9-23 and 9-24). Others are found in the predentinal tubules, usually in the region of pulp horns or roof of the coronal area (see Fig. 9-24). These nerve endings are presumed to function in pain reception. Few nerve endings are located along the larger muscular blood vessels in the central pulp. All these nerve endings have a similar appearance and are highly vascular. They are believed to function in regulation of blood flow, constriction, or dilation of large blood vessels of the pulp. These nerve

Parietal
layer
nerves

Nerve
trunks

Fig. 9-21 Nerve trunks pass from the radicular pulp into the coronal area. These nerves extend to the periphery, where they form a plexus of nerves adjacent to the odontogenic zone above. (From Bhaskar SN, editor: *Orban's oral histology and embryology,* ed 11, St. Louis, 1991, Mosby.)

endings are post-ganglionic, sympathetic nerves with cell bodies located in the superior cervical ganglion.

PAIN AND THE PULP-DENTIN COMPLEX

Pain is a function of the high concentration of nerve endings within the tooth. Pulp is highly sensitive to temperature changes, electrical and chemical stimuli, and

Fig. 9-22 Myelinated nerves extending into the parietal nerve plexus in the peripheral pulp. From this area, they extend between odontoblasts to terminate among them or in dentinal tubules. (From Avery JK: *Oral development and histology,* ed 3, Stuttgart, 2002, Thieme Medical.)

Odontoblasts

Parietal layer nerves

Nerve trunks

Fig. 9-23 Ultrastructure of a nerve ending in close contact with the odontoblastic process in predentin. The nerve contains small vesicles believed to contain a neurotransmitter substance. The nerve terminal interdigitates with the odontoblastic process. (From Bhaskar SN, editor: *Orban's oral histology and embryology,* ed 11, St. Louis, 1991, Mosby.)

Odontoblastic process

Nerve ending containing vesicles

Odontoblastic process

Nerve ending in tubule

Fig. 9-24 Vesiculated nerve terminal in a dentinal tubule making contact with odontoblastic process. The nerve and process are close to each other. Dark-stained mineral of dentin is shown above and below the tubule.

pressure as applied to the inner enamel, dentin, or pulp. Teeth are one of the few body structures that perceive only the modality of pain. The close relationship between nerve endings and the odontoblasts and their processes is significant. Moreover, the nerve endings in the dentinal tubules and the pulp may be some distance from where the pain is perceived, at the dentinoenamel junction and the inner enamel. Several theories attempt to explain this phenomenon.

The first theory is called the **direct innervation theory,** which is based on the belief that the nerves extend to the dentinoenamel junction. However, studies have not shown nerves present at this junction. In a second theory, other scientists believe the odontoblastic process is the receptor and that it conducts the pain to nerve endings in the peripheral pulp and in the dentinal tubules. This theory has been termed the **transduction theory** (Fig. 9-25).

A third theory, the **hydrodynamic theory,** was developed to explain the transmission of pain through the thickness of dentin (see Fig. 9-25). This theory is based on the premise that when dentin is stimulated, fluid

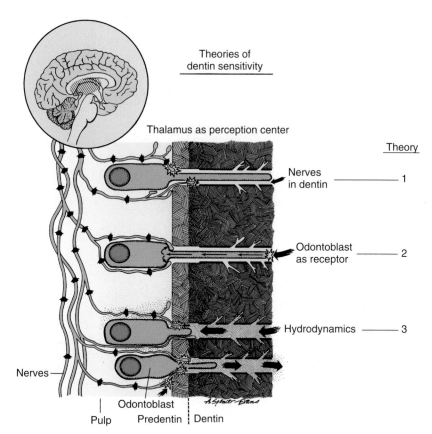

Theories of dentin sensitivity

Thalamus as perception center

Nerves in dentin ——— 1

Odontoblast as receptor ——— 2

Hydrodynamics ——— 3

Theory

Nerves

Pulp   Odontoblast   Predentin   Dentin

Fig. 9-25 Summary of theories on the passage of nerve impulses through dentin. At the top, impulses are shown stimulating nerves in dentin; this is termed the direct stimulation theory. In the center, an odontoblast is depicted as receptor passing impulses to nerves in the peripheral pulp and hence on to the brain, which is the transduction theory. At the bottom, the diagram displays concept of fluid and odontoblast movement. This movement causes pressure on the nerve endings, which stimulates them. The odontoblast thus acts as a mechanoreceptor to nerve endings, which, in turn, conduct impulses to the brain. This is termed the hydrodynamic theory. (Modified from Bhaskar SN, editor: *Orban's oral histology and embryology,* ed II, St. Louis, 1991, Mosby.)

and the odontoblastic process move within the tubules, making contact with the nerve endings in the inner dentin and adjacent pulp. When these nerve endings are contacted, they deform and act as mechanoreceptors to produce an impulse. Several factors support this theory. For example, when a stimulus such as cold is applied to the dentin, the odontoblastic process moves outward, but when heat is applied, the odontoblastic process moves inward. Other evidence is seen in the close relationship of the nerve endings and the odontoblastic process.

The odontoblast is a unique cell that forms dentin throughout life. It forms reactionary or response dentin, for example, in response to various stimuli. In addition, it plays a role in conducting stimuli through dentin and in affecting nerve endings in the peripheral pulp.

FUNCTIONS OF THE PULP

Pulp has several functions, none of which is more important than providing vitality to the teeth with its cells, blood vessels, and nerves. The loss of pulp after a root canal does not mean the tooth will be lost; on the contrary, the tooth will function without pain. The tooth, however, has lost the protective mechanism its pulp nerves provided.

Pulp has several other functions. It is **inductive** because in early development the pulp (papilla) interacts with the oral epithelium and initiates tooth formation. Pulp organs are **formative** because odontoblasts of the pulp form the dentin that surrounds and protects pulp. Pulp is **protective** in its response to stimuli, such as heat, cold, pressure, and operative cutting procedures. The formation of sclerotic dentin, the process of mineral deposition in the tubules, originates in pulp and protects pulp from invasion of bacteria and bacterial products. Pulp is **nutritive** because it carries oxygen and nutrition to the developing and functioning tooth. Finally, pulp has the ability to be **reparative** (Fig. 9-26) through its response to operative cutting or dental caries by the formation of reparative dentin.

 CLINICAL COMMENT

A cracked tooth may result from masticatory impact on a hard object. It can cause a fracture of a restoration margin. As a result, bacterial organisms or their toxins may penetrate the tooth and cause inflammation of the pulp, pain, and eventually pulpal pathosis.

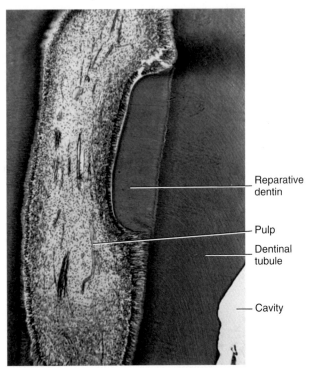

Fig. 9-26 Reparative dentin is deposited underlying areas of stimulation by caries, abrasion, cavity preparation, and restorations. It is limited to area underlying dental tubules leading from the cavity floor. (From Avery JK: *Oral development and histology,* ed 3, Stuttgart, 2002, Thieme Medical.)

REGRESSIVE CHANGES

Numerous regressive changes in the pulp and surrounding dentin are related to environmental stimuli and to aging. It is often difficult to determine which factor has caused the specific change seen. As the tooth ages, pulp decreases in size because of the continued deposition of dentin. This decrease in size usually occurs because of uniform deposition around the entire perimeter of the pulpal border (Fig. 9-27). In addition, changes occur in the dentin with both aging and injury. Areas of dentinal changes, such as dead tracts and mineral deposits, appear in zones of trauma. Reparative dentin usually forms under traumatized areas (see Fig. 9-27). In addition, as a result of both aging and trauma, pulpal cells decrease in general, as do cellular perinuclear cytoplasm and organelles in the cytoplasm, such as mitochondria and endoplasmic reticulum. This indicates that cell activity has decreased. Therefore, aging decreases the ability of the pulp to respond to injury and to repair itself. With injury, however, deposition of dentin appears in a specific location (see Fig. 9-27).

Fibrous Changes

Fibrosis, which is seen in some pulps more than others, is believed to be caused more by injury than by aging.

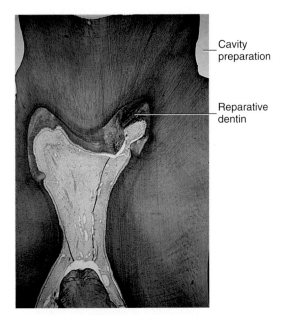

Fig. 9-27 Reparative dentin underlying cavity preparation on the mesial-occlusal-distal aspects of a crown. Reparative dentin on roof and sides of coronal pulp chamber underlie cut dentinal tubules that lead from cavity preparation. (From Avery JK: *Oral development and histology,* ed 3, Stuttgart, 2002, Thieme Medical.)

In some cases, diffuse fibrosis with collagen fibers appears throughout the pulp. Occasionally, the fibers nearly obliterate the pulp. What mechanism causes this condition is not certain, although it is believed to result from pulpal injury, at least in part. Scarring caused by injury is an important factor. One characteristic of aging is an increase in collagen fibers, which become more evident with the decreasing size of the pulp (see Fig. 9-17). Some pulps contain diffuse areas of collagen, and others have bundles of them probably because of injury, as well as unknown systemic factors.

Pulp Stones

Pulp stones or **denticles** are round to oval calcified masses appearing in either the canal or coronal portions of the pulp organ (Fig. 9-28). They appear in teeth that have suffered injury such as microtrauma, as well as in otherwise normal pulps. Pulp stones also occur in unerupted, as well as erupted, teeth. These denticles are noted in most pulps of permanent teeth, especially in individuals more than 50 years of age. They are classified according to their structure as true or false. **True denticles** have dental tubules like dentin. Odontoblasts may be on the surface of these denticles, and their processes are evident in their tubules. **False denticles** are concentric layers of calcified tissue (Fig. 9-29). In the center of these false stones may be a group of cells that

Pulp
stone

Root pulp

Fig. 9-28 Fibrous changes and pulp stone in coronal pulp.
A pulp stone appears in the coronal area of a molar tooth.

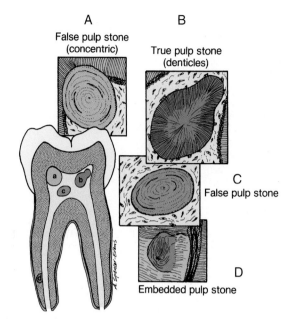

A
False pulp stone
(concentric)

B
True pulp stone
(denticles)

C
False pulp stone

D
Embedded pulp stone

Fig. 9-29 Diagram of types of pulp stones. A, False attached denticle. **B,** True denticle with tubules. **C,** False free denticle. **D,** Embedded denticle.

appear necrotic. These cells are believed to serve as the nidus of denticle formation.

All denticles begin small and grow, sometimes nearly obliterating the pulp. Denticles may appear free in pulp, attached to dentin, or embedded in dentin. Therefore, they are classified as **free, attached,** or **embedded denticles.** One pulp may have all three types (see Fig. 9-29). Investigators believe that a free denticle may become attached and later embedded as dentin is deposited around the denticle. Most denticles are false stones that are free in the pulp.

CLINICAL COMMENT

Pulp stones begin to develop as early as functional occlusion. They normally are asymptomatic unless they impinge on blood vessels or nerves and usually do not present a problem to the dentist. Pulp stones are thought to be a result of microtrauma to the pulp resulting in ectopic calcifications.

Diffuse Calcifications

Diffuse calcifications appear as irregular calcified deposits along collagen fiber bundles or blood vessels in the pulp. This is considered a pathologic condition and usually appears as a sprinkling of or occasionally

large masses of mineral. These calcifications appear more often in the root canal than in the coronal area of the pulp.

Consider the Patient

> ***Discussion:*** This condition can be caused by internal resorption of the root and crown dentin. The crown appears pink because the transparent enamel reveals the blood vessels in the pulp.

SELF-EVALUATION QUESTIONS

1. Describe the characteristics of the odontogenic zone.
2. Compare the odontoblast in coronal pulp with the odontoblast in root pulp.
3. What are the most prominent cells of pulp and what are their functions?
4. What are five other cell types found in normal pulp?
5. Describe the various blood vessels of pulp and how they differ from blood vessels of the periodontium.
6. Give descriptions and locations of nerve endings in pulp.
7. Name five functions of pulp.
8. Name and describe various types of denticles.
9. What are the types of junctional complexes found between odontoblasts?
10. Name and describe the types of reparative dentin.

Suggested Reading

Avery JK: *Oral development and histology,* ed 3, Stuttgart, 2002, Thieme Medical.

Avery JK: Pulp. In Bhaskar SN, editor: *Orban's oral histology and embryology,* ed 11, St. Louis, 1991, Mosby.

Avery JK, Chiego DJ Jr: Cholinergic system and the dental pulp. In Inoki R, Kudo T, Olgart L, editors: *Dynamic aspects of dental pulp: molecular biology, pharmacology and pathophysiology,* New York, 1990, Chapman & Hall, pp 297-332.

Baume LJ: The biology of pulp and dentine. In Myers H, editor: *Monographs in oral science,* vol 8, New York, 1980, S Karger.

Berdal A, et al: Mineralized dental tissues: a unique example of skeletal biodiversity derived from cephalic neural crest, *Morphologie* 84(265): 5-10, 2000.

Boabaid F, et al: Leucine-rich amelogenin peptide: a candidate signaling molecule during cementogenesis, *J Periodontol* 75(8): 1126-1136, 2004.

Chan E, Darendeliler MA: Physical properties of root cementum. Part V. Volumetric analysis of root resorption craters after application of light and heavy orthodontic forces, *Am J Ortho Dentofac Orthop* 127(2):186-195, 2005.

Jin QM, et al: Cementum engineering with three-dimensional polymer scaffolds, *J Biomed Mater Res* 67(1):54-60, 2003.

Nanci A: *Ten Cate's oral histology,* ed 6, St. Louis, 2003, Mosby.

Rex T, et al: Physical properties of root cementum. Part IV. Quantitative analysis of the mineral composition of human premolar cementum, *Am J Ortho Dentofac Orthop* 127(2):177-185, 2005.

Yamamoto T, et al: The structure of the cemento-dentinal junction in rat molars, *Ann Anatomy* 182(2):185-190, 2000.

Zou SJ, et al: Tooth eruption and cementum formation in the Runx2/Cbfa1 heterozygous mouse, *Arch Oral Biology* 48(9): 673-677, 2003.

10

CEMENTUM

LEARNING OBJECTIVES

After reading this chapter the student will be able to:
- describe the development of cementum and its function on the surface of the root
- describe the nature of and the physical properties of intermediate cementum, cellular cementum, and acellular cementum
- discuss the aging of cementum, the formation of cementicles, and the repair of cementum

KEY TERMS

Cellular-acellular cementum
Cementoid layer

Intermediate cementum
OMG

OVERVIEW

Cementum, which is the focus of this chapter, has two major functions. It seals the tubules of root dentin and serves as an attachment for periodontal fibers to keep the tooth in its socket. Cementum has the ability to reverse root resorption by means of deposition as it forms a smooth patch on the cemental surface.

Two types of hard tissue cover tooth roots. The first, called **intermediate cementum,** is a homogenous layer originating from epithelial root sheath cells. The second, called **cellular-acellular cementum,** is a thicker deposit of a bonelike substance produced by cementoblasts that differentiate from the periodontal ligament fibroblasts. The latter is laid down in increments, usually an acellular layer followed by a cellular layer. Cementum simulates bone by displaying cells within lacunae and cell processes within canaliculi. Cementum also exhibits incremental lines but does not have the vascular and neural filament characteristics of bone. As a result, the cementum has unique characteristics, such as lack of neural sensitivity and a greater ability than bone to resist resorption. Both are important clinical features. Aging cementum exhibits a rough and irregular surface caused by resorption of the cemental surface. This cementum also is associated with free, attached, or embedded cementicles. These oval to round stones are similar to the denticles in pulp. They are calcified bodies that may be embedded, attached to cementum, or free in the periodontal ligament.

ROLE OF CEMENTUM ON THE ROOT SURFACE

The hard tissue that covers the entire root surface is very thin but manages to carry out two important functions. First, it seals the surface of the root dentin and covers the ends of the open dental tubules. Second, perforating

fibers of the periodontal ligament become embedded in the cementum. These fibers function as an attachment for the periodontal ligament fibers to the tooth root and aid in maintaining the tooth in its socket. This chapter discusses sealing of the root surface (Fig. 10-1), and Chapter 12 discusses the attachment fibers.

CLINICAL COMMENT

Cementum can aid in maintaining the teeth in functional occlusion if it is deposited at the apical aspect of the root, especially in patients with chronic bruxism. Because cementum is the slowest growing tissue compared with the other periodontal tissues, it will be the last tissue to be added to the root surface after occlusal loss.

DEVELOPMENT OF CEMENTUM

The first cementum deposited on the root's surface is called intermediate cementum and is formed by the inner epithelial root sheath cells that formed during root dentin formation. This deposition occurs before the root sheath cell layer disintegrates (Fig. 10-2). Intermediate cementum is situated between the granular dentin layer of Tomes and the secondary cementum that is formed by the cementoblasts. These cementoblasts arise from the periodontal ligament fibroblasts. The thin layer of intermediate cementum is approximately 10 nm thick. After being deposited, this layer mineralizes to a greater extent than the adjacent dentin or the cellular-acellular cementum. Under proper magnification, a thin line of radiopacity is seen covering the root.

The cellular-acellular cementum is a specialized hard tissue covering the root surfaces of teeth (see Figs. 10-2

Fig. 10-1 Relation of tooth roots to the periodontium. Cementum is shown on the root apex. It covers entire root surface overlying dentin. (From Avery JK: *Oral development and histology*, ed 3, Stuttgart, 2002, Thieme Medical.)

Alveolar bone

Periodontal ligament

Cementum

and 10-3). The initial thin layer of this cementum is acellular and is deposited on intermediate cementum. Subsequent layers alternate between cellular and acellular. Thus, cementum is deposited incrementally. Both grossly and histologically, this cementum resembles bone because it is a hard tissue with cells contained in lacunae that exhibit canaliculi (see Fig. 10-2). However, unlike bone, cementum does not contain blood vessels, nerves, or haversian or Volkmann's canals, which are the nutrient canals containing blood vessels and nerves in bone (see Fig. 10-3).

Cementum is limited to the roots of teeth. In 60% of cases, cementum is formed on the cervical enamel for a short distance; in 30% it stops at the cervical line just meeting the enamel; and in 10% a small gap exists between them. This order of frequency is known as **OMG,** or overlap, meet, and gap (Fig. 10-4 and Table 10-1).

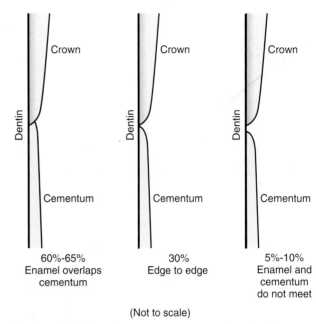

(Not to scale)

Fig. 10-4 Relation of cementum to enamel at the cemento-enamel junction. Overlap, meet, and gap *(OMG)* describe the order of frequency of these conditions. (Modified from Daniel SJ, Harfst SA: *Mosby's dental hygiene: concepts, cases, and competencies,* 2004 update, p. 288, St Louis, 2004, Mosby.)

TABLE 10-1	RELATIONSHIP OF CEMENTUM TO ENAMEL AT THE CEMENTOENAMEL JUNCTION

Relationship of how enamel and cementum meet during development	Percentage of cases
Cementum overlaps enamel	60
Cementum meets enamel	30
Small gap exists between cementum and enamel	10

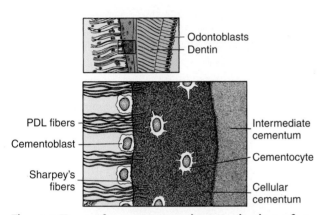

Fig. 10-2 Types of cementum on the root dentin surface. Intermediate cementum on the right overlying dentin cellular cementum in the center of the field and periodontal attachment fibers (PDL) on the left. (From Avery JK: *Oral development and histology,* ed 3, Stuttgart, 2002, Thieme Medical.)

Fig. 10-3 Young cementum deposition on root dentin. Some cementoblasts become enmeshed in cementum matrix and develop into cementocytes living in lacunae. (From Avery JK: *Oral development and histology,* ed 3, Stuttgart, 2002, Thieme Medical.)

INTERMEDIATE CEMENTUM

Intermediate cementum is a thin, noncellular, amorphous layer of hard tissue approximately 10 μm thick. It is deposited by the inner layer of the epithelial cells of the root sheath. Deposition occurs immediately before the epithelial root cells disintegrate as a sheet and migrate away from the root into the periodontal tissue (see Fig. 10-2). Recently, most authors have used the term intermediate cementum, although some prefer **cementoid layer.** The latter term is confusing because the initial layer of cementum is called cementoid, like osteoid in bone.

Intermediate cementum is the first layer of hard tissue deposited, and it seals the tubules of dentin. Because of its epithelial origin, intermediate cementum is composed of enamelin protein rather than collagen, which is the protein typical of cellular or secondary cementum. Intermediate cementum is completely formed before deposition of the secondary cementum begins. As an amorphous, noncellular layer, it is similar to the aprismatic enamel layer on the crown surface of teeth. This cementum calcifies to a greater extent than either the adjacent cellular cementum or the dentin and therefore has a harder consistency (see Fig. 10-2).

 CLINICAL COMMENT

Cementum functions as a covering for the root surface, a seal for the open dentinal tubules, and an attachment for the periodontal fibers that hold the tooth in its socket.

CELLULAR AND ACELLULAR CEMENTUM

Cementum is deposited directly on the surface of the intermediate cementum at a thickness of about 30 to 60 μm at the cervical region of the crown (see Figs. 10-3 and 10-5). It increases gradually to a thickness of 150 to 200 μm at the root apex (Fig. 10-6).

The cementum appears to be more cellular as the thickness increases, probably to maintain its viability (Fig. 10-7). The thin layer near the cervical region requires no cells to maintain viability because fluids bathe its surface.

Cementum forms more slowly than the adjacent dentin (see Fig. 10-5). After the inner epithelial root sheath cells stimulate the formation of the root dentin, they deposit the intermediate cementum on the surface of the dentin. These cells then begin to degenerate and migrate from the root surface into the periodontal ligament. Then the cementoblasts, which originate from the

Cementoblasts

Cementum

Odontoblasts

Dentin

Fig. 10-5 Development of cellular cementum. Epithelial root sheath cells have moved from the root surface of dentin to a position peripheral to the cementum in the periodontal ligament. Cementoblasts are forming cementum along left side of band of dentin and cementum. (From Avery JK: *Oral development and histology,* ed 3, Stuttgart, 2002, Thieme Medical.)

Cementum at root apices

Fig. 10-6 Thick cementum on root apices of an older tooth. Cementum is deposited around apical foramen and is lining the pulpal wall near the apex, constricting the foramen. (From Avery JK: *Oral development and histology,* ed 3, Stuttgart, 2002, Thieme Medical.)

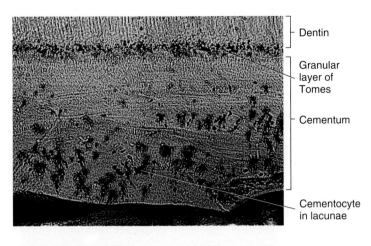

Dentin

Granular layer of Tomes

Cementum

Cementocyte in lacunae

Fig. 10-7 Histology of the granular layer of Tomes and cells in the lacunae in cementum. Cementum near the apex has the greatest number of lacunae. (From Avery JK: *Oral development and histology,* ed 3, Stuttgart, 2002, Thieme Medical.)

Cementoblastic processes

Cementum

Cementoid

Cementoblast

Fig. 10-8 Ultrastructure of cementoblasts on the surface of young cementum. Cementoblasts become cementocytes as their processes (and later their cell bodies) become incorporated in the matrix. (From Avery JK: *Oral development and histology,* ed 3, Stuttgart, 2002, Thieme Medical.)

periodontal ligament, begin to form increments of cementum along the root surface.

Cementum is always thickest at the apex of the root (see Fig. 10-6). Cementum forms through the deposit in increments of a collagenous matrix that then becomes

Lacuna   Cell process

Viable cementocyte

Fig. 10-9 Ultrastructure of cementocyte near the surface of cementum. Cementocytes in this region appear viable and communicate with adjacent cementocytes by gap junctions on their processes. (From Avery JK: *Oral development and histology,* ed 3, Stuttgart, 2002, Thieme Medical.)

secondarily mineralized (see Chapter 5). The young matrix is called cementoid, and its formation is similar to that of bone from osteoid and dentin from predentin.

Some cementoblasts become incorporated in the forming cementum along the developing front as cementum continues to form around the cementoblasts (see Figs. 10-7, 10-8 to 10-11). These cells are then termed cementocytes because they reside in lacunae and appear most notably in the thick apical cementum (see Fig. 10-7). The cementocytes found deep in the cementum are polygonal and have fewer organelles (see Fig. 10-9).

Although many blood vessels are near the surface, none actually enters the cementum. In laboratory tests, cementum is slightly more permeable to dyes than bone or dentin. However, the permeability of viable cementum is unknown. Cementum is deposited in increments, resulting in incremental lines similar to those of bone, dentin, and enamel (Fig. 10-12). Cementum has many characteristics of hard tissue, although some elements are absent. Therefore, cementum is not exactly like any other tissue in the human body. A thin layer of acellular cementum covers the cervical half of the root surface to a distance of approximately 20 μm. A deposit of cellular cementum then covers the acellular layer on the cervical

Fig. 10-10 Ultrastructure of two cementocytes lying deep in cementum. These cells contain few organelles and appear to be inactive. (From Avery JK: *Oral development and histology,* ed 3, Stuttgart, 2002, Thieme Medical.)

Alveolar bone

Attachment fibers | Cemental spike | Reversal lines | Resorption site filled with cementum

Fig. 10-11 Aging cementum showing projection of cemental spikes into ligament. A reversal line indicates root resorption and anatomic repair. Cementum builds up around bundles of periodontal ligament attachment fibers. (From Avery JK: *Oral development and histology,* ed 3, Stuttgart, 2002, Thieme Medical.)

Alveolar bone

Periodontal ligament

Dental cementum

Dentin

Incremental line

Fig. 10-12 Histology of cementum on the root surface. Horizontal incremental lines in cementum appear similar to those of bone, dentin, or enamel.

root to a total thickness of 50 μm. Cellular cementum is then deposited on the apical root dentin to a thickness of 150 to 200 μm.

Without the presence of nerves, cellular cementum is insensitive to pain, which is an important clinical feature. Cementum is also more resistant to resorption than bone, and the lack of cementum vascularity may be part of the reason.

Deep within cementum, many lacunae appear empty, implying that these cells gradually die. Some of these cells have long processes that lie in canaliculi and are in contact with adjacent cementocytes (see Figs. 10-7 to 10-10). Near the surface of cementum, the cells appear active with organelles such as Golgi's apparatus, rough-surface endoplasmic reticulum, and mitochondria, which are all associated with protein secretion (see Fig. 10-10). Layers of cellular cementum may alternate with noncellular layers in their formation, although the reason is unknown. Deeper in the cementum, the cells may be less active (see Fig. 10-9).

The collagen fibers formed within the cementum are associated with the cementum's function on the root's surface. More superficially, cementum has bundles of noncalcified fibers that are associated with the function of attachment of periodontal fibers. These perforating fibers are called extrinsic fiber bundles of cementum.

PHYSICAL PROPERTIES

As one group of hard connective tissues, cementum contains slightly less mineral than dentin or bone (Table 10-2). It is yellow and can be distinguished from enamel because cementum, unlike enamel, has no luster. Cementum is slightly lighter in color than dentin, which makes it difficult to distinguish between the two. It is softer than dentin, however, which aids in its identification.

AGING OF CEMENTUM

With aging, the relatively smooth surface of cementum becomes more irregular (see Fig. 10-11). This is caused

TABLE 10-2	ORGANIC AND MINERAL COMPOSITION OF CEMENTUM, DENTIN, AND BONE	
Substance	Percentage of organic material (collagen)	Percentage of mineral (calcium, phosphorus)
Cementum	50–55	45–50
Dentin	30	65.5
Bone	30–35	60–65

by the calcification of some ligament fiber bundles where they were attached to the cementum. Such occurrences appear on most surfaces of cementum, but to no greater degree near the apical zone. In aging, a continuing increase of cementum in the apical zone may obstruct the apical canal (see Fig. 10-6).

Microscopically, only the lacunae near the surface may have cells that appear viable, whereas deeper lacunae appear empty. Cementum resorption is one characteristic of aging cementum (see Fig. 10-11). Resorption becomes active for a period and then may stop. Deposition of cementum occurs in that period, creating reversal lines. Resorption can also occur in root dentin, and cemental repair can cover this defect (Fig. 10-13).

 Consider the Patient

> An older patient notes that root exposure seems common in her contemporaries. She has also noticed this condition in her son, who has periodontal disease. She asks why this condition is shared by both groups of people.

CLINICAL COMMENT

> Cellular cementum appears similar to bone in structure but does not contain any nerves. Therefore, cementum is nonsensitive. Scaling, when necessary, does not produce pain. However, if cementum is removed, exposure of underlying dentin results in sensitivity.

Alveolar bone

Cementum

Resorption site

Dentin

Fig. 10-13 Cemental and dentin resorption with periodontal soft tissue occupying the area. Alveolar bone develops in this space to compensate for root loss. The length of the periodontal fibers is thus maintained. (From Avery JK: *Oral development and histology,* ed 3, Stuttgart, 2002, Thieme Medical.)

CEMENTICLES

A cementicle is a calcified ovoid or round nodule found in the periodontal ligament. Cementicles may be found singly or in groups near the surface of the cementum (Figs. 10-14 and 10-15). The origin of a cementicle may be a nidus of epithelial cells that are composed of calcium phosphate and collagen in the same amount as

Cementicle (embedded)

Cementum

Fig. 10-14 Cementicle embedded in cementum. Cementicles may be found as free, attached, or embedded cementicles. They may begin free but gradually become attached and then become deeply embedded in the cementum. (From Avery JK: *Oral development and histology,* ed 3, Stuttgart, 2002, Thieme Medical.)

Attachment fibers

Free cementicles

Resorption site

Fig. 10-15 Two groups of free cementicles in the periodontal ligament. A resorption area in the cementum is at the right. (From Avery JK: *Oral development and histology,* ed 3, Stuttgart, 2002, Thieme Medical.)

cementum (45% to 50% inorganic and 50% to 55% organic). Cementicles may be free in the ligament, attached, or embedded in the cementum (see Figs. 10-14 and 10-15). They are more prevalent along the root in an aging person, although they may also be found at a site of trauma.

CEMENTAL REPAIR

Cemental repair is a protective function of the cementoblasts after resorption of root dentin or cementum. These cells are programmed to maintain a smooth surface of the root. Defects arise because of trauma of various kinds, such as traumatic occlusion, tooth movement, and hypereruption caused by the loss of an opposing tooth. Loss of cementum is accompanied by a loss of attachment fibers to the root surface. When this occurs, repair cementum may be deposited by cementoblasts in the defect. After this happens, the attachment fibers readily appear and are found embedded in the repair cementum (see Fig. 10-11). A cemental deposit means the development of a reversal line. This is seen at the point where resorption stops and deposition begins (Fig. 10-16). In an older individual, the surface cementum no longer exhibits a smooth surface (see Fig. 10-15).

Fig. 10-16 Reversal line in cementum *(arrows).* The root surface is again smooth as a result of cementum deposit in the resorption area (anatomic repair). (From Avery JK: *Oral development and histology,* ed 3, Stuttgart, 2002, Thieme Medical.)

 ## CLINICAL COMMENT

Cementum is resistant to resorption in younger tissues. This is the reason that orthodontic tooth movement results in alveolar bone resorption rather than tooth root loss. Cemental repair is an important root protective mechanism.

 ### Consider the Patient

Discussion: Root exposure is common in both aging and periodontal disease. In either condition, when there is an apical migration of the epithelial attachment, exposure of cementum and dentin occurs. Pain is associated with exposed dentin and cementum because dentinal tubules open into pulp, where nerves are located. Also, cementum is thin or nonexistent on the cervical root. Patients with root exposure should be careful. Root caries is also common in root exposure. This occurs because the exposed cementum and dentin are less resistant to caries than is enamel. The pain decreases in time because pulpal odontoblasts respond to the stimuli of exposed dentinal tubules with deposition of reparative dentin in the pulp underlying this area.

SELF-EVALUATION QUESTIONS

1. What is the origin of intermediate cementum?
2. Where on the root is cementum thinnest and where is it thickest?
3. Name three types of cementicles.
4. Describe the appearance of healed root surfaces.
5. Why is cementum insensitive to pain?
6. What is the function of cementum?
7. What is the origin of cementoblasts and cementocytes?
8. Name two characteristics of aging cementum.
9. What are the percentages that cementum overlaps, meets, or gaps enamel?
10. What are some reasons for cemental resorption?

Suggested Reading

Braverman D, Everhardt D, Stoll S: Antigens found in cementum exposed to periodontal disease, *J Periodontol* 59:656, 1979.
Schroeder HE: *Oral structure biology,* New York, 1991, Thieme Medical, pp 187, 290.

PERIODONTIUM: PERIODONTAL LIGAMENT

LEARNING OBJECTIVES

After reading this chapter the student will be able to:

- describe the location and structure of the periodontal ligament
- explain the purpose of the periodontal ligament
- understand the different functions of nerves and blood vessels in and around the ligament and how they interact with one another
- describe the changes that occur in the periodontium as a result of the aging process

KEY TERMS

Aciniform
Alveolar crest fibers
Alveolar crest group
Apical fiber group
Attached gingival fibers
Cementoblasts
Circular or circumferential fibers
Dentoalveolar group

Fibroblasts
Free gingival fibers
Fundic alveolar bone
Gingival fibers
Gingival group
Horizontal fiber group
Interradicular fibers
Interstitial space

Macrophages
Oblique fiber group
Osteoblasts
Osteoclasts
Oxytalan fibers
Transseptal fibers

OVERVIEW

The periodontal ligament is a fibrous connective tissue between the alveolar bone proper and the cementum covering the root. This ligament covers the root of the tooth and connects with the tissue of the gingiva. The periodontal ligament occupies the periodontal space and is composed of fibers, cells, and intercellular substance. The latter consists of collagen fibers and ground substance, which, in turn, contains proteins and polysaccharides. The periodontium develops from dental follicular tissue that surrounds the tooth. The cells forming the ligament fibers, alveolar bone, and cementum develop from the follicle. The periodontium has a thickness of 0.15 to 0.38 mm, is thinnest in the midroot zone, and decreases slightly in thickness with age. The ligament is composed of collagen fiber bundles that attach the cementum to the alveolar bone proper. Interstitial spaces contain the blood vessels and nerve trunks, which communicate freely with vessels and nerves at the apex of the roots and the alveolar bone. This tissue is highly cellular, containing fibroblasts and vascular, neural, bone, and cemental cells. The primary function of the periodontal ligament is support for the teeth.

The ligament also transmits neural input to the masticatory apparatus and has a nutritive function essential to maintaining the ligament's health, which has important clinical implications.

ORGANIZATION OF THE PERIODONTAL LIGAMENT

Two groups of principal fibers are named according to their location with respect to the teeth. The **gingival group** is located around the necks of the teeth, and the **dentoalveolar group** surrounds the roots of the teeth (Fig. 11-1). These principal fibers are bundles of collagen fibers strategically positioned at inclinations important to their functions along the root surface from the cervical region to the tooth's apex (see parts labeled *1* to *6* in Fig. 11-1). The collagen bundles are embedded in the cementum of the root and extend into the alveolar bone. Therefore they act as a suspensor ligament for the teeth.

Between each group of fibers is a space termed the **interstitial space** (Fig. 11-2), which is not actually a space. Interstitial spaces contain a network of blood vessels, nerves, and lymphatics that maintain the vitality

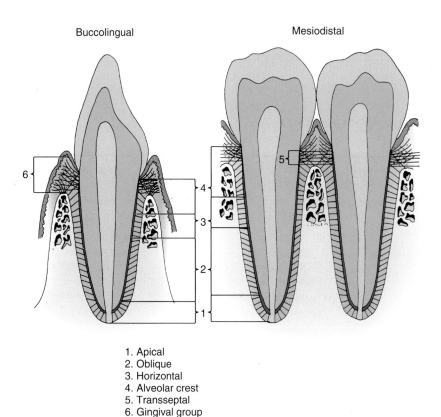

Buccolingual   Mesiodistal

1. Apical
2. Oblique
3. Horizontal
4. Alveolar crest
5. Transseptal
6. Gingival group

Fig. 11-1 Principal fiber groups of the periodontal ligament. All fibers listed in buccolingual plane are also present in mesiodistal plane. The transseptal fiber group number 5, however, is seen only in mesiodistal plane as these fibers are attached tooth to tooth. All other principal fibers are attached tooth to the gingiva or alveolar bone.

Periodontal
ligament
fibers

Tooth
root

Alveolar
bone

Horizontal
principal
fibers of
periodontal
ligament

Interstitial
space

A   B

Fig. 11-2 Appearance of principal fiber bundles and interstitial spaces in the periodontal ligament. A, As they appear in cross-sectional plane. **B,** In plane longitudinal to tooth.

of the periodontal ligament and a network of finer fibers that interlace in the spaces, as well as support the dense collagen fiber bundles. The function of the interstitial space relates to the constant stretching and contraction of the fiber bundles during mastication. Most supporting fibers are collagenous, but a few have been described as elasticlike and of a structure different from that of collagen. These are termed **oxytalan fibers** (Fig. 11-3). Oxytalan fibers are small in diameter and appear to interface with the collagen bundles, supporting the collagen bundles and the blood vessel walls. These fine, elasticlike fibers stain with special stains that reveal their location to be almost longitudinal within the ligament when the fibers are viewed through a light microscope (see Fig. 11-3).

Gingival Fiber Group

The principal fibers of the periodontal ligament in the gingival area are known as the **gingival fibers.** They consist of four groups of fibers, each having a different orientation and all supporting the gingiva (Fig. 11-4). The **free gingival fibers** arise from the surface of the cementum in the cervical region and pass into the free gingiva. The **attached gingival fibers** arise from the

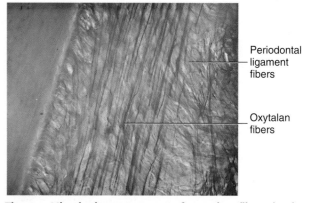

Periodontal
ligament
fibers

Oxytalan
fibers

Fig. 11-3 Histologic appearance of oxytalan fibers in the periodontal ligament oriented parallel to the tooth's surface.

alveolar crest and pass into the attached gingiva. The **circular** or **circumferential fibers** are continuous around the neck of the tooth and resist gingival displacement. The **alveolar crest fibers** arise from the cementum at the neck of the tooth and terminate in the alveolar crest. **Transseptal fibers** originate in the cervical region of each crown and extend to similar locations

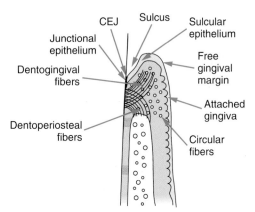

Fig. 11-4 The four groups of gingival fibers. Dentogingival fibers extend from the cervical cementum into free and attached gingiva. Alveologingival fibers extend from the alveolar crest into gingiva. Circular fibers surround the teeth, and the dentoperiosteal group extends from the cervical cementum into the alveolar crest. (Modified from Daniel SJ, Harfst SA: *Mosby's dental hygiene: concepts, cases, and competencies,* 2004 update, p. 288, St Louis, 2004, Mosby.)

on the mesial and distal surfaces of each adjacent tooth (Figs. 11-5 and 11-6). This fiber group functions in resistance to the separation of each tooth. Figure 11-6 shows that transseptal fibers are found in the mesiodistal plane and are not present in the buccolingual plane. All these fiber groups are illustrated in Figure 11-1 and listed in Table 11-1.

Dentoalveolar Fiber Group

The dentoalveolar fiber group consists of five differently oriented principal fiber groups named according to their origin and insertion in the dentoalveolar process. The **alveolar crest group** originates at the cervical area, just below the dentinoenamel junction, and extends to the alveolar crest, as well as into the gingival connective tissue (see Fig. 11-6). These fibers resist intrusive forces. The **horizontal fiber group** extends in a horizontal

Fig. 11-5 Histology of gingival fibers in the interproximal area. The transseptal fiber group extends from mesial of one tooth to distal of an adjacent tooth. Relationship of free gingival and circular fibers to transseptal fibers is shown.

Fig. 11-6 Histology of alveolar crest fibers extending from the cementum of the cervical region to the alveolar bone. Periodontal fibers penetrate alveolar bone, and transseptal fibers extend from the tooth on the left to the right.

direction from the midroot cementum to the adjacent alveolar bone proper. These fibers resist tipping of the teeth, as illustrated in Figure 11-7. The **oblique fiber group** extends in an oblique direction from the area just above the apical zone of the root upward to the alveolar bone (Fig. 11-8), and the fibers resist vertical or intrusive masticatory forces. The **apical fiber group** extends perpendicular from the surface of the root apices to the adjacent **fundic alveolar bone,** which surrounds the apex of the tooth root. Apical fibers resist vertical and extrusive forces applied to the tooth (see Fig. 11-8). Another group of fibers that are located between the

TABLE 11-1 **PRINCIPAL FIBERS**

Fiber group	Location of attachment	Function
GINGIVAL FIBER GROUP		
Transseptal	Cervical tooth to tooth mesial or distal to it	Resist tooth separation mesial distal
Attached gingival	Cervical tooth to attached gingival	Resist gingival displacement
Free gingival	Cervical tooth to free gingival	Resist gingival displacement
Circumferential	Continuous around neck of tooth	Resist gingival displacement
DENTOALVEOLAR FIBER GROUP		
Apical	Apex of root of fundic alveolar bone proper	Resist vertical forces
Oblique	Apical one third of root to adjacent alveolar bone proper	Resist vertical and intrusive forces
Horizontal	Midroot to adjacent alveolar bone proper	Resist horizontal and tipping forces
Alveolar crest	Cervical root to alveolar crest of alveolar bone proper	Resist vertical and intrusive forces
Interradicular	Between roots to alveolar bone proper	Resist vertical and lateral movement

Fig. 11-7 Histologic appearance of horizontal fiber bundles. The bundles are perpendicular to the root and alveolar bone surface; their perforating fibers are embedded in both bone and cemental surfaces.

Fig. 11-8 Histology of horizontal, oblique, and apical fiber groups of the periodontal ligament. The angulation is shown for each of these bundle groups, which resist forces of mastication.

roots of multirooted teeth is termed **interradicular fibers.** Such fibers extend perpendicular to the tooth's surface and to the adjacent alveolar bone (Fig. 11-9) and resist vertical and lateral forces. These fibers are summarized in Table 11-1.

CLINICAL COMMENT

> Healthy periodontal tissues are of significant importance to the health of dental patients. Chronic periodontal disease and dental caries can lead to infusion of bacteria into the bloodstream.

Interstitial Spaces

The principal fibers make up the structural and functional bulk of the periodontal ligament. They are positioned at regular intervals along the gingival-apical extent of the periodontal ligament. Between each bundle of ligament fibers an interstitial space appears. These spaces appear in both the cross-sectional and longitudinal planes of the ligament (see Fig. 11-2). The regularity of these spaces clearly relates to the vascular and neural needs of the functioning ligament. Interstitial spaces appear designed to carry these vascular and neural structures both by encircling the tooth at regular intervals and by connecting with the vessels that run longitudinal to the root (Figs. 11-10 and 11-11). These interstitial spaces are designed to withstand the impact of masticatory forces. The collagenous fiber bundles that surround these spaces are arranged at angles to the surfaces of the spaces, thus providing support for their maintenance. These spaces are compressed during mastication or tension, as noted in Figure 11-12. For this reason, their position and support by fiber bundles are important. A network of fine fibers within these spaces can be seen supporting the nerves and nerve endings that occupy these spaces (Figs. 11-13 and 11-14).

Fig. 11-9 Histology of interradicular fiber groups of principal fibers. These are located between the roots and alveolar bone of multirooted teeth.

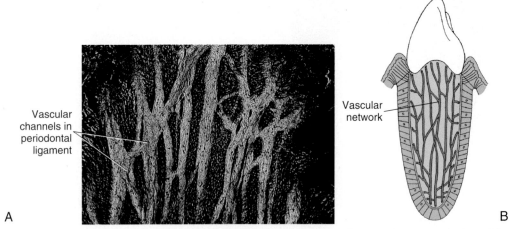

Fig. 11-10 Histology of the periodontal ligament in the longitudinal plane. A shows continuity of the interstitial system in center of ligament with lateral connections throughout the interstitial spaces. **B,** Diagram of organized network of blood vessels in the ligament.

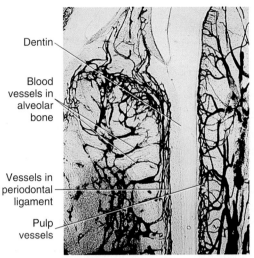

Dentin

Blood vessels in alveolar bone

Vessels in periodontal ligament

Pulp vessels

Fig. 11-11 Vascular supply of alveolar bone, periodontal ligament, and tooth pulp as seen after injection of vessels with carbon and clearing of the tissues. Bone is on the left, the periodontal ligament is in the center, dentin is to the right of center, and pulp is on the right.

Nerve

Artery

Artery

Vein

Fig. 11-13 Interstitial space viewed at high magnification. At the upper left, a nerve enters interstitial space from the ligament. Within the interstitial space are the thick-walled artery and thin-walled veins. Beside the artery and veins are several nerve trunks.

Blood vessel in compressed interstitial space

Interstitial space

Principal fibers and cells

Fibroblasts

Fig. 11-12 Histology of the periodontal ligament illustrating tension. Note diminished interstitial spaces and flattening of cells when the fibers are stretched.

Alveolar bone

Nerve

Nerve terminal

Fig. 11-14 A nerve trunk traversing the periodontal ligament along the surface of alveolar bone on the right. At the lower extremity of the trunk is an encapsulated pressure receptor (modified pacinian). These pressure receptor endings sense the density of food during mastication.

Vascular System

The periodontal ligament has a rich blood supply that arises from the inferior and superior alveolar arteries and from branches of the facial artery from the external carotid. These vessels supply the alveolar bone and anastomose freely with the periodontal ligament. The vascular plexus that extends into the ligament traverses from the apical areas to the gingival areas with loops that surround the teeth at regular intervals (see Fig. 11-10, *B*). Figure 11-10, *A* shows the density and complexity of the ligament. When the alveolar bone and tooth have been sectioned and the vascular plexus has been injected with carbon particles and then cleared, the orientation and relationship of these vessels can be demonstrated (see Fig. 11-11). Both arterioles and venules traverse these tissues, carrying blood to and away from them. Arteriovenous shunts have been demonstrated in the periodontal ligaments that provide direct connections between the arterial and venous blood supply without having to go through a capillary network. Capillaries are evident throughout the principal fiber bundles. The ligament is highly active, undergoing compaction and extension as mastication takes place. Evidence of the ligament activity is seen in cell turnover, in its ability to modify in tooth movement, and in its ability to heal. These conditions relate to the rich vascular supply of the ligament.

 CLINICAL COMMENT

The suspensory apparatus of the teeth is organized to protect the blood vessels from undue compression. Pressure receptors in the ligament are thus protective during mastication.

Neural System

The larger nerve trunks of the periodontal ligament are found in the central zone of the tooth's long axis (Fig. 11-15). Branches of these trunks pass into the ligament and alveolar bone at intervals along the path to the gingival tissues. Most nerve trunks and finer nerves are observed in the interstitial spaces, either in the tracts that traverse the ligament longitudinal to the tooth's surface or within any of the spaces between bundles along the root (see Fig. 11-13). Nerve terminals are noted throughout the ligament and especially in bundles of principal fibers. Encapsulated pressure receptors and **aciniform**, fine pain receptors are in greatest numbers

Interstitial space

Nerve trunk

Fig. 11-15 Nerve trunk passing from the apical region toward the gingival area. Fibers of the periodontal ligament wrap around the interstitial space.

(see Fig. 11-14). These terminals are known to function during masticatory activity.

 CLINICAL COMMENT

Maintaining normal tissue vitality through disease prevention and constant maintenance is important. Oral health is dependent on the combination of professional care and patient participation.

CELLS OF PERIODONTAL LIGAMENT

Fibroblasts, Osteoblasts, and Cementoblasts

Several types of cells located in the ligament have formative, supportive, and resorptive functions. **Fibroblasts** are the most numerous seen in the periodontal ligament because of the high collagen density of this tissue. The abundance of fibroblasts allows rapid replacement of fibers (see Fig. 11-12). Recent investigations show that fibroblasts, in addition to forming new collagen fibers, function in the breakdown of worn-out fibers. Fibers are ingested and broken down into amino acids. These amino acids are taken up by other cells and are recycled into the formation of new collagen fibers. **Osteoblasts** are located along the surface of the alveolar bone. As bone is continually turning over, the osteoblasts are busy forming new bone in the area of the alveolar bone proper. All osteoblasts differentiate locally from mesenchymal cells as the need for osteoblasts arises. **Cementoblasts** appear along the surface of the cementum. Cementum is constantly being formed as new principal fibers are embedded along the root surface. Cemental resorption may also occur for a number of reasons, such as changes in occlusal relationships or tooth movement, resulting in activity of new cementoblasts in the repair of resorbed cementum or dentin of the root.

Macrophages and Osteoclasts

Macrophages found in the ligament are important defense cells in this location. Macrophages have mobility, as well as phagocytic function. They take up dead cells, bacteria, and foreign bodies. Some fibroblasts become macrophagic in the periodontal ligament because they have the ability to destroy collagen, as well as form it (Fig. 11-16). This activity relates to the high metabolic function of the periodontal ligament. Two types of fibroblasts may exist—those that only form collagen and those that form and destroy collagen. Macrophages, lymphocytes, leukocytes, and plasma cells may also appear in the periodontium when it is stressed by disease.

Osteoclasts, in instances of both tooth movement and periodontal disease, may function in bone resorption (Fig. 11-17). They appear as a normal consequence of tipping or bodily movement of a tooth (Fig. 11-18). Osteoclasts originate from monocytes within the blood vascular system and become multinucleated cells seen in lacunae of resorption sites in hard tissue.

Epithelial Rests

Epithelial rests are normal constituents of the periodontal ligament and are seen throughout life. Epithelial cells are scattered throughout the ligament, but in the early life of the tooth they are seen along the root surface. Epithelial rests may appear as resting, proliferating, or degenerating cell masses. They also may be characterized as going through extensive periods of dormancy. These rests are composed of a mass of epithelial cells, some four to six in number, although there may be more in cases where they are proliferating. The cells are believed to originate in the remnants of the root sheath. Epithelial rests can also be induced to proliferate by chronic inflammatory mediators and can form the lining of periapical cysts. Type 2 dendritic cells can also be found lining periapical cysts. However, epithelial rests may continue to proliferate from the epithelial cells lining the gingival crevice. They can be observed along the root surface as seen in Figure 11-19.

Intercellular Tissue

Intercellular tissue surrounds and protects the cells of the periodontal ligament and is the product of these cells. This extracellular matrix (ECM) is composed of water, glycoproteins, and proteoglycans, which surround the collagen fibers. These protein and polysaccharide substances provide the cells with vital substances that arise from the blood capillaries and return unwanted waste products catabolites from these cells to the vessels.

Fig. 11-16 Fibroblasts are present in the periodontal ligament in great numbers. It is probable that some of these cells function in forming as well as destroying collagen fibers as need arises.

Formation of new fibers

Ingestion of collagen fibers and breakdown into amino acids

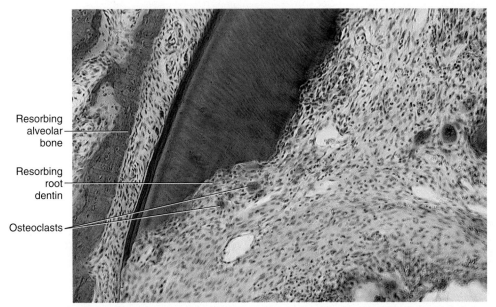

Resorbing alveolar bone

Resorbing root dentin

Osteoclasts

Fig. 11-17 Osteoclastic action on alveolar bone and on root dentin can be seen in this micrograph. Tooth roots *(at left)* and alveolar bone *(at right)* are undergoing resorption in preparation for eruption of tooth in permanent dentition. In the lower right corner is a follicle surrounding erupting permanent tooth crown. Osteoclasts are much larger than any other cell in field.

Fig. 11-18 Diagram of tooth tipping that may occur in orthodontic tooth movement or naturally as a result of malocclusion. As the tooth crown moves to the left, the root moves to the right. As ligament zones marked *A* are compressed, zones marked *B* are stretched. Osteoclasts appear in *A* zones, accompanying bone resorption, and osteoblasts will appear in *B* zones with bone formation.

Sensory

The periodontal ligament is supplied with abundant receptors and nerves that sense any movement in function. When receptors sense pressure, the nerves send signals to the brain, which informs the masticatory apparatus, including the temporomandibular joint and muscles of mastication.

Nutritive

The blood vessels of the ligament provide the essential nutrients for the ligament's vitality and for the hard tissue of cementum and alveolar bone. All cells, such as fibroblasts, osteoblasts, cementoblasts, and even the resorptive osteoclasts and macrophage cells, require the nutrition that is carried by the blood vessels of the ligament (Fig. 11-20).

When an orthodontic appliance or an occlusal problem causes compaction and compression, a constriction of the blood vessels may occur. This results in a lack of vascular continuity, which leads to a diminishing of cells in the area, and the tissue becomes ischemic. The tissue

Dentin

Epithelial rests

Periodontal ligament

Fig. 11-19 Epithelial rests appear in the periodontal ligament near the cementum covering dentin at the top of the micrograph. This is a young specimen; thus, rests are large and distinctive.

FUNCTIONS OF PERIODONTAL LIGAMENT

Supportive

The most important function of the periodontal ligament is support of the teeth. Failure of this function results in tooth loss. Every time the teeth are clenched, as in mastication, the periodontal fibers are stretched and then relaxed. This system is highly efficient to compensate for the thousands of times this ligament is called into action.

then begins to appear glasslike and is described as a "hyalinized" area. Continued pressure usually leads to the appearance of osteoclasts at this site, with the loss of alveolar bone. This condition then may create space for blood vessels to grow back into this area. The periodontium therefore responds as a coordinated unit.

Maintenance

Periodontal tissues function in maintenance of the masticatory apparatus because these tissues heal readily. The interaction of the mesenchymal cells with their intercellular environment is a continuous process. These tissues function for a lifetime if health is maintained and appropriate care is provided.

 Consider the Patient

A patient asks about prevention of periodontal disease. What can the patient do to prevent a future problem?

 CLINICAL COMMENT

Renewal capability is an important characteristic of the periodontal ligament fibers. The periodontal fibroblasts provide maintenance of the system when repair is needed.

AGING OF LIGAMENT

Aging occurs in ligamentous tissue as in all other tissues of the body. Cell number and cell activity decrease as aging takes place. In aging cementum and alveolar bone, scalloping occurs (Fig. 11-21). Some fibers are attached to the peaks of these scallops rather than over the entire surface. This is one of the more remarkable changes that occur in the aging of supporting structures of the teeth. Activity of these tissues is likely to decrease during the aging process because of restricted diets, and therefore normal functional stimulation of these tissues is diminished. With aging, a healthier periodontium can result from general good health of the individual and good oral hygiene. A loss of gingival height related to gingival and periodontal disease promotes destructive changes. Unfortunately, at that time, the presence of a low-grade inflammation may be characteristic of the gingival tissue.

 CLINICAL COMMENT

The four tissues comprising the periodontium are variable in their rate of regeneration—from the fastest, the gingiva, to the slowest, the cementum. The periodontist is aware of these differences and uses these differences in regeneration capacity and rate in the clinical practice of periodontics.

Fig. **11-20** **Ultrastructure of an interstitial space with a nerve bundle containing myelin and unmyelinated nerves** *(lower right)* **and small arterioles** *(above).*

 Consider the Patient

Discussion: The patient's role is very important. Patients assist the dental professional in the maintenance of the periodontal structures. These tissues are very susceptible to poor oral hygiene, and therefore deterioration of the periodontium results.

Fig. **11-21** **Aging periodontal ligament, cementum, and alveolar bone.** The number of fiber bundles has decreased. Cemental spikes are shown, which are caused by excessive deposition around depleted fiber bundles. Resorption sites are also noted.

SELF-EVALUATION QUESTIONS

1. Describe the function and location of the principal fiber groups in the gingival group.
2. Describe the function and location of the principal fiber groups in the dentoalveolar group.
3. Describe the function and location of the interstitial system of the periodontal ligament.
4. Describe the vascular system of the periodontal ligament.
5. Describe the types and locations of the nerves and nerve endings in the periodontal tissues.
6. Name the cells and their functions in the periodontal ligament.
7. What are the three types of epithelial cell rests, and where are they found?
8. Discuss the several functions of the periodontal ligament.
9. What are oxytalan fibers, and what are their function and location?
10. Describe the characteristics of aging in the periodontal ligament.

Suggested Reading

Bonucci E: New knowledge on the origin, function and fate of osteoclasts, *Clin Orthop* 158:252, 1982.

Contos JG, et al: Langerhans cells in apical periodontal cysts: an immunohistochemical study, *J Endodont* 13(2):52-55, 1987.

Marchi F: Secretory granules in cells producing fibrillar collagen. In Davidovich Z, editor: *The biological mechanisms of tooth eruption and root resorption,* Birmingham, AL, 1988, EBESCO Media, pp 53-59.

Marks SC Jr: The origin of osteoclasts; evidence of clinical applications and investigative challenges of an extraskeletal source, *J Oral Pathol* 12:226, 1983.

Melcher AH: Periodontal ligament. In Bhaskar SN, editor: *Orban's oral histology and embryology,* ed 11, St. Louis, 1991, Mosby.

Nakamura TK, Hanal H, Nakamura MT: Ultrastructure of encapsulated nerve terminals in human periodontal ligaments, *J Oral Biol* 24:126, 1982.

Nanci A, Somerman MJ. Periodontium. In *Ten Cate's oral histology: development, structure, and function,* ed 6, St. Louis, 2003, Mosby

Schroeder HE: *Oral structure biology,* New York, 1991, Thieme Medical, pp 187, 290.

Wong RS, Sims MR: A scanning electron-microscopic, stereo-pair study of methacrylate corrosion casts of the mouse palatal and molar periodontal microvasculature, *Arch Oral Biol* 32(8):557-566, 1987.

12

PERIODONTIUM: ALVEOLAR PROCESS AND CEMENTUM

LEARNING OBJECTIVES

After reading this chapter the student will be able to:

- describe the nature of alveolar bone proper and supporting bone
- explain how cementum serves in tooth support
- describe the condition of physiologic tooth movement and the effects of the various types of orthodontic tooth moving devices on the hard tissues of the periodontium
- understand the effects of aging on the tooth supporting structures and the condition of edentulous jaws

KEY TERMS

Alveolar bone proper
Alveolar crest
Area of reversal
Bodily movement
Dehiscence
Extrusion
Fenestration

Haversian bone
Hyalinization
Incisor liability factor
Intrusion
Lamina dura
Leeway space
Mesial drift

Reversal line
Rotation
Sharpey's fibers
Supporting bone
Tipping movement

OVERVIEW

This chapter discusses the hard tissues of the periodontium, which are cementum and alveolar bone. The alveolar process is the bony part of the maxilla and mandible that has the primary function of supporting the teeth. Alveolar bone is composed of alveolar bone proper, which is attached to the fibers embedded in the roots of the teeth. Supporting bone is the bone covering the mandible, and it serves as cortical plates that give support to the alveolar bone proper. This alveolar bone is in the process of continuous turnover, which enables the tissue to be responsive to manipulation, such as tooth movement resulting from normal physiologic function or orthodontic treatment. Cementum functions as the means of fiber attachment to the tooth roots. These fibers have the ability to form and resorb, which are necessary for support during tooth movement. If teeth are moving in a straight line or rotating, all parts of the suspensory apparatus must change simultaneously. This phenomenon first took place during tooth eruption and continues to function for both the primary and secondary dentition. Tooth function is a prerequisite for the maintenance of the alveolar bone and cementum. Bone loss occurs during aging or periods of inactivity, resulting in possible tooth mobilization. With loss of alveolar bone, loss of periodontal fibers occurs as well. Periodontal disease can cause these conditions with possible tooth loss that could result in an edentulous jaw (Box 12-1).

ALVEOLAR PROCESS

The alveolar process is the part of the maxilla and mandible that supports the roots of teeth and is composed of **alveolar bone proper** and **supporting bone** (Fig. 12-1). Alveolar bone proper is the bone lining the tooth socket. In clinical radiographic terms, it is defined as the **lamina dura.** Dense bone serves as the attachment bone that surrounds the roots of the teeth. Supporting bone is, as the name implies, the bone that serves as a dense cortical plate to sustain the alveolar bone proper. This cortical plate covers the surface of the maxilla and mandible and supports the alveolar bone proper. The supporting cancellous bone underlies and supports the dense cortical bone (see Figs. 12-1 and 12-2). The existence of alveolar bone is entirely dependent on the presence of teeth. Alveolar bone develops initially as a

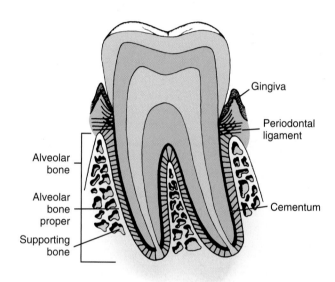

Fig. 12-1 Structures of the periodontium: alveolar bone proper, supporting bone, and cementum.

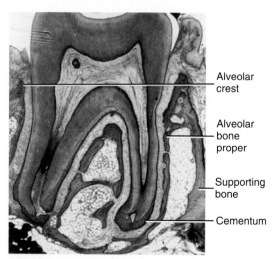

Fig. 12-2 Histology of tooth and its supportive tissues showing relationships among alveolar bone proper, supporting bone, and cementum covering roots.

12.1 | **BOX** | **RATIONALE FOR PERIODONTAL TREATMENT**

The removal of plaque or biofilm and calculus in combination with regular tooth brushing and oral rinses will reduce, if not eliminate, periodontal disease. This is termed nonsurgical therapy and may be all that is necessary if the periodontium is treated early. It may also be necessary to replace defective restorations that may have overhangs before periodontal therapy begins or to adjust the occlusion and/or use a bite splint to help relax tense jaw muscles.

In many cases of more advanced periodontal disease, root planing is needed to smooth the root surfaces and to allow reattachment of the supporting tissues of the teeth. In most cases, the use of antibiotics is recommended to eliminate the bacteria associated with this disease.

protection for the soft developing teeth and later, as the roots develop, as a support to the teeth. Finally, as the teeth are lost, the alveolar bone resorbs. Teeth are responsible not only for the development but also for the maintenance of the alveolar process of the mandible (see Fig. 3-21). The coronal border of the alveolar process is known as the **alveolar crest** (see Fig. 12-2). This crest is normally located approximately 1.2 to 1.5 mm below the dentinoenamel junction of the teeth. It is rounded on the anterior region and nearly flat in the molar area. When teeth are in buccolingual version, the alveolar crest may be thin or missing. The area of bone loss where an apical root penetrates the cortical bone is known as a **fenestration,** and bone loss in the coronal area of the root is termed a **dehiscence** (Fig. 12-3).

 CLINICAL COMMENT

> The lamina dura is an important diagnostic landmark in determining the health of the periapical tissues. Loss of density usually means infection, inflammation, and resorption of this bony socket lining.

Alveolar Bone Proper

The compact or dense bone that lines the tooth socket is of two types when viewed microscopically. This bone either contains perforating fibers from the periodontal ligament or is similar to compact bone found elsewhere in the body. Perforating fibers or **Sharpey's fibers** are bundles of collagen fibers embedded in the alveolar bone proper. These fibers are at right angles or oblique to the surface of the alveolar bone proper and along the root of the tooth (see Fig. 12-1). The fiber bundles inserting in the bone are regularly spaced and appear similar to those that insert into the root surface cementum (Figs. 12-4 and 12-5). These perforating fibers are not limited to periodontal bone. They also appear in the body where ligaments or tendons attach to cartilage or bone.

Because bone of the alveolar process is regularly penetrated by collagen fiber bundles, it can be appropriately

termed bundle bone. Bundle bone, being synonymous with alveolar bone proper or lamina dura, appears more dense radiographically than the adjacent supportive bone (Fig. 12-6). This density is probably the result of the mineral content or orientation of the bone crystals

Fig. 12-4 Histology of alveolar crest area from an older individual illustrating bundle bone with penetrating (Sharpey's) fibers and haversian-type supporting bone.

Fig. 12-5 Histology of perforating fiber bundles (Sharpey's). Uniformity of position of numerous fibers in cemental and bony surfaces is shown. Fiber bundles of bone are larger and less numerous than fibers entering cemental surface.

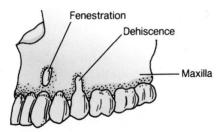

Fig. 12-3 Loss of alveolar bone adjacent to tooth. Loss near root apices is termed fenestration, whereas bone loss in region of cervical root is termed dehiscence.

Fig. 12-6 **Radiograph of alveolar bone illustrating lamina dura, the radiographically dense bone lining tooth sockets.**

Fig. 12-7 **Histology of alveolar bone proper and supporting bone.** Foramina communicate between periodontal ligament and marrow spaces in supporting bone on the left.

surrounding the fiber bundles. Blood vessels and nerves penetrate the lamina dura through small foramina. Because the mineral density is sufficient, this bone appears opaque in radiographs (see Fig. 12-6). Tension on the perforating fibers during mastication is believed to stimulate this bone and is considered important in its maintenance.

Not all alveolar bone proper appears as bundle bone because the bone lining the socket is constantly being remodeled for adaptation to the stresses of occlusal impact. Newly formed bone does not have perforating fibers (Fig. 12-7). Teeth are constantly moving (drifting) within their sockets, resulting in loss of some fibers. Other fibers continually form and initially attach to the bone's surface and later become embedded.

Fig. 12-8 Micrograph of alveolar bone showing a concentric haversian system, interstitial lamellae, and lacunae.

Supporting Compact Bone

Supporting compact bone of the alveolar process is similar to **haversian bone** found elsewhere in the body (Fig. 12-8). Compact bone of the alveolar process extends over the lingual surface of the mandible and maxilla beside the tongue. Compact bone also covers the buccal surface of the mandible or maxilla adjacent to the lining of the cheek. Compact or cortical bone contains osteons with radiating lamellae accentuated by lacunae, which contain the osteocytes in living bone (Fig. 12-9). Haversian and Volkmann's canals form a continuous system of nutrient canals that radiate throughout the bone. The haversian canals extend through the long axis of the bone, and Volkmann's canals enter haversian canals at right angles. These canals form a nutrient network throughout bone. Bone cells or osteocytes are present in many of the lacunae and provide the maintenance and viability of the bone (see Fig. 12-9).

Supporting Cancellous Bone

The cancellous or spongy bone supporting the alveolar bone proper of the alveolar process is composed generally of heavy trabeculae or plates of bone with bone marrow spaces between them. Bone marrow contains blood-forming elements, osteogenic cells, and adipose tissues (see Fig. 12-7). The supporting bone of the maxilla in particular is filled with marrow tissue, which contains immature red blood cells and leukocytes, especially in the molar region posterior to the maxillary sinus. Bone marrow, found in bones throughout the body, is one of the largest organs in the body and represents approximately 4.5% of body weight.

CEMENTAL SUPPORT

Cementum functions as a support by attaching to perforating fibers of the periodontal ligament at the root surface. The surface of cementum functions like bundle

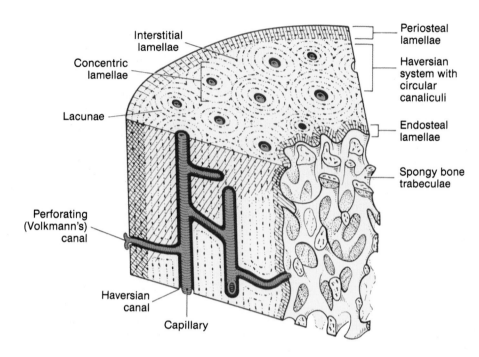

Fig. 12-9 Diagram of haversian systems of compact bone similar to compact bone throughout body. Periosteal lamellae cover the surface of the mandible and numerous haversian systems contain blood vessels interconnected by Volkmann's canals. Lacunae containing osteocytes surround the haversian canals.

Fig. 12-10 **Cemental loss by resorption, which has also destroyed adjacent alveolar bone.**

bone because the perforating fibers cover the entire surface of the roots (see Fig. 12-5). Some areas of the cementum are inactive, with the absence of fiber bundles, or they undergo surface resorption (Fig. 12-10). The collagen fiber bundles of cementum are smaller in size but more numerous than the bundles of alveolar bone proper (see Fig. 12-5). The principal fiber bundle system of the periodontal ligament is balanced in function, although distributed differently on the two surfaces.

Characteristic of the two surfaces, bone and cementum, are their ability to resorb and later to rebuild hard tissue. Cementum is more resistant to resorption than bone, hence the ability to move teeth through bone without the loss of the tooth surface. Some investigators

claim that an autoinvasive factor in cementum contributes to this resistance. Other investigators believe that the absence of a blood supply in cementum, unlike bone, is important to this resistance. The distribution of penetrating fibers over the surface of the cementum could also relate to resorption. Cementum will resorb, as will dentin, in cases of stress caused by traumatic occlusion or of tooth movement resulting from drift or orthodontic treatment (Box 12-2). During exfoliation of primary teeth, root loss is considered a normal process. This process of normal physiologic root and cemental resorption is the result of permanent tooth eruption.

TOOTH MOVEMENT

Physiologic Movement

The eruptive process involves major remodeling of the alveolar process to compensate for root growth and changes in positional relations of the primary and permanent teeth. Repositioning of teeth occurs, for example, during facial growth. Movement occurs in facial and buccal directions as the arches increase in dimension (Fig. 12-11). The height of the alveolus changes in relation to root growth as part of the facial growth process. Accommodation is made for increased dimension of the permanent teeth. In one situation, **leeway space** (Fig. 12-12) is created in the arches by the replacement of larger primary molars by smaller permanent premolars. This important situation helps compensate for the **incisor liability factor,** which is the replacement of the smaller primary incisors with larger

permanent ones (Fig. 12-13). Part of this increase is com-
pensated by the inclination of the permanent incisors
(Fig. 12-13, *B*). Also important is **mesial drift,** a significant occurrence during the mixed dentition period.
When the teeth are clenched during normal masticatory
function, an anterior force is exerted on the teeth
because most cusps are inclined anteriorly and their
occlusal inclined planes therefore produce an anterior
force. This is in part the result of proximal wear.
Summation of these forces defines the principle of
mesial drift of the teeth. The alveolar process compen-
sates for tooth-related factors, such as increased arch
size, as well as effects of occlusal function. The effect of
tooth loss or hypereruption is mesial drift, which can
result in disruption of normal occlusal function.

Permanent premolars

**Fig. 12-12 Radiograph of permanent premolars replacing
primary molars.** A smaller premolar produces a leeway space
in the arch.

**Fig. 12-11 Growth of the face results in migration of teeth
laterally and anteriorly.** This accompanies an increasing
dimension of arch posteriorly as permanent molars develop
and erupt.

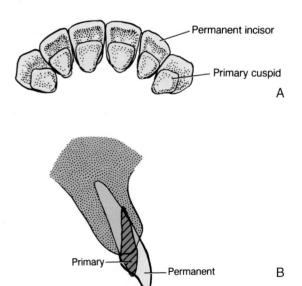

Permanent incisor

Primary cuspid

A

Primary — Permanent

B

Fig. 12-13 A, Comparison of interdental spacing of primary
and permanent incisor teeth. **B,** Inclination comparison of
anterior primary and permanent teeth.

Consider the Patient

A patient asks what would occur if cementum were more easily resorbable than alveolar bone.

CLINICAL COMMENT

The rate of mesial drift varies from 0.05 to 0.7 mm per year. This may be related to dietary factors and age.

Orthodontic Movement

Tooth movement by orthodontics is possible only if bone resorption takes place in the direction in which the tooth is being moved. Such movement causes pressure on the surface of the alveolar bone in the direction of tooth movement. Tooth movement also causes tension on the periodontal ligament on the opposite surface of the root. These stresses cause activation of cells and changes in the vascular and neural tissue along the bone and cemental surfaces that are mediated through the periodontal ligament (Fig. 12-14). The alveolar bone and cementum show remarkable ability to be modified. As bone resorption occurs on one surface of the lamina dura, or bone lining the socket, the tooth is allowed to move in that direction and bone consequently forms on the opposite side of the socket. This stabilizes the tooth in a new position.

For example, if a tooth is tipped, as in Figure 12-15, *A,* several areas of the periodontium are compressed and several exhibit tension. The **tipping movement** is necessary to accomplish the change in occlusion desired. Pressure applied on a specific point on the tooth causes compression in a limited area between the root and the bone. However, a tooth may need to be moved by **bodily movement,** in which case the root is moved in the same direction, affecting the entire surface of the socket. Compression changes occur in the ligament along the advancing root surface, and tension changes occur in the ligament fibers, bone, and cementum along the opposite surface (Fig. 12-15, *B*). The situation is the same whether a single-rooted tooth or a multiple-rooted tooth is involved. In the multiple-rooted tooth, movement is complicated by the bifurcation bone, which has the additional bony surface related to pressure and tension (see Fig. 12-4).

When compression is too great or too rapid, it causes **hyalinization** of the ligament. The vascularity is excluded, and the ligament appears colorless or "hyalinized." Tooth movement is limited by the rate of resorption, meaning that cells that respond to the needs of compression and tension must be mobilized. On the compression surface, bone removal is requisite, so the osteoclasts must become organized. These cells originate from monocytes in the bloodstream. The osteoclasts organize rapidly, appearing within a few hours after tooth movement begins (Fig. 12-16).

Bone loss may occur on the bony surface of the socket, the cementum of the root surface, or both. This action may be reversed by deposition of bone or cementum in the area of resorption. The process of deposition in a resorption zone is known as an **area of reversal.** The area where deposition begins, in this site, is termed a **reversal line.**

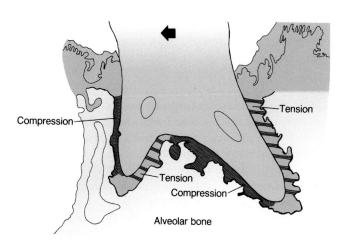

Fig. 12-14 Tooth movement to left with zones of compression along the advancing root surface and tension along the trailing root surface.

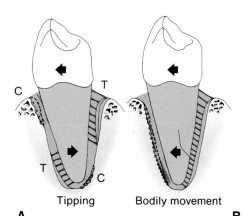

Fig. 12-15 A, Tipping of the tooth crown to the left causes the root to compress the ligament at the upper left and lower right. Tension then occurs at upper right and lower left *(T).* Bodily movement (**B**) of the crown and root to the left causes compression on the ligament (*C*), bone resorption along the entire surface of the advancing root, and formation of a tension surface of bone and cement on the right.

Fig. 12-16 Histology of compression zone of periodontal ligament. Osteoclasts remove bone to relieve compression.

Fig. 12-18 Interproximal zone of two molar teeth. Both teeth moving to the right *(arrowhead)* cause compression of the ligament on the left and tension on the right. Bone formation appears along the alveolar bone on the right as a result.

Fig. 12-17 Histology of tension zone of periodontal ligament. Stretched fibers and a number of osteoblasts and cementoblasts are along surface of hard tissue.

On the tension side of the root, collagen fibers appear stretched and the cells become oriented in the direction of the tension (Fig. 12-17). As this occurs, the force of tension is transmitted into a biologic force characterized by the appearance of cells that are responsive to these needs. Fibroblasts, osteoclasts, and cementoblasts arise from mesenchymal cells in this area and begin to function. Many fibroblasts are present that function in collagen renewal. Osteoblasts, in turn, synthesize bone proteins necessary for producing osteoid. These osteoblasts also mineralize the bone matrix. As tension

continues, bone develops along the alveolar bone and cemental surfaces around the stretched perforating fibers (Fig. 12-18).

Other types of tooth movement include **rotation** and a combination of tipping and rotation. In addition, **intrusion** or **extrusion** of a tooth may be necessary. Figure 12-19 illustrates a case of tooth movement over the long term. Fingerlike projections of bone follow the path of tooth movement. This bone growth is a result of tension. The principles of compression and tension are similar in all cases. The plasticity of the alveolar process is remarkable.

CLINICAL COMMENT

Patients may be concerned about tooth mobility even when it is within normal limits. The mobility of individual teeth varies. Teeth are slightly more mobile in the morning than later in the day.

AGING OF ALVEOLAR BONE AND CEMENTUM

A comparison of young and old alveolar bone reveals a shift with age from dense bone and smooth-walled sockets to osteoporotic bone and sockets with rough, jagged walls. Aging brings bone loss with fewer fiber bundles inserted in the bone and cementum. Hard tissue then forms around the fibers in support of these bundles, thus creating a scalloped surface (Fig. 12-20). During aging, fewer viable cells are in the lacunae, and the marrow spaces become infiltrated with fat cells. Osteoporosis then becomes more apparent, and the support of the teeth is further diminished.

A   B

Fig. 12-19 Rotation of a maxillary molar. A, Large lower root moves less than upper two roots. Bone forms along trailing root surfaces, and resorption occurs on the advancing bony surface. **B,** Histology of rotation of a maxillary molar illustrating loss of bone along the advancing surfaces and bone formation along the tension (trailing) surfaces. In addition to rotation, the tooth is moving away from the zone of tension.

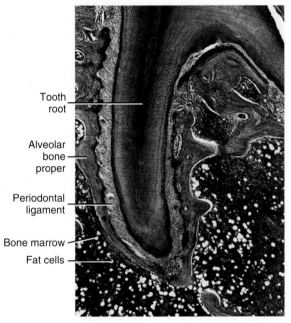

Fig. 12-20 Histology of aging alveolar bone illustrating scalloping of alveolar bone proper and infiltration of fat cells in marrow spaces.

Fig. 12-21 Histology of an edentulous ridge after loss of tooth-bearing alveolar bone. The compact bone of the mandible is dense. This bone shows little evidence of osteoporosis.

EDENTULOUS JAWS

Several facts are known about the loss of teeth, although much remains to be learned about changes in the bony alveolar process after tooth loss. First, it is recognized that alveolar bone volume decreases. This is evident from the general loss of the alveolar process with tooth extraction. Next, some loss of the internal structure of the bone occurs, resulting in open spaces and fewer trabeculae in the cancellous supporting bone (Fig. 12-21). Osteoporosis may then become more evident. Little change occurs in the location of blood vessels, nerves, glands, and fatty zone in the aging edentulous jaws or in dense compact bone of the mandible beneath the alveolar bone (see Fig. 12-21).

 CLINICAL COMMENT

As in development, the interactions between the tooth and its supporting tissues are critical and ongoing throughout life. Loss of the teeth results in loss of the surrounding tissues including the alveolar process.

CLINICAL COMMENT

Tooth movement can be monitored through radiographic examination, and changes in the interproximal bone density or dimension can also be evaluated. The orthodontist depends on this type of information to follow bone formation and resorption. Radiographs of the hard tissues are also useful in evaluating aging changes. Recognizing changes in the color of the gingival and alveolar mucosa is another valuable index of tissue health.

Consider the Patient

Discussion: Tooth movement, such as mesial drift or orthodontic treatment, could not occur. With tooth movement, cemental and root loss would occur.

SELF-EVALUATION QUESTIONS

1. The cortical plates are described as what type of bone?
2. What is the origin of osteoclasts and osteoblasts, and how rapidly can they be mobilized?
3. Define mesial drift and describe some consequences of its occurrence.
4. What is a reversal line, and how is it evidenced?
5. Describe an aging periodontium, and list the features seen.
6. Describe the difference in tipping and bodily movement.
7. Supporting bone comprises what parts of the mandible?
8. Describe the cells that function in compression and tension.
9. What is the life span of the alveolar bone?
10. In what manner do masticatory stress forces placed on bundle bone differ from those placed on haversian bone?

Suggested Reading

Bosshardt DD, Schroeder HE: Cementogenesis reviewed: a comparison between human premolars and rodent molars, *Anatom Record* 245(2):267-292, 1996.

Bosshardt DD, Schroeder HE: How repair cementum becomes attached to the resorbed roots of human permanent teeth, *Acta Anatomica* 150(4):253-266, 1994.

Grzesik WJ, Narayanan AS: Cementum and periodontal wound healing and regeneration, *Crit Rev Oral Biol Med* 13(6):474-484, 2002.

Ripamonti U, et al: Induction of cementogenesis by recombinant human osteogenic protein-1 (hop-1/bmp-7) in the baboon, *Arch Oral Biol* 41(1):121-126, 1996.

Schroeder HE: *Oral structure biology,* New York, 1991, Thieme Medical, pp 197-200.

Seo BM, et al: Investigation of multipotent postnatal stem cells from human periodontal ligament, *Lancet* 364(9429): 149-155, 2004.

Wikesjo UM, et al: Periodontal repair in dogs: effect of recombinant human bone morphogenic protein-12 (rhBMP-12) on regeneration of alveolar bone and periodontal attachment, *J Clin Periodontol* 31(8):662-670, 2004.

Wikesjo UM, et al: Periodontal repair in dogs: gingival tissue occlusion, a critical requirement for GTR? *J Clin Periodontol* 30(7): 655-664, 2003.

13

TEMPOROMANDIBULAR JOINT

CHAPTER OUTLINE

LEARNING OBJECTIVES

After reading this chapter the student will be able to:

- describe the structure of the temporomandibular joint, the condyles and the temporal fossa, the articulating disk, and the capsule
- discuss the function of the temporomandibular joint and the role of the masticatory muscles

KEY TERMS

Anterior tympanic artery
Ascending pharyngeal artery
Auriculotemporal
Deep auricular artery
Deep temporal
Gliding action
Hinge action

Lateral ligament
Lateral pterygoid
Lingula
Masseter
Masseteric
Medial pterygoid
Sphenomandibular ligament

Stylomandibular ligament
Superficial temporal artery
Synovial membrane
Temporalis
Temporomandibular ligament

OVERVIEW

This chapter discusses articulation between the condyles of the mandible and temporomandibular fossa of the temporal bone. The temporomandibular joint (TMJ) allows the mandibular condyles to move in both gliding and hinge actions. Therefore, instead of being a stationary hinge, the joint slides along the inclined plane while functioning also as a hinge joint. The complex motion of the joint can be observed during mastication. TMJ problems can be associated with pain in the related muscles of the jaws and neck.

The anatomy, histology, and function of the various structures related to jaw function are described in this chapter. The TMJ includes (1) the right and left condylar heads of the mandible, (2) the articulating surfaces of the mandibular condyles and the temporal fossae, (3) a disk that intervenes between the fossa and condyle, and (4) a capsule and supportive ligaments. The capsule enclosing this joint serves as a stabilizer, making complex function possible.

The fibrous articular disk divides the joint in two. The upper half is involved in sliding action, and the lower functions as a hinge action. The joint is supported anteriorly by a tendinous attachment of the capsule and the lateral pterygoid muscle, laterally by the lateral or temporomandibular ligament, medially by the sphenomandibular ligament, and posteriorly by the stylomandibular ligament. The TMJ functions as a ginglymoarthrodial joint, indicating that it moves as a sliding and hinge joint.

Myofascial pain dysfunction (MPD) is a syndrome that has received attention. It has been defined as a complex problem relating to neuromuscular concepts, occlusal concepts, muscle balance, tooth morphology, and guidance and psychophysiologic factors. Much remains to be learned about the normal and abnormal stomatognathic system.

CLINICAL COMMENT

Because of the complexity of the TMJ, there are many ways to irritate it. Many different diseases can result in TMD including bone and collagen disorders, neuromuscular diseases, and chronic inflammatory diseases such as fibromyalgia and lupus erythematosus.

STRUCTURE

Mandibular Condyle

The right and left heads of the mandibular condyles articulate in the temporomandibular or glenoid fossae. At birth, the heads of the condyles are round and covered with a thick layer of cartilage. The cartilage front is uneven with spikes of cartilage projecting into the underlying marrow space. Bone forms around these spikes of cartilage, so the head of the condyle is porous (Fig. 13-1, *A*). During development, the condyle grows in a lateral direction, changing into an ovoid shape by maturity, which is attained at age 25 (Fig. 13-1, *B*). The oval condyle consists of a smooth, bony surface, which is covered with a layer of fibrous connective tissue in the adult. The cartilage serves as a growth site in the condyle.

New cartilage cells arise from near the surface of the perichondrium, which covers the condyle. The cartilage cells grow and divide, and the cells deeper in the cartilage die as the cartilage that surrounds these cells calcifies (Fig. 13-2, *A*). The calcified cartilage is then replaced by bone from the underlying ramus (Fig. 13-2, *B*). This process continues during development with a gradual thinning of the cartilage layer, and at maturity the cartilage has been replaced by bone (Fig. 13-2, *C*).

The heads of the condyles and the heads of the long bones differ in that long bones form secondary

Fig. 13-1 A, Condyle *(C)* of a 6-year-old child. Perforations on surface are created by cartilage cap, which is missing because of tissue preparation. **B,** In the adult, smooth bony surface of condyle *(C)* illustrates lateral growth.

ossification centers (Fig. 13-3). Secondary ossification centers produce cartilage-bone junctions termed epiphyseal lines, where the lengthening of long bone occurs. No epiphyseal line is formed in the condyles. The heads of the condyles, however, accomplish growth much like that of long bones. Differentiation of new cartilage cells first appears, then cartilage matrix around these cells develops, which is then replaced by bone. Another difference in long bones is that the cartilage cells are organized in long rows as they approach the bony junction, whereas in the condyles the chondroblasts are scattered. The chondroblasts go through similar changes of cell enlargement, cartilage matrix calcification, and bony replacement (see Fig. 13-3). This ability to modify the shape of the condyles through cartilage-bone remodeling allows adaptation to functional stress.

Temporomandibular Fossa

The fossa is composed of an anterior part in the form of an eminence and a posterior part, a depression or cavity

Fig. 13-2 Histology of condylar cartilage A, Showing the wide band of cartilage that appears during the postnatal period. *EC,* Reserve cartilage zone; *HC,* hypertrophy cartilage zone; *MC,* multiplication cartilage zone. **B,** Cartilage has thinned considerably. *OB,* Bone formation. **C,** Thin cartilage zone underlying the perichondrium in an 18-year-old patient.

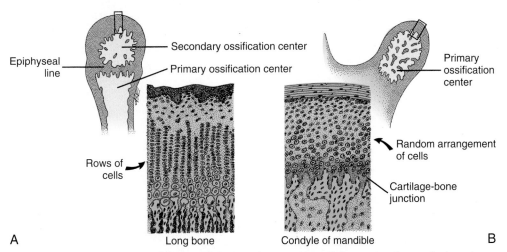

Fig. 13-3 Diagram comparing the head of a long bone and condyle. A, Cartilage of a long bone showing straight vertical rows of cartilage cells, young cells to maturing ones, top to bottom. Bone replaces cartilage at the junction of these two tissues. **B,** Random arrangement of cells in a condyle, which accomplishes same result as rows of cells. As in long bone, at the conclusion of this process in the condyle, bone replaces cartilage at the junction shown.

on the inferior part of the temporal bone. This fossa is located at the posterior medial aspect of the zygomatic arch (Fig. 13-4). The anterior wall of the fossa is smooth and forms a tubercle in which the condyles slide during articulation. On the posterior wall of the fossa is the petrotympanic fissure. This is the junction of the temporal and parietal bones. Some authors report that the origin of elastic fibers, which insert into the posterior part of the disk, is on the posterior wall of this fissure. These elastic fibers may function in retraction of the disk. The temporomandibular fossa is where the condyles are positioned at rest (see Fig. 13-4).

Upper and Lower Compartments

The TMJ cavity is divided into upper and lower compartments by the articular disk (Fig. 13-5). The upper compartment is bound by the articular fossa above and by the disk below. The lateral, medial, and posterior boundaries are enclosed by the capsule that outlines the TMJ. The lower compartment is bound superiorly by the disk and inferiorly by the head of the disk. The two compartments differ in action.

In the upper compartment is a gliding action between the condylar head and the articular eminence, and in the lower compartment is a hinge action between the undersurface of the disk and the rotating surface of the head of the condyle (see Figs. 13-5 and 13-6).

Articular Disk

The articular disk is a dense, collagenous, fibrous pad between the condylar heads and the articular surfaces (see Figs. 13-5 and 13-6). When the jaw opens, each condylar head moves from the articular fossa and slides along the articular plane to the articular eminence while resting on the intervening articular disk (Fig. 13-7, *A*).

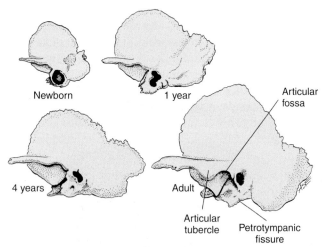

Fig. 13-4 Development of the glenoid (temporomandibular) fossa from birth to maturity. The articular fossa deepens during development to accommodate the growing condylar head as it enlarges laterally.

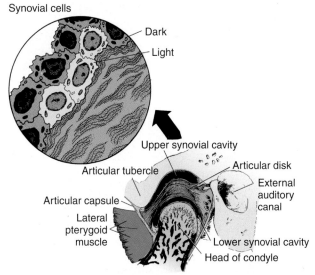

Fig. 13-5 Temporomandibular joint with a thin anterior and thicker posterior articular disk. Observe the position of the capsule anteriorly and posteriorly and the upper and lower synovial compartments in relation to the lateral pterygoid muscle and external auditory canal. The upper and lower compartments that are not under shearing or compressive forces are lined with synovial cells. In the upper diagram are examples of light and dark synovial cells, which function to lubricate movements of condyles.

Fig. 13-6 Lateral view of the gross appearance of the temporomandibular joint at 17 years of age. This figure shows the size of the articular fossa and attachment of muscles to the condyle. (From Avery JK: *Oral development and histology,* ed 3, Stuttgart, 2002, Thieme Medical.)

The head of the condyle rotates during the sliding action (Fig. 13-7, *B*). This allows the two movements of the TMJ, which are a smooth, **gliding action** and a **hinge action.** The articular disk is a soft pad of fibrous tissue. It is thin and avascular in its center, but thicker and vascular around the margin (Fig. 13-8). The articular disk attaches to the inner wall of the capsule anteriorly and posteriorly, but not medially and laterally, which is where it attaches to the head of the condyle. This structural design requires the disk to be immobile when the head of the condyle moves.

The disk is covered with a thin layer of synovial cells and is known as a **synovial membrane.** This membrane secretes a synovial fluid, which moistens both the upper and lower surfaces of the articular pad and the lining of both compartments (Fig. 13-9). The synovial membrane lining is associated with numerous capillaries and lymphatics along the surface of the disk, especially in the periphery. Synovial fluid is a distillate of the blood, having a high viscosity that provides lubrication and allows freedom of condylar movement. The disk can perforate in its center, or the center can contain a few cartilage cells and islands of cartilage, especially in older age.

 CLINICAL COMMENT

The TMJ is a complex and precisely integrated bilateral joint that functions in speech, mastication, and deglutition. You can perceive the downward and forward sliding action of the condylar heads by placing the fingers on them as you open the jaw. This sliding action can also be felt during symmetric protrusion and retrusion or asymmetric lateral shift.

Capsule and Ligaments

A fibrous capsule encloses the TMJ like a cuff. This capsule is composed of an inner lining, or synovial layer, and an outer loose ligamentous layer that is fibrous and tough and supports articulatory movements. The attachment superiorly is to the temporal bone around the limits of the articular eminence and the fossa, and the capsule attaches around the neck of the condyle (Fig. 13-10, *A*). Fibers of the capsule fuse with the fibers of the lateral pterygoid muscle anteriorly, and laterally the capsule is strengthened by the **lateral ligament** or **temporomandibular ligament** (Fig. 13-10, *B*). Medially, the **sphenomandibular ligament** supports the joint (Fig. 13-10, *C*). This ligament arises superiorly from the spine of the sphenoid bone and extends downward on

Fig. 13-8 Articular disk with vascular channels injected with latex and surrounding tissue removed. This preparation illustrates that the vascular network is only in the periphery of the disk and not to any extent in the center of the disk. (From Avery JK: *Oral development and histology,* ed 3, Stuttgart, 2002, Thieme Medical.)

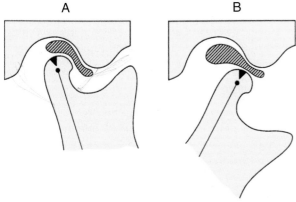

Fig. 13-7 The two actions of the temporomandibular joint. A, Pathway of movement of the condylar head along the slope of the articular eminence. **B,** Rotary movement of the condyle as the mouth is opened. Actions occur simultaneously.

Synovial cells

Fig. 13-9 Histology of lateral posterior aspects of the disk illustrating dark-stained synovial cells that line the joint cavity and disk.

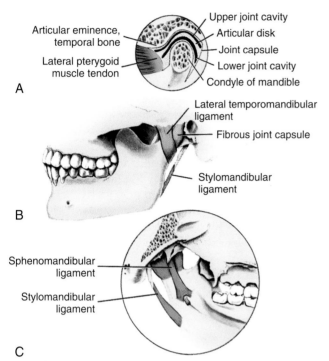

Fig. 13-10 Components of the temporomandibular joint (TMJ). A, Relationship of various TMJ compartments and the capsular ligament. **B,** Lateral view of the lateral fibrous joint capsule showing the relationship of the stylomandibular ligament to the mandible. **C,** Medial view illustrating the location and attachment of the sphenomandibular ligament of the TMJ.

the medial side of the ramus to insert on the **lingula,** which is a spine of bone arising from the rim of the mandibular foramen (Fig. 13-10, *C*). Posteriorly, the **stylomandibular ligament** arises from the styloid process and inserts on the posterior border of the ramus (see Fig. 13-10, *B* and *C*). The lateral ligament and the capsule work in concert to support the joint and limit excursions of the condyles to the normal range. The other two ligaments, the sphenomandibular and stylomandibular, also serve as support. Mandibular movements involve interplay of the morphology of the teeth and the action of muscles and ligaments surrounding the TMJ.

Vascular Supply

The blood supply to the TMJ is from four arteries, including (1) branches of the **superficial temporal artery,** (2) **deep auricular artery,** (3) **anterior tympanic artery,** and (4) **ascending pharyngeal artery** (Fig. 13-11). All these vessels converge on the joint, penetrate the capsule, and send branches into the network of vessels in the periphery of the disk and the posterior area of the joint. Figure 13-8 shows that the disk is oval and has more blood vessels in the anterior and posterior

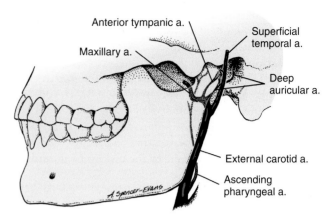

Fig. 13-11 Vascular supply of the temporomandibular joint (TMJ). The external carotid artery serves the TMJ through branches of the ascending pharyngeal and superficial temporal arteries. From the maxillary artery come the auricular and anterior tympanic arteries, which also supply the joint.

areas than the lateral or medial surfaces. Interestingly, the blood vessels do not enter the fibrous covering of the head of the condyle (see Fig. 13-11), as do blood vessels in some other joints.

Innervation

The nerve supply to the TMJ arises from the branches of the mandibular division of the trigeminal nerve, specifically the **auriculotemporal, masseteric,** and **deep temporal** branches (Fig. 13-12). These are the same nerves supplying the muscles of mastication that function with this joint movement, and they help to ensure coordination of function of the muscles and joint. Both large myelinated and smaller nonmyelinated nerves enter the capsule and disk, and they supply all surfaces of the condylar head, fossa, disk, and capsule (see Fig. 13-12). Pain, temperature, touch, and deep pressure nerve terminals are found within the joint. Elaborate encapsulated terminals have been found in the connective tissue associated with the synovial folds and in the disk. Figure 13-13 shows four types of nerve terminals located in the TMJ.

Muscles of Mastication

The eight powerful muscles of mastication include four on each side of the jaw. Each muscle has a different location, and therefore the direction of fiber contraction results in a different functional relationship. Three of the muscles on each side—the medial pterygoid, the masseter, and the temporalis—exert vertical forces in closing the jaw, whereas the lateral pterygoid muscles protract the mandible and stabilize the joint. These muscles do not function alone but work as a group with the suprahyoid muscles and tongue muscles. Free movements of the mandible relate to the interplay of masticatory muscles

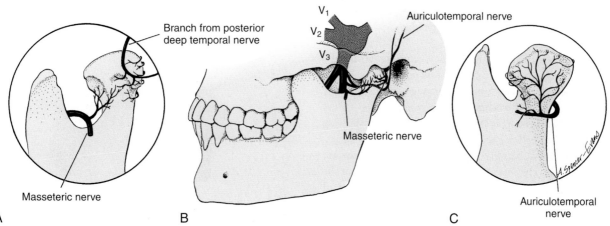

A   B   C

Fig. 13-12 Nerve supply to the temporomandibular joint (TMJ). Mandibular division of the fifth nerve supplies all surfaces of the TMJ through the auricular, temporal, masseteric, and deep temporal nerve branches. **A,** Anterolateral view. **B,** Lateral view. **C,** Posterior view.

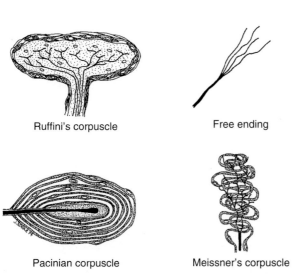

Fig. 13-13 Types of nerve endings in the temporomandibular joint. The four types are Ruffini's or temperature endings; the pacinian, which is a deep pressure receptor; free nerve endings, which are pain endings; and Meissner's corpuscles, which are touch receptors. These are representative of the variety of mechanoreceptors found in capsule, disk, and soft tissues of the joint that are also involved in proprioception.

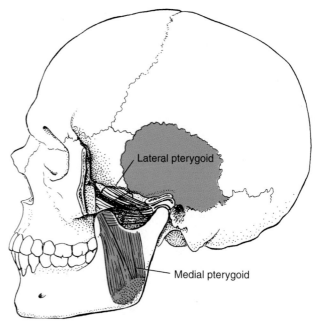

Fig. 13-14 Lateral view of the medial pterygoid muscle of mastication. The medial pterygoid functions in elevation and protraction of the condyle. This muscle functions in concert with the masseteric muscle, forming a sling.

and the morphology of the teeth, whereas masticatory movement is the synergistic action of the three groups of muscles—the elevators, depressors, and protractors—that function together and at different times during mastication of food.

Following are more details about the muscles of mastication:

1. The **medial pterygoid** arises from the medial surface of the lateral pterygoid plate and inserts on the inferior surface of the ramus and on the angle of the mandible.

The blood supply is from the maxillary artery, and the nerve supply is from the mandibular division of the trigeminal nerve. This muscle protracts and elevates the mandible (Figs. 13-14 and 13-15).

2. The **lateral pterygoid** has two heads, the upper arising from the greater wing of the sphenoid and the lower from the pterygoid plate. They insert into the front of the neck of the condyle and the capsule. The blood supply is from the maxillary artery, and the nerve supply is from the pterygoid branch of the

mandibular nerve. Both heads of this muscle protrude the mandible and pull the articular disk forward (see Figs. 13-14 and 13-15).

3. The **temporalis** muscle fibers originate from the floor of the temporal fossa and temporal fascia. These muscle fibers insert on the anterior border of the coronoid process and anterior border of the ramus of the mandible (Fig. 13-16). The blood supply is from the superficial temporal and maxillary arteries, and the nerve supply is from the deep temporal branches of the mandibular nerve. The temporalis muscle elevates and retracts the mandible and clenches the teeth.

4. The **masseter** muscle has a deep and superficial part. The superficial fibers originate from the anterior two thirds of the lower border of the zygomatic arch, and the deep fibers originate from the medial surface of the same arch. The superficial fibers are at right angles to the occlusal plane of the posterior teeth, and the deep fibers are directed downward and slightly anteriorly. This muscle inserts into the lateral surface of the coronoid process of the mandible, the upper half of the ramus, and the angle of the mandible. The blood supply is from the superficial temporal and the maxillary arteries, and the nerve supply comes from the mandibular division of the trigeminal nerve. The masseter muscle elevates the jaw and clenches the teeth (Fig. 13-17).

Fig. 13-16 Temporalis muscle of mastication. The temporalis muscle functions in elevation of the jaw, retraction of the mandible, clenching of the teeth, and side-to-side movements of the jaw.

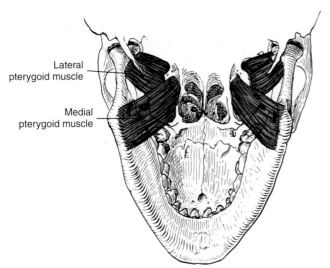

Fig. 13-15 Inferior view of the medial and lateral pterygoids to illustrate attachments to the mandible and base of the skull. The medial pterygoid arises from the lateral pterygoid plate and inserts in the inferior angle of the mandible. The lateral pterygoid arises from the greater wing of the sphenoid and the lower head from the lateral pterygoid plate. These muscles insert in the neck of condyle and capsule.

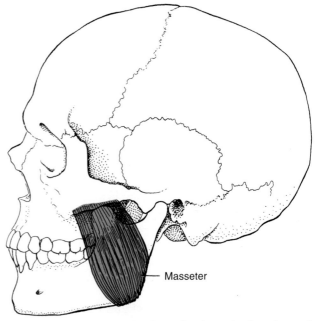

Fig. 13-17 Masseter muscle of mastication. The functions of the masseter muscle are to elevate the jaw, clench the teeth, and assist in side-to-side movement of the jaw.

Fig. 13-18 Histologic view of the head of the condyle and the overlying articular disk. The head of the condyle exhibits a perichondrium and zones of cartilage formation and resorption. The reserve cartilage cell zone overlies the multiplication zone, zone of cartilage cell hypertrophy, and zones of cartilage resorption and bone replacement. (From Avery JK: *Oral development and histology,* ed 3, Stuttgart, 2002, Thieme Medical.)

CLINICAL COMMENT

A functional relationship of the occlusion of the teeth is expressed through the muscles of mastication. A detailed history and physical examination help the clinician provide an accurate diagnosis. Clinicians must rely on their own judgment in the treatment of patients with TMJ pain.

Consider the Patient

A patient is experiencing severe TMJ discomfort. What treatment is needed? What methods of pain alleviation could be employed during treatment?

REMODELING OF TEMPOROMANDIBULAR JOINT ARTICULATION

Articular remodeling is the morphologic adaptation of the joint in response to environmental stress. The articular surfaces of the TMJ have been shown to adapt to minimize the effects of the stressful mandibular function.

Presence of cartilage on the condyle and the fossa allows the TMJ to withstand stress better than other fibrous joints. Progressive remodeling occurs with proliferation of the articular cartilage and production of intercellular matrix followed by its mineralization. The cartilage is then resorbed as it is replaced by bone (Fig. 13-18). This may happen in one or both of the condylar heads and articular eminences and may relate to any changes in structure of the articular surfaces. In some cases, remodeling may begin in the proliferative zone, causing an increase of cartilage on the surface, which may then become mineralized and be replaced by bone at the zone of resorption. Functional adaptation is the response of chondrogenesis and osteogenesis to withstand the effects of mastication resulting from compression. In aging, with decreased proliferation, these changes may be degenerative.

CLINICAL COMMENT

Myofascial pain dysfunction (MPD) continues to be an area of concern because of varying opinions about treatment. Because much remains to be learned about both the normal and abnormal functions of the TMJ, more progress in the treatment of MPD is expected.

Consider the Patient

Discussion: Several approaches exist, but occlusal adjustment is usually the treatment of choice because of the prevalence of malocclusion. The administration of a mandibular anesthetic could help alleviate the pain. During this injection, the needle pathway is through the mucosa and the buccinator muscle and lateral to the medial pterygoid muscle, and the anesthetic is deposited near the mandibular foramen.

SELF-EVALUATION QUESTIONS

1. Name the three supporting ligaments of the TMJ.
2. What is the role of the TMJ capsule?
3. Describe the two different functions of the upper and lower compartments of the TMJ.
4. How do the heads of the condyles change as a person grows and matures?
5. What are the functions of the two heads of the lateral pterygoid muscle?
6. What is the significance of the sling muscles, and is this a function of the muscles' location and innervation?
7. What are the location and function of the temporalis muscle?
8. What is the significance of the TMJ's and the masticatory muscles' having the same innervation?
9. What are the major blood vessels supplying the TMJ?
10. What is the function of the synovial cells?

Suggested Reading

Bravetti P, et al: Histological study of the human temporomandibular joint and its surrounding muscles, *Surg Radiologic Anatomy* 26(5):371-378, 2004.

Dimitroulis G: The role of surgery in the management of disorders of the temporomandibular joint: a critical review of the literature. Part 2, *Int J Oral Maxillofac Surg* 34(3):231-237, 2005.

Honda K, et al: Relationship between sex, age, and the minimum thickness of the roof of the glenoid fossa in normal temporomandibular joints, *Clin Anatomy* 18(1):23-26, 2005.

Kubein-Meesenburg D, et al: Functional conditions of the mandible: theory and physiology, *Ann Anatomy* 181(1):27-32, 1999.

Nitzan DW, Kreiner B, Zeltser R: TMJ lubrication system: its effect on the joint function, dysfunction, and treatment approach, *Compend Cont Educ Dent* 25(6):437-438, 440, 443-444, 449, 471, 2004.

Nozawe-Inoue K, et al: Synovial membrane in the temporomandibular joint—its morphology, function, and development, *Arch Histol Cytology* 66(4):289-306, 2003.

Toure G, Duboucher C, Vacher C: Anatomical modifications of the temporomandibular joint during aging, *Surg Radiol Anatomy* 27(1):51-55, 2005.

14

ORAL MUCOSA

CHAPTER OUTLINE

LEARNING OBJECTIVES

After reading this chapter the student will be able to:

- describe the various types of oral mucosa including lining, masticatory and specialized
- describe the location and characteristics of each type of mucosa as well as the characteristics of nonkeratinocytes
- explain the various changes in oral mucosa that occur with aging

KEY TERMS

Attached gingiva
Basal cell
Basal lamina
Circumvallate papilla
Col
Desmosomes
Eleidin
Filiform papillae
Foliate papillae
Fordyce's spots
Free gingival groove
Free or marginal zone
Fungiform papillae

Hemidesmosomes
Interdental papilla
Interdental zone
Langerhans' cells
Lining mucosa
Macula adherens
Masticatory mucosa
Median raphe
Melanocytes
Merkel's cells
Mucogingival junction
Papillae
Rugae

Specialized mucosa
Stratum basale
Stratum corneum
Stratum granulosum
Stratum intermedium or stratum
  spinosum
Stratum superficiale
Supporting or sustentacular cells
Sweet, salty, sour, and bitter
Taste cells
Tonofibrils
Traction bands
Vermilion border

OVERVIEW

The structure of stratified squamous epithelium of the oral mucosa includes both the nonkeratinized lining mucosa of the cheeks, lips, soft palate, and floor of the mouth and the keratinized epithelium covering the palate and alveolar ridges. Masticatory mucosa consists of multiple layers of epithelial cells associated with the lamina dura layer, which contains blood vessels, nerve endings, and serous, mucous, or mixed glands. A third type of mucosa found on the surface of the tongue is specialized mucosa, consisting of four types of papillae, which are filiform, fungiform, foliate, and circumvallate.

Taste is associated with the latter three types of papillae, which are located on the tongue, soft palate, and pharynx. Four types of taste are regionally associated with the tongue. At the tip, sweet and salty tastes are perceived; sour taste is associated with the sides of the tongue; and bitter taste is at the back of the tongue.

Masticatory mucosa includes the gingiva, which is composed of the tissue surrounding the necks of the teeth. The gingiva consists of three areas, which are free, attached, and interdental. The free gingiva is characterized by the gingival sulcus. The attached gingiva has junctional epithelium, which binds the gingiva to the necks of the teeth. The interdental area is that tissue between the teeth below their contact point. The hard palate is covered by masticatory mucosa, which is firmly attached to the underlying bone.

Cells of the oral mucosa are termed keratinocytes and can be distinguished from the nonkeratinocytes, which are Langerhans' cells, Merkel's cells, and melanocytes. In case of inflammation, lymphocytes and leukocytes may appear in the mucosa. They are commonly found in gingival epithelium.

Four types of nerve receptors—heat, cold, pain, and touch—are located in the lips and oral cavity. They are most numerous in the lips and in the tip of the tongue. With age, the oral mucosa becomes thinner and may be lower on the necks of the teeth. Also, it can become less moist because of the decrease in activity of the salivary glands.

STRUCTURE OF ORAL MUCOSA

The oral cavity is lined with stratified squamous epithelium, which is divided into three types of tissue. **Lining mucosa** covers the floor of the mouth and the cheeks, lips, and soft palate. It does not function in mastication and therefore has little attrition. **Masticatory mucosa** covers the hard palate and alveolar ridges and is so named because it comes in primary contact with food during mastication. **Specialized mucosa,** which covers

the surface of the tongue, is quite different in structure and appearance from the two previous tissues.

Each type of tissue has structural differences: the lining mucosa is soft, pliable, and nonkeratinized; the masticatory mucosa is keratinized, indicative of the attrition that takes place during mastication. Specialized mucosa on the tongue surface is composed largely of cornified epithelial papillae, which function in mastication. The mucosa of the oral cavity has several features common to epithelium elsewhere in the body. One of these features is the lamina propria, the connective tissue layer immediately below the epithelium. It is composed of the papillary layer and deeper reticular layer (Fig. 14-1). In the papillary layer, the connective tissue extends into pockets in the epithelium. This increases the surface of the epithelium for contact with vascular supply and nerves. The reticular layer contains the deeper plexus of vessels and nerves supported by the connective tissue. These two layers, papillary and reticular, contribute the lamina propria or dermis. Beneath this zone is the submucosa or subcutaneous tissue.

Consider the Patient

A patient mentions that she heard the oral cavity is a logical location to place medication because the medication can be absorbed and taken into the bloodstream. She asks whether this is true for all medications.

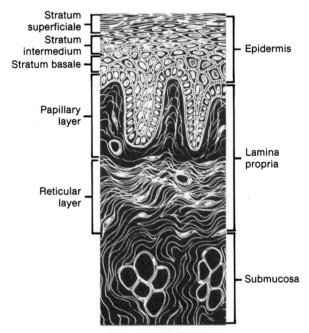

Fig. 14-1 Relationships among oral epidermis, dermis (lamina propria), and submucosal tissue. The names of layers of epidermis and dermis are noted on the left.

Lining Mucosa

Lining mucosa is composed of a thin layer of epithelium and an underlying lamina propria. The epithelium is composed of a basal layer of cuboidal cells, termed the **stratum basale.** The next cell layer is called the **stratum intermedium** or **stratum spinosum.** The cells in this layer appear oval and somewhat flattened. The third or superficial layer is termed the **stratum superficiale,** and its cells are flattened, with many containing small oval nuclei (see Fig. 14-1). These three cell layers of the epidermis form the nonkeratinized epithelium of the oral mucosa and appear similar to the lining of the pharynx. Another component of the mucosa is the dermis or lamina propria, composed of the papillary and reticular connective tissue layers.

Lips

The inner oral surface of the lips is lined with moist surface, stratified squamous cells, and nonkeratinized epithelium and is associated with small, round sero-mucous glands of the lamina propria. These glands are part of the minor salivary glands found throughout the oral cavity. Beneath the lamina propria is the submucosa, in which fibers of the orbicularis oris muscle are located (Fig. 14-2). Nonkeratinized mucosa of the lips is distinguished by a red border known as the **vermilion border.** This area is at the junction between the oral mucosa and the skin of the lips, becoming modified into keratinized epithelium, which is different from skin or mucosa. There are three reasons that the vermilion border is red, including the following: the epithelium is thin; this epithelium contains **eleidin,** which is transparent; and the blood vessels are near the surface of the papillary layer, revealing the red blood cells' color (Fig. 14-3). Also observable in the skin of the lips are hair follicles and

their associated sebaceous glands, erector pili muscles, and sweat glands. Sebaceous glands can be seen at the angles of the mouth. They are not associated with hair follicles. These glands are known as **Fordyce's spots** (Fig. 14-4).

Soft palate

Lining mucosa of the highly vascularized soft palate is more pink than the mucosa of the keratinized epithelium of the hard palate (Fig. 14-5). This tissue is pink because the lamina propria contains many small blood vessels. Beneath the connective tissue of the lamina

Fig. 14-2 Histology of the lip and alveolar bone, which contains functioning primary and developing permanent teeth.

Fig. 14-3 Vermilion border of the lip illustrating the thin and lucent stratum corneum and the presence of capillaries in the papillary layer. Observe the close relationship of the blood supply to the surface of vermilion border epithelium.

Fig. 14-4 **Fordyce's spots, sebaceous glands not related to hair follicles, are found at the angles of the mouth.**

Fig. 14-5 **Sagittal plane of the soft palate** *(anterior on left);* **the nasal cavity is above, and respiratory epithelium covers the superior part of the soft palate.** The oral cavity is below this tissue and is covered with squamous epithelium. Observe the glands underlying the oral mucosa and muscle throughout the submucosa.

Fig. 14-6 **Histology of cheek tissues.** Skin is on the far left, and oral mucosa on the far right. Observe the glands intermingling with muscle fibers in the subcutaneous zone of the cheek.

propria is the submucosa, which contains muscles of the soft palate and mucous glands.

Cheeks

The mucosa of the cheeks is like that of the lips or soft palate because each has stratified squamous epithelium that is nonkeratinized, lamina propria, and underlying submucosa. In the cheeks, however, the submucosa contains fat cells and mixed glands (seromucous)

located within and between the muscle fibers. The presence of these glands and fat cells is a unique feature of the cheeks (Fig. 14-6).

Ventral surface of the tongue

Lining mucosa also contains a lamina propria and submucosa. In the submucosa, muscle fibers are located under the surface of the tongue. The entire area exhibits dense, interlaced muscle and connective tissue fibers.

Limits of the submucosa are not distinct because the submucosa continues with the deep muscles of the tongue along with connective tissue fibers (Fig. 14-7).

 CLINICAL COMMENT

The ventral surface of the tongue is an area of well vascularized lining mucosa of the oral cavity. This area is used for drug delivery in patients who suffer from cardiovascular disease and other systemic diseases.

Floor of the mouth

Nonkeratinized mucous membrane covers the floor of the mouth and appears loosely attached to the lamina propria. In contrast, the adjacent undersurface of the tongue mucosa is firmly attached. In the floor of the mouth are minor salivary glands (Fig. 14-8) and the right and left major mucous glands, the sublingual glands.

Masticatory Mucosa

Masticatory mucosa is the epithelium covering the gingiva and hard palate. This mucosa is thicker than the

Fig. 14-7 Histology of the ventral surface of the tongue showing the density of muscle fibers intermingling in the lamina propria.

Muscle

Mucosa of ventral surface of tongue

Epithelium of floor of mouth

Connective tissue fibers

Salivary gland (minor)

Fig. 14-8 Histology of mucosa lining the floor of the mouth. Observe the lack of muscle fibers and the delicate appearance of the connective tissue fibers. Scattered glands of minor serous and mucous salivary glands are near the tip of the tongue.

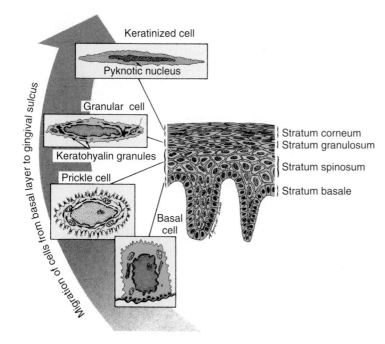

Keratinized cell

Pyknotic nucleus

Granular cell

Keratohyalin granules

Prickle cell

Basal cell

Migration of cells from basal layer to gingival sulcus

Stratum corneum
Stratum granulosum

Stratum spinosum

Stratum basale

Fig. 14-9 Keratinized stratified squamous epithelium of the oral cavity. Observe the characteristics of four cell types of this epithelium, from basal to surface layers.

nonkeratinized mucosa with the addition of a keratinized surface of flat, hornified cells offering resistance to attrition. The basal and intermediate stratum (stratum spinosum) layers are the same as those of nonkeratinized epithelium. The granular layer **(stratum granulosum)** and the surface layer **(stratum corneum)** are the two other layers (Fig. 14-9). The cells of the basal layer are cuboidal or columnar. Their nuclei are irregularly oval and exhibit numerous mitotic figures as they undergo constant cell division. These basal cells gradually migrate to the surface of the mucosa. Figure 14-9 shows the differences in each cell layer. The second layer, stratum spinosum, is several cells thick. These cells are oval to polygonal, and mitotic figures can be seen in this layer.

Basal cells interface with a membrane separating the epithelium and connective tissue. This membrane is called the **basal lamina.** The basal cells are attached to the basal lamina by minute disks termed **hemidesmosomes** (Fig. 14-10). These thickenings of the cell membrane are supported by filaments from within the cells, anchoring fibrils that attach the basal lamina and the epithelial cells to the collagen fibers of the lamina propria. Figure 14-11 shows these structures.

The next layer of cells superficially is the stratum granulosum, so named because the cells contain many keratohyalin granules (Fig. 14-12). The surface layer of cells, the stratum corneum, is characterized by thin, flattened, nonnucleated cells. These cells are filled

Fig. 14-10 Ultrastructure of the junction of epithelium and lamina propria, as seen in an electron micrograph. Extending across the field from left to right is basal lamina, to which epithelial cells are attached by hemidesmosomes.

Epithelial cells

Hemidesmosome

Basal lamina

Dermis

Fig. 14-11 Diagram of hemidesmosomes of oral mucosa showing how hemidesmosomes of epithelial cells attach to the basal lamina membrane. Anchoring collagen fibers of connective tissue attach to the basal lamina and fibers of the hemidesmosome.

Epidermis

Filaments

Hemidesmosome

Basal lamina

Anchoring fibrils

Collagen fibers

with a soft keratin that replaces the cell cytoplasm. This soft keratin may be compared with hard keratin of the nails and hair. Keratin is tough, nonliving material that is resistant to friction and impervious to bacterial invasion.

To permit cell movement and loss of individual cells along the surface, the superficial layers have surface

CLINICAL COMMENT

Recognition of change in a patient's mucosa is based in part on knowledge of the individual's normal characteristics and on evaluation of the patient's history. Among the basic conditions of the mucosa to be considered are variations in tissue color, dryness, smoothness, or firmness and whether the gingiva bleeds easily.

Stratum corneum —

Stratum granulosum —

Stratum spinosum —

Stratum basale —

Lamina propria —

Fig. 14-12 An electron micrograph of oral epithelium. This is a view of keratinized oral epithelium that shows the relative thickness of each cell layer from stratum basale to stratum corneum and lamina propria beneath the epithelium.

interdigitations rather than desmosomes. These cells are continually becoming lost and replaced by cells of the underlying layers.

As each cell moves to the surface of the epithelium, it does so by means of cell attachments to neighboring cells that hold until the cell has reached a specific stage of development. When that stage occurs, the cell attachment releases, which allows that cell to move to a higher level where it reattaches. All epithelial cells function with **desmosomes.** In the oral mucosa, desmosomes are discoid and are called **macula adherens** (Fig. 14-13). The junctions are composed of thin protein adhesion disks located between the cells. These disks are anchored by means of intracellular filaments, termed **tonofibrils,** which arise in the cell and project to the surface, where they attach to the cell junction. The disks temporarily hold the cells in contact but later release them, allowing the cells to move superficially and reattach to a cell in another location (see Figs. 14-12 and 14-13).

— Desmosome

— Tonofibrils

Fig. 14-13 Electron micrographs of cell junctions of oral epithelial cells; these are termed desmosomes or macula adherens. A, At low magnification, *arrows* indicate attachments between each cell. **B,** At higher magnification, multilayer arrangement of desmosomes can be seen. Tonofibrils of cell attach to these platelike junctions.

A

B

Gingiva and epithelial attachment

In the oral mucosa, the gingiva surrounds the necks of the teeth and extends apically to the mucogingival junction (Fig. 14-14). The gingiva develops as a coalescence of the oral and reduced enamel organ epithelium when the tooth first emerges into the oral cavity (Fig. 14-15, *A* to *C*). The reduced enamel organ epithelium makes contact with the undersurface of the oral epithelium, and the two fuse. Then the tooth penetrates this combined layer to enter the mouth and produces the gingiva as the epithelium continues to separate from the enamel surface (Fig. 14-15, *C*) until occlusion of the teeth is reached (Fig. 14-15, *D*). At this point, the gingiva covers only the cervical area of the enamel where it is attached (Fig. 14-15, *D*).

The gingiva is divided into three zones. They are as follows: (1) the **free** or **marginal zone,** which encloses the tooth and defines the gingival sulcus; (2) the **attached gingiva,** that portion of the epithelium attached to the neck of the tooth by means of junctional epithelium; and (3) the **interdental zone** (groove), the area between the two adjacent teeth beneath their contact point (see Fig. 14-14). The free and attached gingivae have an indistinct groove on the surface of the epithelium separating them. This groove is termed the **free gingival groove** (see Figs. 14-14 and 14-16).

Free and attached gingiva

The free or marginal gingiva is bound on its inner margin by the gingival sulcus, which separates it from the tooth; on its outer margin by the oral cavity; and apically at its free surface by the free gingival groove (Fig. 14-17). This groove separates the free and attached gingivae. Therefore, the attached gingiva lies adjacent to the free gingiva and is separated from the alveolar mucosa by the **mucogingival junction** (see Fig. 14-17). The free and attached gingivae are keratinized, but the alveolar mucosa is not. The attached gingiva is stippled, but

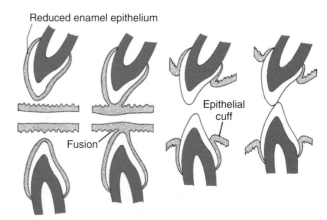

Fig. 14-15 Diagram of gingiva developing from reduced enamel epithelium (including the developmental cuticle) of the tooth combined with oral epithelium. The two meet, fuse, and rupture to allow the tooth to erupt.

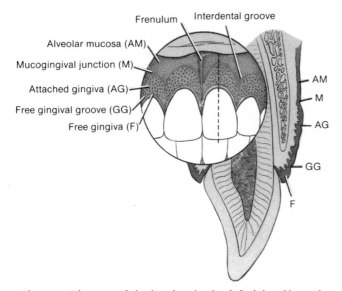

Fig. 14-14 Diagram of gingiva showing both facial and lateral views. Shown are free gingiva *(F)* along the crest of gingiva; free gingival groove *(GG)* at junction between free and attached gingiva; stippled attached gingiva *(AG);* mucogingival junction *(M),* which separates gingiva from alveolar mucosa; and alveolar mucosa *(AM)* above attached gingiva. The frenulum and interdental zones (grooves) are also shown.

Fig. 14-16 Histology of gingiva illustrating the gingival sulcus, junctional epithelium, and free gingiva. Enamel space is created by loss (decalcification) of enamel.

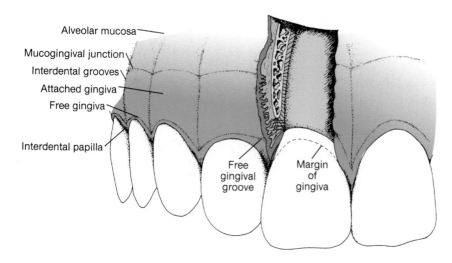

Fig. 14-17 Location of free and attached gingivae and location of the mucogingival junction. This junction separates keratinized gingiva from nonkeratinized alveolar mucosa.

Fig. 14-18 View of normal gingiva, illustrating free and attached (stippled) gingivae.

the free gingiva has a smooth surface (Fig. 14-18). In some instances, the free gingiva may be covered with parakeratinized mucosa, which contains keratinized cells modified by the presence of nuclei in the cells of the surface layer. The unique feature of attached gingiva is the junctional epithelium.

Junctional epithelium

Junctional epithelium provides attachment for the gingiva to the tooth in the cervical area and forms the epithelium-lined floor of the gingival sulcus (Fig. 14-19). Cells of the attached epithelium are cytologically different from other cells of the gingival epithelium. They have fewer desmosomes (cell attachment buttons). This indicates a higher rate of turnover than occurs in the other gingival epithelial cells (see Fig. 14-19). These cells have

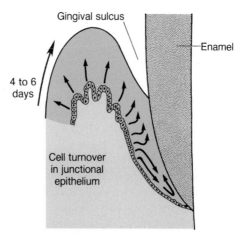

Fig. 14-19 Epithelial cell turnover in gingiva. Note the direction of epithelial cell maturation from basal cell to surface in attachment zone and in the margin of gingiva.

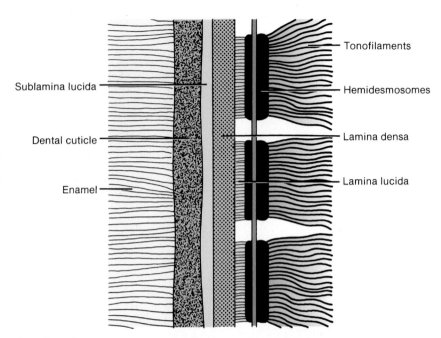

Fig. 14-20 **The means of gingival attachment with tooth's surface.** Diagram of a hemidesmosome, which is a specialized attachment plaque that attaches cell to protein of cuticle or pellicle on tooth's surface. Protein of enamel surface is composed of dense and lucent layers. If the hemidesmosome is disturbed, reattachment can occur.

been reported to turn over in approximately 6 days, from the time of their appearance in the stratum basale to the time when they are sloughed in the free surface. The cells have many organelles, such as rough-surface endoplasmic reticulum, Golgi's apparatus, and mitochondria, indicating high metabolic activity.

Stratum basale cells also contain hemidesmosomes, the mechanism for the attachment of cells to the salivary protein layer, which covers the cervical area of the enamel (Fig. 14-20). The half of a desmosome in these junctional epithelial cells is like the hemidesmosome of the basal cells of the squamous epithelium, which attaches to the basal lamina and lamina propria of the gingiva (see Fig. 14-12). Disturbance of this attachment to the tooth by infection, food impaction, calculus, or other irritants results in a deepening of the gingival sulcus.

 CLINICAL COMMENT

In examining the gingiva, keep in mind its normal appearance. From this viewpoint, conditions other than normal ones can be more easily recognized.

Interdental papilla and col

Gingiva located between the teeth and extending high on the interproximal area of the crowns on the labial and lingual surfaces is known as the **interdental papilla** (see Fig. 14-18). This tissue fills the space created by the constricted cervical areas of the adjacent crowns. In the interproximal area, between the lingual and vestibular papilla, is a concave zone of the gingiva that follows the contour of each crown (Fig. 14-21). The junctional

Fig. 14-21 **Clinical view of gingiva showing free and attached gingiva and the interdental groove *(arrow)*.** The col is found in the interdental area.

☐ Inflamed
☐ Normal
▨ Contact point

Fig. 14-22 **Positional relationship of the col in health and disease.** The col is accentuated in inflammation and swelling of gingiva. The col is found to be pointed in anterior teeth and flat or concave posteriorly. The contact point on each crown is represented by an oval above the col.

epithelium of this zone is known as the **col.** The col is characterized as a thin, nonkeratinized epithelium. These basal epithelial cells invade the connective tissue where inflammatory cells of the lamina propria may appear (Figs. 14-22 and 14-23). The col is more inclined in a peak between anterior teeth and more flattened or concave between posterior teeth. When the interproximal gingiva becomes inflamed or hyperemic, the col is exaggerated and is positioned higher on the neck of the tooth (see Fig. 14-22).

Hard palate

The roof of the mouth, or hard palate, is covered with keratinized stratified squamous epithelium. This epithelium is similar to that of the gingiva in the middling area, where there is no submucosa. The midline is known as the **median raphe,** which may only be barely discernible, except anteriorly, where an incisive papilla can be seen. On each side of the median raphe are ridges of tissue called **rugae** (Fig. 14-24). These folds of epithelium are supported by dense lamina propria (Fig. 14-25). In the anterior lateral palate a zone of fatty tissue is located in the submucosa. However, in the posterior lateral hard palate is mucous glandular tissue (see Fig. 14-24). Both the hard and soft palates have mucous glands. **Traction bands** (Fig. 14-26) exist in the lamina propria of the rugae. These bands also exist between the lobules of fatty tissue and glands of the anterior and

Fig. 14-23 **Histology of a col, a concave, nonkeratinized epithelial lining of gingiva between teeth.**

Fig. 14-25 **Histologic section of the anterior palate showing rugae.** Rugae are epithelium-covered ridges in the lamina propria of the anterior palate.

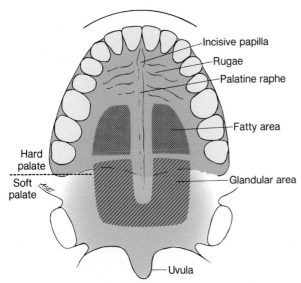

Fig. 14-24 **Diagram of the palate indicating location of the fatty zone anteriorly and the glandular zone posteriorly.** These tissues are found in subcutaneous tissue underlying the lamina propria. In the midline of the palate there is no subcutaneous zone; only lamina propria exists, as in the gingiva of the lateral palate.

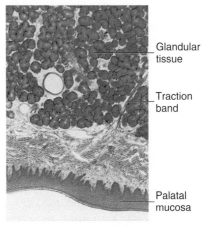

Fig. 14-26 **Histologic section of the palate in the glandular zone.** Traction bands of collagen fibers bind palatal epithelium to the underlying bone.

posterior hard palate. Traction bands are bundles of collagen fibers that insert into the papillary fibers of the lamina propria and extend into the bony palate. These collagen fibers anchor the palatal mucosa to the underlying bone, and the hard palate assists in mastication.

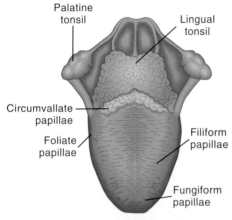

Fig. 14-27 Diagram of the dorsal surface of tongue showing papillae. Filiform papillae are scattered over the surface of the tongue body. Fungiform papillae are few in number, round, and pink, but larger than filiform papillae. Foliate papillae are 4 to 11 in number along the posterior sides of the tongue. Circumvallate papillae are 8 to 10 in number along the junction of body and base of the tonsillar area of the tongue.

Fig. 14-28 A scanning electron micrograph of the tongue's surface showing filiform papillae (arrows). These pointed papillae are directed toward the throat and assist in moving food in that direction as the tongue moves.

Specialized Mucosa

Types of papillae

The dorsum or superior surface of the tongue (anterior two thirds) is covered with a specialized mucosa. This mucosa consists of four types of epithelial structures called **papillae** (Fig. 14-27). Most of these papillae are **filiform papillae,** which are slender, threadlike keratinized extensions of the surface epithelial cells. The entire roughened surface of the tongue is covered with these papillae (see Figs. 14-27 to 14-29). They project

Fig. 14-29 Histologic picture of the filiform papillae of the tongue's dorsal surface. Pointed keratinized projections are shown.

Fig. 14-30 Histologic section of the fungiform papilla, with a connective tissue core and epithelial covering. Two taste buds are located on the superior surface of the papilla.

about 2 to 3 mm high from the surface of the tongue. These papillae facilitate mastication and movement of the food on the surface of the tongue.

Interspersed between the filiform papillae are the **fungiform papillae,** which are few in number but more numerous near the tip of the tongue. The fungiform papillae are mushroom shaped, with the cap usually larger than the stalk (Fig. 14-30). The covering epithelium of the fungiform papillae is thin and nonkeratinized, so the papillae appear pink or reddish because blood vessels are near the surface. Taste buds are occasionally found on the superior surface of the fungiform papillae (see Figs. 14-30 and 14-31, *B*). A third type of papilla is the **circumvallate papilla.** Only 10 to 14 in number, the circumvallate papillae are located along the V-shaped sulcus between the body and base of the tongue (see Fig. 14-31). These papillae are level with the surface of the tongue, and each has a surrounding groove. They are large—3 mm in diameter.

Ducts of the underlying serous glands (von Ebner's glands) are seen opening into the grooves surrounding these papillae. Taste buds line the walls of the papillae (see Fig. 14-31, *B*). The watery secretion of these glands washes out substances so that new tastes can be perceived. On the lateral posterior sides of the tongue are 4 to 11 vertical grooves or furrows containing taste buds (see Fig. 14-31, *A*). These furrows are termed **foliate papillae.** Like circumvallate papillae, they contain serous glands underlying the taste buds, which cleanse the trenches of the foliate papillae.

Taste buds

Taste buds are microscopically visible, barrel-shaped bodies found in the oral epithelium. These discrete sense organs contain the chemical sense of taste. They are generally associated with the papillae of the tongue—the circumvallate, foliate, and fungiform—although some are distributed in the soft palate, epiglottis, larynx, and pharynx (Figs. 14-32 to 14-34 and Box 14-1).

Taste buds are easily recognized under the microscope as barrel-shaped structures; their epithelial cells appear ovoid (see Fig. 14-32). Although they have been

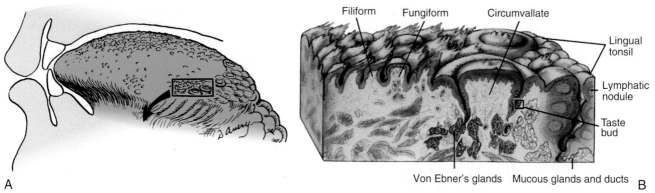

A

B

Filiform   Fungiform   Circumvallate

Lingual tonsil

Lymphatic nodule

Taste bud

Von Ebner's glands   Mucous glands and ducts

Fig. 14-31 Circumvallate papillae. A, Note the large (2-mm) papillae with trench around each and underlying serous (von Ebner's) glands, which wash out tastable substances from the area of the taste buds. **B,** Rectangle in **A,** enlarged. Dorsal appearance of the tongue with filiform, fungiform, and circumvallate papillae. A taste bud is shown within a *small,* rectangular area.

Dark cells

Taste pore

Light cells

Fig. 14-32 Light microscope picture of a taste bud with its dark and light cells. The taste pore on the left opens into the wall of a trench, as seen in Figure 14-33.

Taste buds

Duct of gland

Serous glands

Duct of gland

Fig. 14-33 Histology of the circumvallate papilla with taste buds located in its walls in a trench. Von Ebner's gland (pure serous secretion) and its ducts are emptying into a trench located in the lower left and right.

referred to as neuroepithelial structures, they are more correctly referred to as epithelial cells closely associated with club-shaped sensory nerve endings. These nerves arise from the chorda tympani and come to lie among the taste cells.

CLINICAL COMMENT

The distribution of nerve endings in the oral cavity is greatest in the lips and anterior oral mucosa and least in the more posterior regions of the oral cavity. Therefore, the mouth tastes food and beverages before they are taken farther into the alimentary canal. The one exception to this anterior sensitivity is that of cold and pain nerve endings, which are numerous in the posterior palate.

14.1 | NUMBER OF TASTE BUDS IN THE HUMAN ADULT

BOX

Tongue: 10,000
Soft palate: 2,500
Epiglottis: 900
Larynx and pharynx: 600
Oropharynx: 250

Several types of taste cells are found among the 10 to 14 cells in a taste bud. Each taste bud contains a few **supporting** or **sustentacular cells** (several types) that lie in the periphery of the taste bud. Most **taste cells** bear either elongated microvilli that project into the taste pore or ones with shortened villi that open into the base of the pore. Each cell is associated with nerves that penetrate the taste bud. Another type of cell found in the taste bud is the **basal cell.** These basal cells are in close contact with the basal lamina (see Fig. 14-34). There is a rapid turnover of these cells, approximately every 10 days. They are believed to arise from the surrounding epithelial cells.

Four types of taste sensation can be detected, and evidence of regional sensitivity for these tastes is on the tongue and palate. The four taste sensations are **sweet, salty, sour,** and **bitter.** Sensations of sweet and salty are perceived at the tongue's tip, sour on the sides, and bitter in the region of the circumvallate papillae (Fig. 14-35). These areas overlap, and evidence indicates that all papillae respond to all four types of taste sensations. However, the levels of sensitivity differ. For example, with higher concentrations of a bitter taste, the sensation is perceived most notably on the posterior segment of the tongue. This indicates a regional selectivity of taste in the mouth, which may be caused in part by the origin of the nerve supply.

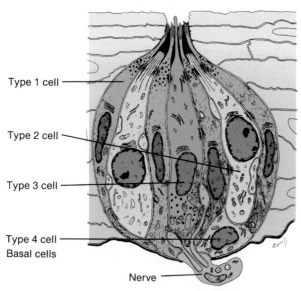

Fig. 14-34 Diagram of typical taste bud with four types of cells. Type 1, dark cells, represents 60% of the cells; type 2, light cells, represents 30%; type 3 represents 7%; and type 4, basal cells, represents 3%.

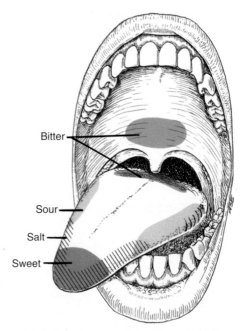

Fig. 14-35 Location of taste perception on the tongue and soft palate. The tip of the tongue has sweet receptors; along the front sides are salty receptors; on the posterior sides are sour receptors; and on the posterior center of the tongue and soft palate are bitter receptors. (Courtesy of Dr. R. Murray, University of Indiana School of Medicine.)

Nerves for taste buds of the anterior two thirds of the tongue pass to the chorda tympani branch of the facial nerve; those of the posterior one third pass to the glossopharyngeal nerve; and those from the epiglottis and larynx pass to the vagus nerve.

Mixing the four basic modalities of taste cannot explain all the flavors that humans are capable of experiencing. Factors such as odors and temperature also contribute to flavors. In addition, taste buds can discriminate between subtleties in flavor, such as the difference between citric or acetic acid. This enables taste buds to identify specific substances even when they are mixed.

Umami Taste Modality

Early in the twentieth century, a new taste modality was suggested and called umami. This distinctive taste was associated with the amino acid glutamate (glutamic acid). Glutamate is an amino acid and a building block of protein. Commonly, this molecule is combined with sodium to make monosodium glutamate (MSG), and is used to flavor foods in many restaurants and kitchens. However, some people can develop severe allergies to MSG and, at least in the United States, many restaurants have discontinued its use.

NERVES AND BLOOD VESSELS

The nerves and blood vessels appear in the lamina propria. Terminal endings of nerves and loops of blood vessels appear in the dermal papillae. There blood vessels consist of a deep plexus of larger vessels in the submucosa underlying the lamina propria, and capillary loops extend into a secondary plexus in the dermal papillae. The overlying epithelium is avascular, and its metabolic needs come from the vessels of the lamina propria. Nutrition passes from these vessels through the connective tissue and basal lamina and then enters the epithelium. Throughout the gingiva, nerves and nerve endings

TABLE 14-1	LEVELS OF SENSITIVITY OF THE ORAL REGION	
Sensation	**Greatest sensitivity**	**Moderate sensitivity**
Pain	Lips, pharynx, base of tongue	Anterior tongue
Heat	Lips	Tip of tongue
Cold	Lips, posterior palate	Base of tongue, ventral tongue
Touch	Lips, tip of tongue	Gingiva

are prevalent. The encapsulated touch and temperature endings are located in the papillary tissue of the lamina propria and axons associated with Merkel's cells (Fig. 14-36). Free endings associated with pain can be seen entering the epithelium between the cells. Table 14-1 shows the areas and levels of sensitivity.

EPITHELIAL NONKERATINOCYTES

In contrast to the epithelial cells or keratinocytes, the nonkeratinocytes constitute about 10% of the mucosal cell population. These cells have a clear halo around their nuclei and have been called "clear cells." The three types of these cells are **Langerhans' cells, Merkel's cells,** and **melanocytes.** Two other nonkeratinocytes, lymphocytes and polymorphonuclear leukocytes, appear in the epithelium in cases of inflammation.

Langerhans' Cells

Langerhans' cells are found in the stratum spinosum and are believed to function in the processing of antigenic material. They are therefore in an ideal location to make contact with invading bacteria and establish response mechanisms to protect the body. The cells

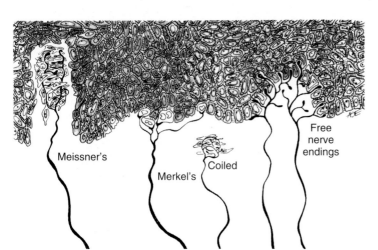

Fig. 14-36 Nerve endings in oral mucosa showing the location of various types in epithelium or lamina propria.

Fig. 14-38 Merkel's cells that are located in basal cell layer and are associated with a nerve ending *(MS).* They function as touch receptors. The *inset* shows nerve terminals *(T)* and secretory granules in Merkel's cell *(G).*

Fig. 14-37 Three histologic views of a nonkeratinocyte. A, In an electron micrograph of Langerhans' cell, the rodlike granules are indicated by *arrows.* **B,** Appearance of cell under light microscopy. **C,** Diagram of Langerhans' cell.

Fig. 14-39 Histology of another type of nonkeratinocyte. A dendritic melanocyte is in the stratum basale of the oral epithelium.

appear to have processes but do not have desmosomes or tonofilaments. This type of cell has unique, racket-shaped organelles (Fig. 14-37).

Merkel's Cells

Merkel's cells are located in the basal layer of the gingival epithelium. Unlike keratinocytes, these cells are associated with the terminal axon. However, they may contain round, electron-dense granules in their cytoplasms adjacent to their axons. These cells and their axons are believed to function as touch receptors (Fig. 14-38).

Melanocytes

Melanocytes are melanin-producing cells in the basal layer of the gingival epithelium. Melanocytes lack desmosomes and tonofilaments and are dendritic. A characteristic feature of the melanocyte is the melanin granules

(melanosomes) in the cytoplasm. Such cells may inject melanosomes into nearby keratinocytes (Fig. 14-39).

Lymphocytes and Leukocytes

Lymphocytes, leukocytes, and mast cells, which are associated with gingival inflammation, may be found in the gingival epithelium and connective tissue. They may be found in the gingival epithelium and underlying connective tissue. They may be located anywhere in the gingiva but most often underlie the junctional epithelium. Their appearance is different from keratinocytes because they have no desmosomes, tonofilaments, or organelles. These lymphocytes appear typical, with a large oval nucleus occupying most of the cytoplasmic space (Fig. 14-40). Granule-bearing mast cells may also be seen in the gingival mucosa during inflammation.

Leukocytes and lymphocytes

Fig. 14-40 Inflamed gingiva with many leukocytes and lymphocytes in the connective tissue of the gingiva.

 CLINICAL COMMENT

> Halitosis can be caused by multiple factors. If the ingestion of offensive foods is ruled out as a cause, possible food impaction, plaque, or the need for oral prophylaxis should be considered. Disease of tooth origin or the periodontium is another factor. Diseased tonsils or sinuses and systemic factors, such as lung problems, are also possible causes.

CHANGES WITH AGING

Recognition of changes in the oral mucosa associated with aging is important. With age, the oral epithelium becomes thinner and more fragile. A flattening of the surface ridges and surface cells causes the oral mucosa to appear smoother. Because of gradual atrophy of the minor salivary glands and less activity of the major glands, the oral mucosa appears less moist. In aging, cellular activity decreases and fibrosis increases. Also, calcifications appear in the lamina propria of the gingiva and the periodontal ligament. The ability to repair is reduced, and the length of healing time is increased. Apical migration of the gingiva usually is associated with periodontal disease but appears routinely in the aging oral mucosa. Some patients may be taking blood thinners or other medications that affect gingival bleeding. Compare Figures 14-41 and 14-42.

Fig. 14-41 Healthy gingiva in a 25-year-old person showing normal color, form, and density.

Fig. 14-42 Healthy gingiva of an 80-year-old person differs from that of the 25-year-old person shown in Figure 14-41. Normal form and contours are altered in older persons.

 Consider the Patient

> ***Discussion:*** The floor of the mouth is an appropriate area for absorption of some medications, such as for the relief of angina, because it is a rapid route. The epithelium is thin and nonkeratinized, with capillaries present in the dermis, which are near the surface of the mucosa.

SELF-EVALUATION QUESTIONS

1. Describe the three areas of the gingiva and the characteristics of each.
2. Name the areas covered with lining mucosa and masticatory mucosa.
3. Where are taste buds most numerous in the oral cavity, and in what other areas are they located?
4. What are the locations and functions of traction bands?
5. Describe junctional epithelium and state its turnover time.

6. What are the location and function of Langerhans' cells?
7. Name four types of nerve sensation found in the oral cavity and their location.
8. What taste sensations are located on the tip, anterior sides, posterior sides, and posterior center of the tongue?
9. What is the name and type of gland found at the corners of the mouth?
10. Describe the structure and function of a hemidesmosome.

Suggested Reading

Bhaskar SN, editor: *Orban's oral histology and embryology,* ed 11, St. Louis, 1991, Mosby.

Kessler HR: Herpes virus infections: a review for the dental practitioner, *Texas Dent J* 122(2):150-165, 2005.

Nunzi MG, Pisarek A, Mugnaini E: Merkel cells, corpuscular nerve endings and free nerve endings in the mouse palatine mucosa express three subtypes of vesicular glutamate transporters, *J Neurocytol* 33(3):359-376, 2004.

SALIVARY GLANDS AND TONSILS

CHAPTER OUTLINE

LEARNING OBJECTIVES

After reading this chapter the student will be able to:

- discuss the classification of the major and minor salivary glands
- explain the composition and function of saliva
- describe the location and purpose of salivary gland duct systems
- discuss the classification of tonsillar tissue
- explain the function of the tonsils

KEY TERMS

Alveolus or acinus
Amylase
B cells
Buccal and labial glands
Epidermal growth factor
Excretory portion
Germinal centers
Glossopalatine glands
Intercalated ducts
Interlobular excretory ducts
Intralobular duct system
Lingual glands
Lingual tonsils
Lobes
Lobules

Major glands
Memory cells
Merocrine glands
Minor glands
Mixed glands
Mucin
Palatine glands
Palatine tonsils
Parotid glands
Pharyngeal tonsil or adenoid
Pure mucous glands
Salivary corpuscles
Secretory end piece or intercalated
   duct
Secretory portion

Serous demilunes
Serous glands
Serous or mucous cells
Stensen's duct
Striated duct
Sublingual glands
Submandibular glands
T cells
Waldeyer's ring
Wharton's duct
Zymogen granules

OVERVIEW

This chapter discusses the structure and function of the salivary glands, saliva, and tonsils. Despite different structures and functions, these soft tissues all contribute significantly to oral health. Saliva is a balanced secretion resulting from both (1) the composition of the secretion and (2) the location of the salivary gland secretions into the oral cavity. The two cell types are serous, which is high protein and low carbohydrate, and mucous, which is low protein and high carbohydrate. Glands of the lips, cheeks, and anterior floor of the mouth produce a watery mixture of a serous and mucous secretion, whereas other glands of the posterior palate, pharynx, and tongue contribute a viscous mucous solution that protects the membranes in those regions. The major salivary glands contribute 85% to 90% of the saliva into the more anterior area of the mouth. In addition to protein and carbohydrate, the parotid, which is the largest gland, secretes the enzyme amylase, which aids in digestion of carbohydrates. Therefore, the buffering ability of saliva results from ionic secretions by the salivary glands. These secretions are collected and modified through an elaborate secretory duct system.

Tonsils, like the salivary glands, have locations that maximally affect and protect the oral environment. These lymph node–like organs are positioned in the oropharynx at the entrance to the alimentary canal. They produce lymphocytes and, with the assistance of macrophages, protect against microbes, foreign cells, and cancer cells. Lymphocytes can recognize foreign cells and respond to them either by becoming T cells, which destroy the foreign cells directly, or by forming B cells, which transform into plasma cells that secrete antibodies to eliminate the foreign cells.

CLASSIFICATION OF SALIVARY GLANDS

Salivary glands are classified as either major or minor depending on their size and the amount of their secretion. The **major glands** carry their secretion some distance to the oral cavity by means of a main duct. The smaller **minor glands** empty their products directly into the mouth by means of short ducts. Both are composed, however, of the same type of cells, either **serous** or **mucous cells** or a combination of the two called **serous demilunes** (Fig. 15-1).

"combo of serous + mucous

CLINICAL COMMENT

The salivary glands are also important for the production of growth factors including nerve growth factor and epidermal growth factor.

The functional unit of the salivary gland is the **alveolus** or **acinus**. An acinus is a cluster of pyramidal cells, either mucous or serous or a combination of the two, that secretes into a terminal collecting duct (see Fig. 15-1). The collecting duct is termed the **secretory end piece** or **intercalated duct**. Both the large and small glands are composed of many acini, although the larger glands contain more acini or units arranged in lobules and lobes (Fig. 15-2). Each cell type provides a different type of

Fig. 15-1 Salivary acinar cells. The serous, mixed, and mucous alveoli are displayed. Observe cell size, shape, and position relative to collecting tubules and intercalated duct.

Fig. 15-2 Histology of the developing salivary gland at a stage in which lobules can be seen outlined by connective tissue fibers (septa).

secretion. Serous cells secrete mostly proteins and small amounts of carbohydrates. Their secretion also contains **zymogen granules,** precursors of the enzyme **amylase,** which functions in the breakdown of carbohydrates. Serous cell secretion has a watery consistency. Mucous cells are high in carbohydrates and low in proteins and discharge a viscous product called **mucin** (Fig. 15-3). When mucin mixes with watery oral fluids, it becomes mucous, causing the saliva to be thick and viscous.

Both types of acinar cells are pyramidal. The nucleus of the serous cell is oval to round, and that of the mucous cell is oval to spindle shaped (see Fig. 15-1). In each of these cell types, the nuclei appear in the basal part of the cell. The cytoplasm of the serous cell stains deeply because it is filled with albumin, whereas the mucous cell appears light and foamy because of the presence of carbohydrates in mucin (see Figs. 15-3 and 15-4).

Ultrastructurally, the serous cell is filled with secretory granules in the apical region, rough-surface endoplasmic reticulum, Golgi's apparatus, mitochondria, and an oval nucleus (Fig. 15-5). The mucous cells contain larger droplets of mucin apically and a prominent Golgi's apparatus and rough endoplasmic reticulum around the flattened nucleus (Fig. 15-6). A third cell-type arrangement is a terminal alveolus of mucous cells with a cap of serous cells (see Fig. 15-4). This configuration is termed a serous demilune, with the secretion of the serous cells passing down a duct between the terminal mucous cells to the lumen of the alveolus (see Fig. 15-1).

Salivary glands are termed **merocrine glands** because the basic mode of product excretion is through membrane vesicles passing to the cell's apex. These vesicles fuse with the cell plasma membrane and are then exteriorized (see Fig. 15-6).

 CLINICAL COMMENT

> The serous and mucous cells of the major glands secrete 85% to 90% of saliva. Their combined secretions produce the viscosity as well as the important buffering actions of saliva. These properties result from the actions of protein, carbohydrate, carbonate, and phosphate that are contributed by the secretory ducts of the glands.

MAJOR SALIVARY GLANDS

The major salivary glands are present as three bilateral pairs. The **parotid glands** are located on the sides of the face in front of the ears; the second pair, the **submandibular glands,** are inside the angle of the mandible; and the third pair, the **sublingual glands,** are on either side of the midline beneath the mucosa of the anterior floor of the mouth (Fig. 15-7 and Table 15-1).

Each major gland secretes a different product. The parotids produce a nearly pure serous secretion, the submandibular a mixed serous and mucous secretion, and the sublingual nearly pure mucous.

The parotids are the largest glands, although they contribute only 25% of the total saliva. The submandibular glands are intermediate in size, but they produce 60% of the saliva. The sublingual glands are the smallest, contributing only about 5% of the saliva. The minor salivary glands located throughout the oral cavity contribute about the same amount as the sublingual.

These salivary glands are organized like grapes on a vine. The acini are the grapes, and they are arranged in

Fig. 15-3 Histologic features of the submandibular gland. Serous cells are at the upper left, and mucous cells are at the lower left. A few mucous cells are capped with serous cells (serous demilunes).

Serous cells

Serous demilunes

Mucous cells

Fig. 15-4 Histology of a serous demilune *(sd)* cap on mucous cells in mixed acinus of the submandibular gland.

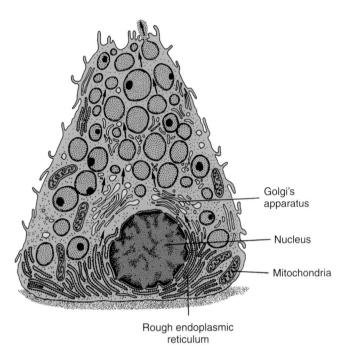

Golgi's apparatus

Nucleus

Mitochondria

Rough endoplasmic reticulum

Fig. 15-5 Ultrastructure of a serous cell with vesicles developing and migrating to the cell apex above. Note the round nucleus, Golgi's apparatus, and rough endoplasmic reticulum that are characteristic of a protein-secreting cell. *Arrows* point to vesicles arising from Golgi's zone and migrating to the cell surface.

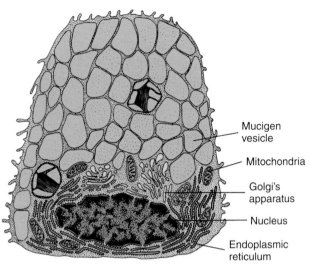

Mucigen vesicle

Mitochondria

Golgi's apparatus

Nucleus

Endoplasmic reticulum

Fig. 15-6 Ultrastructural design of a mucous cell. Compare the shape of this cell and its nucleus with those of the serous cell. Shown are Golgi's apparatus, rough-surface endoplasmic reticulum, and mucous accumulation (mucigen vesicles) in the cell.

Fig. 15-7 Location of major glands—parotid, submandibular, and sublingual. The diagram demonstrates the relationship of facial nerves and blood vessels to oral structures.

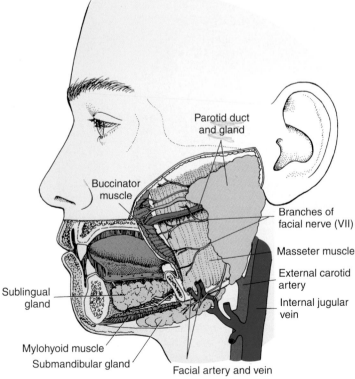

Parotid duct and gland

Buccinator muscle

Branches of facial nerve (VII)

Masseter muscle

External carotid artery

Internal jugular vein

Sublingual gland

Mylohyoid muscle

Submandibular gland

Facial artery and vein

TABLE 15-1 MAJOR SALIVARY GLANDS AND CONTRIBUTION TO SALIVA

Gland	Size	Location	Type cells	Amount secretion (%)	Duct type: striated/intercalated
Parotid	Largest	Anterior ear	Serous	25	Long/long
Submandibular	Intermediate	Angle of mandible	Mixed serous demilune	60	Long/short
Sublingual	Smallest	Anterior floor of mouth	Mucous	5	Short/none

Intralobular excretory duct

Blood vessel

Lobule

Connective tissue septa

Adipose tissue

Fig. 15-8 Histology illustrating the lobular nature of the parotid gland. Blood vessels can be seen within the lobule. *Light lines* that surround each lobule are connective tissue fibers that support lobules. The parotid gland contains many adipose cells *(light-stained cells).*

groups or **lobules** invested in connective tissue. These groups of lobules form larger **lobes.** In turn, the lobes are surrounded by connective tissue containing the ducts that drain the glands and the blood vessels that supply the glands (Fig. 15-8).

The parotid ducts extend anteriorly across the masseter muscles and then bend toward the mouth, opening adjacent to the crowns of the maxillary molar teeth (see Fig. 15-7). The ducts of the submandibular and sublingual glands have a common opening in the anterior floor of the mouth, located at the sublingual papillae on either side of the frenulum and at the tongue's tip (see Fig. 15-7).

MINOR SALIVARY GLANDS

The minor salivary glands are classified as serous, mucous, and mixed types, the same as the major glands (Table 15-2). These glands are located throughout the oral cavity and are named for their location. The glands of the cheeks and lips are termed the **buccal** and **labial glands.** They contain a combination of serous and mucous secretions and are thus known as **mixed glands.** The glands of both the posterior hard palate and soft palate are called **palatine glands,** and those of

TABLE 15-2 MINOR SALIVARY GLANDS AND CONTRIBUTION TO SALIVA

Name	Location	Type secretion
Labial	Lips	Mixed
Buccal	Cheeks	Mixed
Palatine	Hard and soft	Pure mucous
Lingual	Anterior	Mixed
	Middle	Serous
	Posterior	Pure mucous

the tonsillar folds are the **glossopalatine glands.** These glands are referred to as **pure mucous glands.** The tongue contains **lingual glands,** which are mixed glands at the tongue's tip. **Serous glands** are located at the junction of the tongue's body and base, where the watery secretion washes out the taste buds of the circumvallate papillae. The tongue also has mucous glands in the posterior region under the lingual tonsillar tissue. Figure 15-9 shows all these minor glands. Each minor gland is small, consisting of a cluster of acini, and each is drained by a short duct.

Serous

Mucous

Mixed

Fig. 15-9 Location of the minor salivary glands in the oral cavity. Serous glands are located in the midtongue, mucous glands in the palate, and mixed glands in the lips, cheeks, and tongue tip.

CLINICAL COMMENT

The locations of various minor glands in the oral cavity are important to oral functions. In the palate, where keratinized epithelium is present, mucous glands provide adequate lubrication to the epithelium. The lips and cheeks have similar mixed glands that assist in mastication, swallowing, and speech. These minor glands assist in swallowing and speech. Contributions of the three bilateral major glands provide the other 90% of oral fluids.

SALIVA

Composition

All of the major and minor salivary glands contribute to the composition of saliva. This composition varies according to the rate of secretion, which is low during

sleep and high (1 ml per minute ±) during stimulation. Secretion is controlled by the salivary center in the brain, and flow is generated by taste (gustatory). Masticatory function is controlled through receptors in the periodontium and muscles of mastication. Oral and pharyngeal pain and irritation can also induce secretion.

Saliva has fewer proteins and ions than blood. Saliva contains potassium, sodium chloride, calcium, magnesium, phosphorus, carbonate, urea, and traces of ammonia, uric acid, glucose, and lipids. The major salivary protein is amylase, which is present in the parotid gland and to a lesser extent (20%) in the submandibular gland. The sublingual or minor glands do not have any amylase. Saliva also contains the proteins lysozyme and albumin. The viscous nature of saliva results from the presence of salivary mucin, which is a mixture of glycoproteins. Saliva contains epithelial cells shed by the oral epithelium as well as leukocytes from the gingival crevices and lymphocytes from the tonsils. The latter two are known as **salivary corpuscles.**

 ### CLINICAL COMMENT

Saliva is important in mastication, swallowing, and speech. In addition, saliva contains amylase, an important enzyme that functions in the breakdown of carbohydrates and initiates digestive action in the oral cavity.

Functions

The three pints of saliva secreted each day serve several important functions, some of which are the following:
1. To wash the surfaces of the teeth and reduce the possibility of acid etching's leading to dental caries
2. To keep the oral tissues moist and protect against irritants and desiccation
3. To aid in mastication and swallowing of food
4. To provide antibacterial action
5. To assist in the formation of the pellicle, which is a protective membrane on the tooth's surface
6. To provide protection in acid-neutralizing and acid-buffering actions, which prevent dissolution of enamel

The presence of calcium and phosphate ions in saliva increases enamel surface hardness of newly erupted teeth and may assist in enamel remineralization. Through the action of amylase, starches are broken down to more easily digestible carbohydrates. Saliva also enhances taste by breaking down food molecules into a solution that is then brought into contact with the taste buds.

Saliva has numerous proteins—such as lysozymes, lactoperoxidase, and lactoferrin—that have antimicrobial properties. Additionally, saliva has antibodies or immunoglobulin, such as immunoglobulin A (IgA).

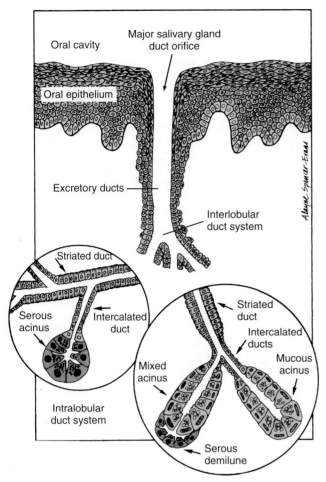

Fig. 15-10 Duct system of the salivary glands. Circles show the duct system of intralobular ducts, that is, intercalated and striated secretory ducts located within the lobule. Above are interlobular and multicelled excretory ducts located outside the lobules and lobes.

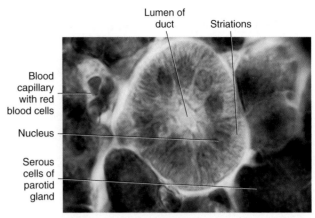

Fig. 15-11 Histology of a striated duct in center of field surrounded by parotid acinar cells. In the duct cell is the centrally located nucleus with basal striations on the periphery of each cell. These striations result from enfolding of the outer cell membrane, which provides a larger area for exchange of nutrients with adjacent vascular supply. A blood capillary can be seen on the left.

Saliva also contains an **epidermal growth factor,** which may assist in the healing of injured oral mucosa.

During most of the day and night, salivary flow is minimal. Secretion depends on gustatory and masticatory stimulation. Both taste and smell perform a major role in determining salivary flow, as do the nerve endings in the periodontal ligament and the muscles of mastication.

Duct Systems

Ducts of the smallest diameter are in direct contact with salivary acini. They become much larger as other acini empty into a collecting duct, which continues increasing in size until it enters the oral cavity. The ducts of the major glands are long, and various types of ducts are within the glands. Many of these ducts are so small that it is difficult to visualize them microscopically.

The duct system consists of a **secretory portion,** which lies among the acinar cells, and an **excretory portion,** which lies in the connective tissue septa between the lobules and lobes of the glands. These ducts continue beyond the glands, emptying into the oral cavity (Fig. 15-10). The difference between the secretory and excretory ducts is that substances enter and leave the cells of the secretory duct by ion exchange with the adjacent blood vessels, whereas the excretory duct is simply a saliva-collecting tube. Acinar cells drain directly into **intercalated ducts,** which are low cuboidal cells (see Fig. 15-10). These secretory cells have metabolic function and contain mitochondria, rough endoplasmic reticulum, and secretory granules.

The intercalated duct opens directly into a larger duct called the **striated duct.** The cells of the striated duct are slightly taller and more columnar than those of the intercalated duct (see Fig. 15-10). These cells have striations caused by enfolding of the basal membrane, which increases the surface area of the cell and allows increased exchange of ions with the nearby blood vessels (Fig. 15-11). Sodium resorption and potassium secretion occur in these cells, causing changes in the saliva composition.

Both intercalated and striated ducts are part of the **intralobular duct system,** located inside the lobules. In contrast, the remaining **interlobular excretory ducts** are located in the connective tissue septa between the lobules and lobes of the gland (see Fig. 15-10). As the ducts enlarge, their walls contain larger and more numerous cells, such as stratified columnar cells. Near its orifice, the duct becomes lined with stratified squamous epithelium, which is continuous with the oral epithelium. **Stensen's duct** drains the parotid gland, and **Wharton's duct** drains the submandibular gland.

CLINICAL COMMENT

The action of saliva provides an important protective function on the tooth's surface and the oral epithelium, where acids contribute to changing conditions. Saliva also contains calcium and phosphate, which may aid in the demineralization of the enamel surface and reverse the action of dental caries.

Consider the Patient

A patient complains of pain and tenderness on the right side of the floor of the mouth. What is the best approach in determining the cause?

Innervation of the Salivary Glands

Salivary gland secretion is regulated mostly by the sympathetic and parasympathetic autonomic nervous system. Stimulation of the salivary glands by sympathetic nerves results in an organic secretion (protein-rich), and stimulation by the parasympathetic nerves results in a watery secretion.

MYOEPITHELIAL CELLS

Myoepithelial cells originate from the oral epithelium at the time that the oral epithelial cells of the salivary gland grow into the mesenchyme. The cells remain on the outside of the secretory end pieces and function as muscle cells to contract and squeeze the acinus, facilitating secretion. Therefore, the term *myoepithelial cells* is used because these cells have an epithelial origin and a muscle function. These cells have long processes that wrap around the acinar and intercalated duct cells (Figs. 15-12 and 15-13). Their large nuclei and cytoplasms, containing microfilaments, enable them to act as muscle cells.

CLINICAL COMMENT

THE USE OF GENE THERAPY IN SALIVARY GLANDS

Because the salivary glands can secrete proteins directly into the bloodstream and/or, using the ducts, into the mouth or gut, they provide an ideal model for showing how the insertion of a gene, that turns on a hormone for example, into the glandular tissue will allow the cells to synthesize a protein that the glands do not normally secrete.

CLINICAL COMMENT

Drugs such as tranquilizers, barbiturates, and antihistamines decrease salivary flow. In some older patients, who may already have deficient salivary flow, this could be a cause of dry mouth (xerostomia).

Fig. 15-12 Histology of a light-stained mucous acinus that contains mucous cells. The mucous acinus is surrounded by a myoepithelial cell.

CLASSIFICATION OF TONSILLAR TISSUE

Tonsillar tissue surrounds the oropharynx in a ring called **Waldeyer's ring.** In the oropharyngeal midline is the single **pharyngeal tonsil** or **adenoid;** adjacent to the posterior molars are the bilateral **palatine tonsils;** and in the floor of the mouth are the bilateral **lingual tonsils** (Fig. 15-14). Tonsils are part of the lymphatic system, which also includes lymph nodes, thymus, spleen, and diffuse lymphatic tissue. Each tonsil is composed of lymphatic tissue or nodules. The lymphatic nodules, in turn, may have **germinal centers,** which are active sites of lymphocyte formation. These centers are common in the lingual and palatine tonsils. The tonsils are covered with epithelium. In the pharyngeal tonsil, the epithelium is respiratory because the tonsil is in the nasopharynx. In the orally located palatine and lingual tonsils, it is stratified squamous epithelium. This epithelial covering lines the grooves or clefts of each gland. Tonsils, unlike lymph nodes, have no afferent lymphatic vessels that lead to them. However, both tonsils and lymph nodes do have efferent lymphatic vessels draining them. Each tonsil is supported by connective tissue and has associated glands underlying it.

Palatine Tonsils

The palatine tonsils are large in children, and these structures are best recognized when they become infected and bulge into the throat, causing difficulty in swallowing. When the tonsils are infected and swollen, they appear red with streaks of white purulent material on their surfaces (Fig. 15-15). They become infected largely as a result of their structure. Because palatine tonsils have deep, branching crypts in which oral bacteria may become lodged, these crypts may become plugged with lymphocyte discharge and desquamated epithelial cells. Beneath the palatine tonsils are seromucous glands, which assist in flushing out these crypts. Their ducts, however, do not open into the tonsillar crypts but onto the surface of the glands. This lack of flushing action in the crypts may account for the accumulation of foreign debris and bacteria that causes tissue inflammation. Structurally, these are the largest tonsils of the three types and are divided into lobules by the crypts. Each lobule contains numerous lymphatic nodules, which contain germinal centers (Fig. 15-16). Septa of connective tissue support the nodules of lymphatic tissue and invest the gland in a capsule.

Myoepithelial cell processes

Fig. 15-13 Scanning electron micrograph of a myoepithelial cell and its cytoplasmic processes wrapping around the acinus of the submandibular gland.

Pharyngeal tonsil

Palatine tonsil
Lingual tonsil

Fig. 15-14 Location of three tonsillar groups. The palatine tonsil is in the lateral wall of the oropharynx, the lingual tonsil is in the posterior of the tongue, and the pharyngeal tonsil is in the midline of the posterior pharyngeal wall.

Fig. 15-15 Oral view of palatine tonsils *(arrows).* These inflamed, swollen tonsils project into the oropharyngeal cavity.

Lingual Tonsils

Lingual tonsils are located on the surface of the posterior third of the tongue (see Fig. 15-14). The tonsillar mass is bilateral because it is divided in the midline, reflecting the bilateral origin of the tongue. The lingual tonsils are composed of wide-mouthed crypts and are

Fig. 15-16 Histology of the palatine tonsil, showing the investing squamous epithelium, deep branching crypts, and organized lymphatic nodules.

nonbranching. They form rows of lymphatic nodules supported by connective tissue septa that are present in each lobule of the gland (Fig. 15-17). These tonsils also have a connective tissue capsule investing them. The capsule is covered with nonkeratinized stratified squamous epithelium. Underlying these tonsils, between the mucous glands, are skeletal muscles and adipose tissue of the tongue. These mucous glands, with their ducts opening into the crypt, function in a cleansing action. Also, because these tonsils are located in the posterior floor of the mouth, the washing action of saliva provides effective cleansing. Therefore, this tonsillar mass is rarely inflamed.

Pharyngeal Tonsil

The pharyngeal tonsil, or adenoid, is located in the posterior wall of the superior portion of the nasopharynx. It is subject to infection in childhood. The pharyngeal tonsil may grow laterally from the midline location to surround the opening of the eustachian tubes. Tonsillar tissue at this location is called the tubal tonsil and can be the source of infection to the eustachian tubes. The pharyngeal tonsil is unlike the other tonsils in that it is an aggregation of lymphocytes that does not have crypts but has occasional folds that appear as clefts in the mucosa (Fig. 15-18). This tonsil is variable in structure because only occasionally are there lymphoid nodules, which are usually only on a surface accumulation of diffuse lymphoid tissue. The covering epithelium is transformed either into respiratory or into stratified

Fig. 15-17 Histology of the lingual tonsil on the posterior tongue. Observe the investing squamous epithelium, short crypts, and lymphatic nodules. *Arrows* denote underlying mucous glands.

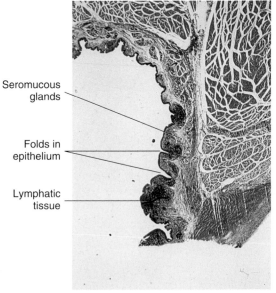

Fig. 15-18 Histologic appearance of the pharyngeal tonsil. Observe the folds in the epithelium rather than crypts in tissue, diffuse lymphatic tissue rather than nodules, and seromucous glands underlying the tonsillar tissue.

squamous epithelium. Underlying the tonsil are mixed glands that drain the surface of the epithelium overlying the gland tissue. This tonsil overlies the muscles of the pharynx.

FUNCTION OF TONSILS

The most notable function of tonsils is the production of lymphocytes that protect the body from foreign microorganisms inhaled or swallowed. Allergens may be sensed by these cells, which start the complex process of coding for antibody production. Because of their ability to retain this information, the lymphocytes have been called **memory cells.** Some lymphocytes transform into **T cells** and engulf bacteria or discharge substances to destroy them. Other lymphocytes become **B cells,** which differentiate into plasma cells. Plasma cells secrete antibodies that destroy antigens. Plasma cells and lymphocytes are found in chronic infections, such as periodontal disease. Plasma cells found in the area of the salivary glands produce IgA, which joins in the end piece of the intercellular area to form secretory IgA. Some foreign substances are absorbed from the crypts of the glands into the gland proper and are then destroyed.

CLINICAL COMMENT

Tonsils are ideally positioned around the entrance to the alimentary canal to aid in protecting the body from invasion of microorganisms. They are important in the antibacterial action of the B and T lymphocytes and in the action of the plasma cells in the formation of secretory IgA, which neutralizes viruses and can be an antibody to food antigens.

Consider the Patient

Discussion: The dentist must examine the mouth carefully, and radiographs should be taken. Radiographs may reveal a stone in the submandibular duct, which is the most common site for a stone. Such a stone will interfere with salivary gland function and should be removed. Palpation by the dentist could assist the stone in passing through the duct.

SELF-EVALUATION QUESTIONS

1. Discuss the location and function of the myoepithelial cells.
2. Describe the types of secretory duct cells and their functions.
3. What are the contributions of the major and minor salivary glands to the total volume of saliva?
4. Compare the appearance and function of serous and mucous cells.
5. Where are most serous demilune cells found?
6. What is the origin of secretory IgA?
7. Name and describe the various types of minor salivary glands.
8. Describe the gland type underlying each tonsil.
9. How does gland structure relate to the causes of tonsillitis?
10. What is the function of B and T cells in the tonsils?

Suggested Reading

Arens R, Marcus CL: Pathophysiology of upper airway obstruction: a developmental perspective, *Sleep* 27(5):997-1019, 2004.

Arvidsson A, et al: Characterisation of structures in salivary secretion film formation. An experimental study with atomic force microscopy, *Biofouling* 20(3):181-188, 2004.

Bradley RM: Salivary secretion. In Getchell TV, et al, editors: *Smell and taste in health and disease,* New York, 1991, Raven Press, pp 127-144.

Castle D: Cell biology of salivary protein. In Dobrosielski-Vergona K, editor: *Biology of the salivary glands,* Boca Raton, FL, 1993, CRC Press, pp 81-104.

Drummond JR, Chrisholm DM: A quantitative and qualitative study of the aging human salivary glands, *Arch Oral Biol* 29: 151, 1984.

Field A, Scot J: Changes in the structure of salivary glands with age. In Dobrosielski-Vergona K, editor: *Biology of the salivary glands,* Boca Raton, FL, 1993, CRC Press, pp 397-439.

Fukami H, Bradley RM: Biophysical and morphological properties of parasympathetic neurons controlling the parotid and von Ebner salivary glands in rats, *J Neurophysiol* 93(2):678-686, 2005.

Gasser RF: Surgical anatomy of the parotid duct with emphasis on the major tributaries forming the duct and the relationship of the facial nerve to the duct, *Clin Anatomy* 18(1):79, 2005.

Haberman AS, Isaac DD, Andrew DJ: Specification of cell fates within the salivary gland primordium, *Devel Biology* 258(2):443-453, 2003.

Jaskoll T, et al: Embryonic submandibular gland morphogenesis: stage-specific protein localization of FGFs, BMPs, Pax6 and Pax9 in normal mice and abnormal SMG phenotypes in FgfR2-IIIc(+/Delta), BMP7 (−/−) and Pax6(−/−) mice, *Cells Tissues Organs* 170(2-3):83-98, 2002.

Joraku A, et al: Tissue engineering of functional salivary gland tissue, *Laryngoscope* 115(2):244-248, 2005.

Ozbilgin MK, et al: Antigen-presenting cells in the hypertrophic pharyngeal tonsils: a histochemical, immunohistochemical and ultrastructural study, *J Invest Allerg Clin Immunol* 14(4): 320-328, 2004.

Passali D, et al: Structural and immunological characteristics of chronically inflamed adenotonsillar tissue in childhood, *Clin Diagn Lab Immunol* 11(6):1154-1157, 2004.

Quissell DO: Stimulus exocytosis coupling mechanism in salivary gland cells. In Dobrosielski-Vergona K, editor: *Biology of the salivary glands,* Boca Raton, FL, 1993, CRC Press, pp 105-127.

Rice DH, Becker TS: *The salivary glands,* New York, 1994, Thieme Medical.

Riva A, et al: Serous and mucous cells of human submandibular salivary gland stimulated in vitro by isoproterenol, carbachol and clozapine: an LM, TEM, and HRSEM study, *Eur J Morphol* 41(2):83-87, 2003.

Ship JA, Hu K: Radiotherapy-induced salivary dysfunction, *Semin Oncol* 31(6 suppl 18):29-36, 2004.

Skinner LJ, et al: Helicobacter pylori and tonsillectomy, *Clin Otolaryngol Allied Sci* 26(6):505-509, 2001.

Turner RJ: Mechanisms and secretion by salivary glands, *Ann NY Acad Sci* 694:24-35, 1993.

Webb CJ, et al: Tonsillar size is an important indicator of recurrent acute tonsillitis, *Clin Otolaryngol Allied Sci* 29(4):369-371, 2004.

Zhang PC, et al: Comparison of histology between recurrent tonsillitis and tonsillar hypertrophy, *Clin Otolaryngol Allied Sci* 28(3):235-239, 2003.

16

BIOFILMS

CHAPTER OUTLINE

Overview
Cuticle
Acquired Pellicle

Plaque
Calculus
Self-Evaluation Questions

Consider the Patient Discussion
Suggested Reading

LEARNING OBJECTIVES

After reading this chapter the student will be able to:

- define the origin and components of cuticle
- discuss the composition of acquired pellicle and plaque
- describe the location and composition of calculus
- explain why saliva is important in determining oral health

KEY TERMS

Cuticular protein
Disclosing solution
Hydroxyapatite
Pellicle or acquired pellicle

Plaque
Primary or developmental cuticle
Prismless zone of enamel
Reduced enamel epithelium

Salivary corpuscles
Serumal calculus

OVERVIEW

This chapter describes substances that form on the surface of the teeth and explains how they develop. Microbial biofilms are a major concern today because they are also associated with implantable medical devices. The dental plaque is characterized as a biofilm. It is important that we characterize this biofilm as it exists on the surface of the body and is capable of being analyzed and characterized and treated with known agents. The primary cuticle is of cellular origin and is formed before tooth eruption. All other products originate from saliva. The primary cuticle forms the zone of junctional epithelium; the remaining epithelium is lost soon after the teeth erupt into incisal or occlusal contact. Saliva contains salivary proteins and glycoproteins that attach to enamel or exposed cementum or dentin. Saliva then deposits a thin protein coat or membrane, called a pellicle, on the surface of the tooth. The pellicle, although protective to the tooth, allows plaque to form on the surface of the tooth. This plaque is composed of bacteria and salivary proteins that will become a dense layer that gradually accumulates on the tooth's surface if not removed. The bacteria in plaque may produce acid that can cause etching and disintegration of the tooth's surface. This leads to the initiation of dental caries. Dental caries therefore develops in areas where brushing or washing of the tooth's surface does not occur. In other instances, plaque may not produce acid but may become mineralized into calculus. Calculus forms by mineralization of the remaining plaque bacteria into a hydroxyapatite deposit on the enamel and exposed cementum surfaces. Continuous acquisition of calculus forms a thick deposit that should be removed because the potential for inflammation or infection of gingival tissue could lead to destructive periodontal disease.

CUTICLE

The **primary** or **developmental cuticle** is deposited on the enamel's surface by the ameloblasts as their last function, shortly before the tooth crown erupts into the oral cavity. At this time, the formed enamel has reached a thickness of 2 to 2.5 mm over the cusps and is fully mineralized. In their final action, the ameloblasts secrete a thin, structureless protein membrane on the tooth's surface. On the outer surface of this cuticle is the remainder of the enamel organ cells, termed the **reduced enamel epithelium.** This cellular membrane on the tooth's surface includes the ameloblasts and other remnants of the enamel organ. Ameloblasts form the primary cuticle.

The reduced enamel epithelium is lost during eruption of the teeth in the oral cavity (Fig. 16-1). Only the developmental cuticle remains on the surface of the tooth as it erupts into occlusal function. However, this cuticle is not present long on the enamel because abrasion from contact of the opposing teeth causes it to wear away. Only that part covering the enamel in the

Fig. 16-1 Histology of an erupting crown. Enamel is covered with a developmental cuticle at that time.

Clinical crown

Developmental cuticle

Junctional epithelium

gingival crevice remains (Fig. 16-2). This membrane serves as an attachment of the gingival junctional epithelial cells to the tooth. The sulcular epithelium is continually forming protein, which renews the gingival attachment throughout its life. **Cuticular protein,** which initiates attachment of the junctional epithelium to enamel, is the most important function of the primary cuticle.

ACQUIRED PELLICLE

 CLINICAL COMMENT

> The acquired pellicle provides an ideal location for attachment of bacteria. During early adherence, the bacteria are mostly aerobic cocci, but over time the ecology changes to rods and filamentous forms.

When the tooth's surface is cleansed, salivary proteins and glycoproteins are quickly deposited with their strong attraction for the enamel surface. The resulting layer forms a thin, structureless membrane about 0.5 to 1.0 μm thick, which is in contrast to the previously formed cuticular layer. This membrane is termed the **pellicle** or **acquired pellicle** (Fig. 16-3). Although the pellicle is bacteria free when formed, bacteria rapidly attach to its surface. The pellicle covers the entire free surface of the enamel and may penetrate any convenient defect in the tooth's surface, such as a crack, a pit, or an overhanging restoration (Fig. 16-4). Normally, surface layers of enamel rods are straight and at right angles to the tooth surface. The zone is about 30 μm thick, with

the long axis of the apatite crystals oriented nearly perpendicular to the enamel surface. This area is termed the **prismless zone of enamel.** The acquired pellicle overlying this zone has a fine, granular appearance and is approximately 500 Å thick when viewed in ultrastructure (Fig. 16-4). If the pellicle is lost as a result of an oral prophylaxis, it forms again in a few minutes. Although the acquired pellicle is considered protective

Fig. 16-3 Histology of an enamel surface and structureless organic pellicle, which covers enamel rods, in this case at the cervical area.

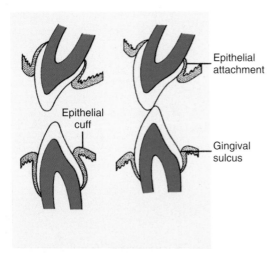

Fig. 16-2 Diagram of an erupting tooth showing the position of the gingiva and epithelial attachment on the cervical enamel.

Fig. 16-4 Electron micrograph showing two areas of newly formed bacteria-free acquired pellicle on the enamel's surface (prismless zone of enamel).

to the enamel surface, it does provide an attachment site for bacteria, which form plaque.

CLINICAL COMMENT

The bathing of the tooth's surface with saliva causes formation of a thin organic membrane, the pellicle, which in part protects the tooth's surface from the action of oral bacteria. Oral bacteria lodge anywhere there is a crevice or other defect and can attach and penetrate the pellicle, causing enamel dissolution by acid production.

PLAQUE

The central fissure of a molar, premolar, or cervical margin of any tooth is the site for accumulation and colonization of oral organisms (Fig. 16-5). In addition to bacteria that

Plaque in central fissure

Fig. 16-5 Incipient carious lesion in a central fissure of enamel in a human molar. Plaque has accumulated in this area.

attach to the pellicle, lymphocytes, leukocytes, desquamated epithelial cells, and clumps of mucin may lodge in any of these sites (Figs. 16-6 and 16-7). Organisms attach to the pellicle and utilize the presence of debris in acid formation.

In gingival or tonsillar inflammation, the number of lymphocytes and leukocytes increases (Fig. 16-8). If microscopic analysis of a saliva sample reveals many lymphocytes, tonsillitis is present. However, an increase in leukocytes in saliva is indicative of gingival inflammation. These cells are called **salivary corpuscles** (Fig. 16-9). At first, only a few bacteria are on the pellicle, but they rapidly grow into a thick **plaque** that contains a variety of microorganisms. The initial plaque quickly changes in composition to include rods and filamentous organisms. These appear after a few days, as shown in Figure 16-10.

The composition of plaque depends also on the extent of gingival disease and whether the location of the plaque is supragingival or subgingival. The initial carious lesions affect the prismless zone of enamel because plaque bacteria cause dissolution of these surface crystals. A breakdown of enamel crystals is seen clinically as a brown spot on the tooth's surface. Figure 16-11 shows a microscopic view of the loss of enamel rod structure. The enamel pellicle may overlie the area of an early lesion on the tooth's surface and may be covered by plaque bacteria. Such a lesion may become filled with organic debris and bacteria (Fig. 16-12). Crystals appear to dissolve in one area and be intact in an adjacent area of enamel. Plaque can best be seen when a **disclosing solution** (0.2% basic fuchsin or erythrosin red No. 3 dye) is used to determine whether all the plaque

Epithelial cells

Fig. 16-6 A salivary smear viewed microscopically showing the presence of desquamated epithelial cells.

Fig. 16-7 Clumps of mucin from saliva that may adhere to crevices or imperfections in enamel's surface.

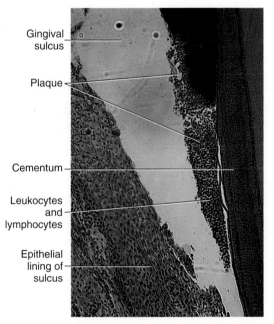

Gingival sulcus

Plaque

Cementum

Leukocytes and lymphocytes

Epithelial lining of sulcus

Fig. 16-8 **The gingival sulcus viewed microscopically.** Leukocytes and lymphocytes appear along the surface of the sulcus and tooth.

Bacteria in and on the surface of salivary corpuscle

Fig. 16-9 Salivary corpuscle: lymphocyte with bacteria on its surface as present in saliva.

has been removed. The advantage of using No. 3 dye is that it does not permanently discolor composite restorations or clothing. The stain left after a quick rinsing reveals any remaining plaque deposits, as observed in Figure 16-13. These visible deposits can be removed by further polishing.

Consider the Patient

A patient appears who is suffering from tonsillitis. The dentist also finds a high level of lymphocytes in the saliva. Why is saliva important in determining oral health?

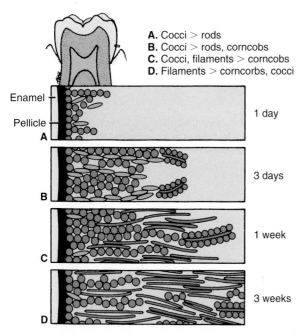

A. Cocci > rods
B. Cocci > rods, corncobs
C. Cocci, filaments > corncobs
D. Filaments > corncorbs, cocci

Enamel

Pellicle

A — 1 day

B — 3 days

C — 1 week

D — 3 weeks

Fig. 16-10 Changes in plaque composition over a 3-week period. A, At 1 day. **B,** At 3 days, the cocci and a few filaments characterize the plaque. **C,** After 1 week, the filamentous organisms increase in number. **D,** By 3 weeks, the filamentous organisms predominate in the plaque. (Modified from Avery JK: *Oral development and histology,* ed 3, Stuttgart, 2002, Thieme Medical.)

Bacteria   Pellicle   Enamel dissolution   Normal enamel

Defect in enamel surface

Fig. 16-12 Electron micrograph of a penetrating carious lesion appearing in the enamel *(left).* Initial enamel dissolution and normal enamel under the pellicle and plaque are shown *(upper right).* (From Avery JK: *Oral development and histology,* ed 3, Stuttgart, 2002, Thieme Medical.)

Bacteria

Site of lesion   Normal enamel

Fig. 16-11 Electron micrograph of bacterial effects on the enamel surface. An initial lesion is shown in the enamel surface *(at left).* Notice the loss of enamel crystals. (From Avery JK: *Oral development and histology,* ed 3, Stuttgart, 2002, Thieme Medical.)

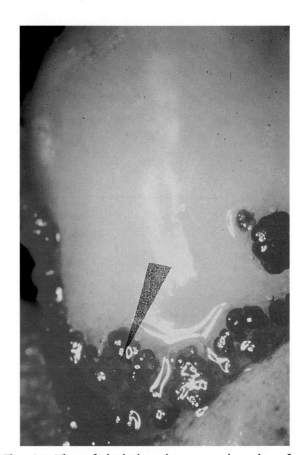

Fig. 16-13 View of gingival crevice area and tooth surface after use of disclosing solution with areas of stained plaque indicated by the *arrowhead.*

CALCULUS

Calculus is a stonelike concretion that forms on teeth or dental prostheses. It is primarily composed of calcium phosphate in the form of **hydroxyapatite,** which develops on the organic cell walls of bacterial plaque. Calculus formation is the reverse of enamel surface demineralization.

CLINICAL COMMENT

Deposition of calculus can occur when the bacteria become calcified, forming a stonelike deposit. A disclosing agent can expose plaque bacteria to facilitate their removal, but plaque will reappear unless appropriate preventive oral hygiene is practiced. The removal of plaque is therefore important in the prevention of gingival and periodontal disease.

Calculus appears on the teeth most often near the opening of the parotid excretory duct on the buccal surfaces of maxillary molars and on the lingual surfaces of the lingual incisors near the openings of the submandibular and lingual ducts. After plaque accumulates, mineralization begins in the inner layer of the pellicle and then spreads into the overlying plaque. Plaque continues to thicken with further deposition of plaque protein. The calcified bacteria appear as circular profiles (Fig. 16-14) and are known as bacterial ghosts.

CLINICAL COMMENT

Salivary calculus is damaging to the gingival tissues and should be removed by scaling. This scaling is frequently accompanied by bleeding of the gingival tissues. The gingiva heals rapidly, however, and the bleeding soon abates.

Calculus deposition follows any surface irregularity of the tooth, such as enamel or cementum (Fig. 16-15). Therefore, calculus forms in a calcospherite manner as the calcium salts derived from saliva organize in the organic skeletons of plaque bacteria. As the plaque calcifies, it loses its ability to produce an acid environment.

Calculus varies in both composition and hardness. Harder calculus contains more mineral matter. Calculus may develop above the gingival margin or within the gingival crevice. Subgingival calculus is much harder and forms more slowly than supragingival calculus. Subgingival calculus is referred to as **serumal calculus** and is usually darker because it contains serum and blood pigments.

Typical bacteria and calculus appear in the gingival crevice (Fig. 16-16). Gram-positive organisms appear in the supragingival area, and gram-negative organisms

Fig. 16-14 Calculus formation viewed by electron microscopy. Minute mineral crystals fill circular bacterial ghosts on enamel surface. (From Avery JK: *Oral development and histology,* ed 3, Stuttgart, 2002, Thieme Medical.)

Fig. 16-15 Calculus on an irregular surface of dentin. Minute mineral crystals are in calculus *(above)* with larger crystals in dentin *(below)*. (From Avery JK: *Oral development and histology,* ed 3, Stuttgart, 2002, Thieme Medical.)

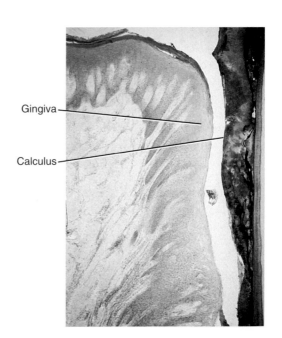

Fig. 16-16 Calculus appearing in this gingival crevice will relate to pocket formation.

Fig. 16-17 Diagram comparing the composition of supragingival plaque organisms with subgingival organisms. Deep in the pocket are gram-negative rods and motile spirochetes. Gram-positive rods are in the area of the supragingival and gingival margin. (Modified from Avery JK: *Oral development and histology,* ed 3, Stuttgart, 2002, Thieme Medical.)

A Supragingival plaque
Predominantly gram-positive rods and cocci
Very few gram-negative rods and motile forms

B Subgingival plaque
Marginal plaque
Mostly gram-positive rods and cocci
Some gram-negative rods and motile forms

Pocket plaque
Predominantly gram-negative rods and motile forms

Calculus

are in the subgingival area (Fig. 16-17). This is because gram-positive organisms are aerobic or live in air, whereas gram-negative organisms are anaerobic or function best without air. Bacterial action and the deposits result in gingival inflammation, affecting the location of the gingival attachment to the cementum rather than the cervical enamel.

Consider the Patient

Discussion: Saliva may reveal other information, such as the presence of bacterial flora, lymphocytes, and leukocytes. Microscopic examination of saliva will disclose the health of the oral tissues. This condition can be indicative of infection in the gingival crevice, especially if bacterial plaque is present.

SELF-EVALUATION QUESTIONS

1. Describe the changes that occur in plaque from 1 day to 3 weeks.
2. Define salivary corpuscles.
3. On what matrix does calculus form?
4. Name and characterize the outermost layer of enamel.
5. What types of bacteria are seen supragingivally and subgingivally?
6. Where does plaque usually form?
7. What are the components of a pellicle?
8. How long does it take an acquired pellicle to form?
9. What is one way to determine if all plaque has been removed from the teeth?
10. What is the difference between serumal and salivary calculus?

Suggested Reading

Li J, et al: Identification of early microbial colonizers in human dental biofilm, *J Appl Microbiol* 97(6):1311-1318, 2004.

Rudney JD: Saliva and dental plaque, *Adv Dent Res* 14:29-39, 2000.

Rudney JD, Pan Y, Chen R: Streptococcal diversity in oral biofilms with respect to salivary function, *Arch Oral Biol* 48(7):475-493, 2003.

Tackuchi, Bachine PC. Anti-plaque agents in the prevention of biofilm-associated oral diseases, In *Oral diseases,* Blackwell Munksgaard, 9 suppl, 2003, pp 23-29.

Vats N, Lee SF: Active detachment of *Streptococcus mutans* cells adhered to eponhydroxylapatite surfaces coated with salivary proteins in vitro, *Arch Oral Biol* 45(4):305-314, 2000.

Zaura E, ten Cate JM: Dental plaque as a biofilm: a pilot study of the effects of nutrients on plaque pH and dentin demineralization, *Caries Research* 38(suppl 1):9-15, 2004.

GLOSSARY

absorption   The passage of substances across and into tissues; a vital process carried out by cells in the body.

accessory root canal   Secondary canal extending from the pulp to the surface of the root, usually found near apices of the root.

acellular cementum   That part of the cementum covering one third to one half of the root of a tooth adjacent to the cementoenamel junction. It consists of collagenous fibers and ground substance.

aciniform   Fine pain receptors in the periodontal ligament.

acinus (alveolus)   A small, terminal, saclike dilation particular to glands such as the salivary glands.

acquired pellicle   An acellular, organic, thin skin or film deposited on the surface of teeth from salivary proteins (saliva) that bathe the surface of the teeth after eruption.

actin   Protein of the myofibril, localized in the I band; acting along with myosin particles, it is responsible for the relaxation and contraction of muscle.

adventitia   Outer layer of vessels within the pulp organ.

afferent (sensory) system   Nerve processes that carry information and convey it from the peripheral nervous system in muscles and glands to the central nervous system.

agranulocyte   A non-granular leucocyte.

alveolar bone   Ridge of bone; refers to tooth-bearing part of the mandible and maxilla because it contains the tooth sockets.

alveolar bone proper   A thin lamina of bone that lines the tooth sockets, supports the roots of the teeth, and gives attachment to principal fibers of the periodontal ligament.

alveolar crest fibers   Principal fibers of the periodontal ligament extending between the crest of the alveolar bone and the neck of the tooth.

alveoli *See dental alveoli.*

ameloblast   One of the differentiated cells of the inner layer of the enamel organ; from these cells comes the enamel of the teeth.

amelogenesis   The process of production and development of enamel.

amelogenin   Protein found in newly deposited enamel matrix. Amelogenins are lost during maturation of enamel.

amylase   Enzyme that catalyzes the hydrolysis of starch into smaller water-soluble carbohydrates.

anaphase   That stage in mitosis and meiosis following the metaphase in which the centromeres divide and the chromatids lined up on the spindle begin to move apart toward the poles.

anatomic crown   That portion of the tooth covered by enamel.

angioblast   The mesenchymal cells of an embryo that form blood cells and vessels.

angiogenic clusters   Origin of angioblasts located in the visceral mesoderm during the third week of prenatal life.

angstrom   Unit of wavelength equivalent to 0.1 millimicron (10^{27} mm). Abbreviated Å.

anterior tympanic artery   One of the main vessels supplying blood to the temporomandibular joint.

antibody   A protein that is produced in the body in response to invasion by a foreign agent or antigen and that has a specific reaction.

aortic arches   A series of arterial channels encircling the embryonic pharynx within the mesenchyme of the branchial arches.

aortic arch vessel   Vessel contained in each of the five pharyngeal arches that leads from the heart through the arches to the face, brain, and posterior regions of the body.

apical fiber group   Part of the dentoalveolar fiber group that extends perpendicular from the surface of the root apices to the adjacent fundic alveolar bone.

apical foramen   Opening at the apex of the tooth's root giving passage to the nerves and blood vessels.

appositional growth (exogenous)   Deposition of successive cell products laid down upon those already present.

area of reversal   The process of deposition in a resorption zone.

articular disk (of the temporomandibular joint)   The fibrous disk that separates the upper and lower joint cavities.

ascending pharyngeal artery   One of the main vessels supplying blood to the temporomandibular joint.

assimilation   The transformation of food into living tissue.

astral rays/asters   Those fibers that form around the centrioles during the prophase step of mitosis.

attached gingiva   The part of the oral mucosa that is firmly bound at the neck of the tooth and the alveolar process.

attached pulpal stones or denticles   Mineralized tissues that are partly fused with the dentin of the coronal pulp or root canal.

auditory capsule   The cartilage of the embryo that develops into the bony labyrinth of the inner ear.

auditory tube   The ear canal.

auricular hillocks   Six small hillocks of tissue grouped around the external ear canal.

auriculotemporal   Branch of the trigeminal nerve supplying the temporomandibular joint.

autonomic nervous system   That part of the afferent system that produces responses involuntarily and is divided into sympathetic and parasympathetic divisions.

axon   That process of a neuron by which impulses travel away from the body of the neuron.

axon terminals   Synaptic end bulbs at the branch ends of axons.

basal cell   Type of cell found in the taste bud, in close contact with the basal lamina, that has a turnover rate of approximately 10 days. They are believed to arise from the surrounding epithelial cells.

basioccipital cartilages   One of the earliest formed skeletal elements in the craniofacial area, located behind the sphenoid cartilage.

basion   A craniometric landmark located at the midpoint of the anterior border of the foramen magnum in the midsagittal plane.

basophilic   Related to basophils.

basophils   Granulocytic white blood cells found in pulp blood vessels.

B cells   Lymphocytes that have differentiated into plasma cells. Plasma cells secrete antibodies that destroy antigens.

basal lamina   Membrane separating the epidermis and dermis that is a product of both.

bell stage   Developmental stage of the tooth characterized by the differentiation of inner enamel epithelial cells into ameloblasts and the formation of the outline of the future crown by these cells.

blastocyst   The postmorula stage of development; a blastula with a fluid-filled cavity.

bone   Mineralized animal tissue consisting of an organic matrix, cells, and fibers of collagen impregnated with mineral matter, chiefly calcium phosphate and calcium carbonate. *See also* **bundle bone**, **cancellous bone**, **compact bone**, and **haversian bone**.

branchial   Barlike; resembling the gills of a fish.

branchial arch   One of a series of mesodermal bars located between the branchial clefts. During embryonic stages, the arches contribute to the formation of the face, jaws, and neck. They appear in higher forms only vestigially.

branchial arch cartilages   The cartilages found in the branchial arches of the embryo.

buccal and **labial glands**   The minor salivary glands of the cheeks and lips.

bud stage   Initial stage of tooth development; the enamel organ develops from this structure. The dental papilla lies adjacent to the epithelial bud, and the dental sac encloses both.

bundle bone   Specialized bone lining the tooth socket into which the fibers of the periodontal ligament penetrate. The radiographic term lamina dura is synonymous with bundle bone.

calcification   *See* **diffuse calcification**.

calcospherite   One of the small globular bodies formed during the process of calcification by chemical union between the calcium particles and the albuminous organic matter of the intercellular substance.

calculus   An abnormal concretion within the body, usually formed of mineral salts and often deposited around a minute fragment of inorganic material, the nucleus. *See also* **dental calculus**, **serumal calculus**.

canals   *See* **haversian canals**.

cancellous bone   Spongy or latticelike structure composed mainly of bone tissue.

capillaries   Endothelium-lined tubes that form a network among the odontoblasts.

cap stage   Part of tooth development; an early stage in enamel organ formation following the bud stage.

cardiac muscle   Involuntary muscle of the heart that pumps blood through some 50,000 miles of blood vessels.

cartilage   Fibrous connective tissue characterized by nonvascularity and a firm consistency. Forms most of the temporary skeleton of the embryo. *See also* **hyaline cartilage**.

cell   Smallest unit of living structure capable of independent existence.

cell body   Part of the neuron that contains the nucleus and the cytoplasm.

cell cycle   A series of discrete steps by which the cell component divides.

cell-free zone   Relatively cell-free layer of the dental pulp adjacent to odontoblasts and overlying the cell-rich zone. Composed of delicate fibrils in ground substance.

cell-rich zone   Layer of the dental pulp situated between the pulp core and the cell-free zone that is richly supplied with cellular elements, blood vessels, and nerves.

cell signaling   A system of effectors, modulators, and receptors through which cells interact.

cellular cementum   That part of the cementum covering the apical one half to two thirds of the root of a tooth. This cementum is most abundant on the root tip.

cementicles   Calcified spherical bodies composed of cementum lying free within the periodontal ligament, attached to the cementum, or embedded within it.

cementoblast   A large cuboidal cell lying on the surface of the bone that is active in cementum formation.

cementocyte   A cell found in the lacuna of cellular cementum. Numerous cytoplasmic processes extend from its free surface.

cementoid layer   *See* **intermediate cementum**.

cementum Bonelike connective tissue that covers the tooth from the cementoenamel junction to and surrounding the apical foramen. *See also* **acellular cementum**, **cellular cementum**.

central nervous system (CNS)   Composed of the brain and spinal cord.

centriole   Either of two short cylinders appearing near the nucleus that migrate to opposite poles of the cell during cell division.

centromere   The constricted portion of the chromosome where the chromatids are found.

cerebellum   The part of the brain located behind the brainstem, responsible primarily for coordinating voluntary muscular activity.

cerebral hemispheres   The two halves of the cerebrum.

cervical loop   Growing free border of the enamel organ. Here, the outer and inner enamel epithelial cell layers are continuous with each other.

chondroblasts   Cells that arise from the mesenchyme and form the cartilage.

chromatids   The paired chromosome strands, joined at the centromere, that make up a metaphase chromosome.

chromosomes   In animal cells, a rodlike structure in the nucleus containing a linear thread of DNA that transmits genetic information.

circular or circumferential fibers   Type of fiber within the gingival fiber group that is continuous around the neck of the tooth and resists gingival displacement.

circumpulpal dentin   Inner portion of the dentin located near the pulp organ of the tooth.

circumvallate papilla   10 to 14 large, 3-mm-diameter papillae located along the V-shaped sulcus between the body and base of the tongue.

cleft lip   The most common facial malformation, affecting one or both sides of the lip.

clinical crown   That portion of the crown exposed and visible in the oral cavity.

CNS   *See* **central nervous system (CNS)**.

col   Valleylike depression in the facial lingual plane of the interdental gingiva. It conforms to the shape of the interproximal contact area.

collagen   White fibers of the corium of the skin, tendon, and other connective tissue. The fiber is composed of fibrils bound with interfibrillar cement.

collagen fiber   High-molecular-weight protein composed of several structural types that vary in diameter and usually are arranged in bundles.

common carotid arteries   Third aortic arch vessels that later supply the neck, face, and brain with blood.

compact bone   Dense bone more highly calcified than cancellous (spongy) bone.

conductivity   The ability of an electric or other system to transmit sound, heat, light, or electromagnetic energy; a vital process carried out by cells in the body.

condyle   *See* **mandibular condyle**.

connective tissue proper   Tissues composed of cells, fibers, and intercellular material that function in tissue support and protection of the body parts, in areas of fluid exchange, and in storage of adipose (fat) tissue.

coronal pulp   Pulp present in the crown of a tooth.

coronoid process   Unit of the mandible that responds to the temporalis muscle development and attachment.

cranial   Pertaining to the cranium, specifically those bones covering the brain.

cranial base   Lower portion of the skull constituting the floor of the cranial cavity.

cranial base cartilages   Cartilages that arise to support the brain, from which come the auditory and olfactory sense capsules.

crypts   Pitlike depressions or tubular recesses on a free surface.

cuticle   *See* **primary cuticle**.

cuticular protein   The most important function of the primary cuticle, which initiates attachment of the junctional epithelium to enamel.

cytoplasm   Protoplasm of a cell located in the area surrounding the nucleus.

cytosol   Semifluid part of cytoplasm in which organelles are suspended and solutes dissolved.

dead tracts   Empty tubules resulting from loss of the odontoblastic processes.

deciduous dentition   Primary teeth that function during the first 8 years of life and then exfoliate, providing space for the permanent teeth.

deep auricular artery   One of the main vessels supplying blood to the temporomandibular joint.

deep temporal   Branch of the trigeminal nerve supplying the temporomandibular joint.

dehiscence   Alveolar bone loss in the coronal root.

demilune   A crescent-shaped structure or cell. *See also* **serous demilune**.

dendrite   Component of the neuron that receives impulses and conducts them to the cell body.

dental alveoli   The alveoli or sockets in which the roots of teeth are embedded.

dental calculus   Stonelike concretion formed on the teeth, on a prosthesis, or in salivary ducts. It varies in color from creamy yellow to black and is composed mostly of calcium phosphate.

dental lamina   Horseshoe-shaped epithelial bands that traverse the upper and lower jaws and give rise to the ectodermal portions of the teeth.

dental papilla   Part of the formative organ of the teeth that forms the dentin and the pulp.

dental plaque   Organic deposit on the surface of teeth. Site of bacterial growth and formation of dental calculus.

dental pulp   The soft tissue contained within the pulp chamber. Consists of connective tissue, blood vessels, nerves, and lymphatics.

dental sac (follicle)   Area of mesenchymal cells and fibers that surround the dental papilla and the enamel organ of the developing teeth. It produces the periodontal ligament, alveolar bone, and cementum.

denticles   Pulp stones.

dentin   Yellowish body of the tooth. It surrounds the pulp and underlies the enamel on the crown and the cementum on the roots of the teeth. Composed of 20% organic matrix, which is mostly collagen, and 10% water. The inorganic fraction (70%) is hydroxyapatite, with some carbonate, magnesium, and fluoride. *See also* **intratubular or peritubular dentin** and **mantle dentin**.

dentinoenamel junction   Interface of the enamel and dentin of the crown of a tooth.

dentinogenesis   The process of dentin formation in the development of teeth.

dentoalveolar group   Principal fiber group that surrounds the roots of the teeth.

deoxyribonucleic acid (DNA)   The nucleic acid constituting the primary genetic material of all cellular organisms.

dermatomes   Dorsal lateral portion of the somite of the embryo. These cells form the dermis, subcutaneous tissue, and supporting tissue of the gastrointestinal tract.

dermis   Arises from the mesoderm underlying the epidermis. The dermis and the epidermis together form the skin.

desmosome   Cell junction. It consists of a dense plate near the cell surface that relates to a similar structure on an adjacent cell, between which are thin layers of extracellular material.

diaphysis   The shaft of the long bone.

differentiation   Process by which cells acquire individual cellular characteristics from an undifferentiated state, that is, specialization.

diffuse calcification   Irregular calcified deposits along collagen fiber bundles or blood vessels in the pulp or elsewhere. It is considered a pathologic condition.

diphyodont   Species that develops two separate dentitions during a lifetime.

direct innervation   Theory based on the belief that nerves may extend to the dentinoenamel junction from the pulp.

disclosing solution   Formula of 0.2% basic fuchsin or erythrosin red #3 dye used to determine if all plaque has been removed from teeth.

drift   Movement of a tooth to a position of greater stability.

duct   Tube with well-defined walls for passage of excretions or secretions.

dystrophy   A disorder arising from defective or faulty nutrition.

ear   Organ composed of three parts: the external ear receives sound waves; the middle ear translates these waves into mechanical vibrations; and the internal ear receives the vibrations and changes them into specific impulses that are transmitted by the acoustic nerve to the brain.

ectodermal cells   Cells that will form the outer body covering (epithelium) of the embryo.

ectomesenchyme   Neural crest cells, mesoderm. Forms spinal ganglia.

edentulous jaw   Alveolar bone without teeth.

efferent (motor) system   Nerve process consisting of neurons that convey responses from the central nervous system to muscles and glands.

elastic or **fibrous cartilage**   Cartilage containing elastic fibers.

eleidin   A protein allied to keratin and protoplasm but more transparent than protein keratin.

embryonic disk   A small disk, to become the embryo, formed after implantation when two small cavities develop on either side of the inner cell mass and meet in the center.

embryonic period   The second to eighth weeks of prenatal life.

enamel   *See* **gnarled enamel**.

enamel crystals   Hydroxyapatite crystals found in enamel rods. They are formed during tooth mineralization.

enamel lamellae   Thin, leaflike spaces that extend from the enamel surface toward the dentinoenamel junction. They represent defects or organically filled spaces in the enamel.

enamel organ   Originates from the dental lamina and consists of four distinct layers.

enamel pearls   Enameloma, a developmental anomaly in which a small nodule of enamel is formed near the cementoenamel junction, usually at the bifurcation zone of molar teeth.

enamel rod   One of the structural units of enamel, extending from the dentinoenamel junction to the surface of the tooth and normally having a translucent crystalline appearance.

enamel spindles   Tubular spaces in enamel found at the dentinoenamel junction in which a terminal extension of the odontoblastic processes can be found.

enamel tuft   Narrow, ribbonlike structures whose constricted inner end arises at or near right angles to the dentinoenamel junction and extends a third of the way into the thickness of the enamel. Tufts consist of hypocalcified spaces that may be filled with organic substance.

enamelin   The organic protein component of enamel.

enameloid   A thin, structureless layer of substance that may be a form of enamel that is deposited by the root sheath.

endochondral   Relating to the type of bone formation that occurs within cartilage and replaces it.

endocrine   Refers to glands of internal secretion that release their secretory product(s), hormones, directly into the bloodstream rather than through a duct system.

endoderm (entoderm)   The innermost of the three primary germ layers of the embryo.

endometrium   The mucous membrane lining the uterus.

endomysium   Individual muscle fiber covering.

endoplasmic reticulum (ER)   An ultrastructural organelle consisting of membrane-bound cavities in the cytoplasm of the cell.

eosinophils   Granulocytic bilobed leukocytes, somewhat larger than a neutrophil, that constitute 1% to 3% of the body's white blood cells.

epidermal growth factor   Element in saliva that may assist in the healing of injured oral mucosa.

epidermis   The surface nonvascular cell layer of the skin that develops from the surface ectodermal cells. It consists of five layers; they are, from the inner to the outer layer, (1) basal, (2) spinous, (3) granular, (4) clear (lucidum), and (5) horny (corneum).

epimysium   Muscle fascicle (a group of muscle fibers) covering.

epiphysis   The extremity of a long bone as opposed to the shaft (diaphysis).

epithelial attachment   Attachment of the gingival epithelium to the tooth's surface at the dentogingival junction.

epithelial cell rests   Origin from the epithelial root sheath that covers the roots during root development. As the sheath develops further, it breaks up into epithelial cell rests, which migrate into the periodontal ligament. Occasionally they may develop into dental cysts. The cell groups are of these types: (1) resting, (2) proliferating, and (3) degenerating.

epithelial diaphragm   Formed by the root sheath at the beginning of root development, important during root formation. It narrows the width of the cervical opening of the root.

epithelial pearls   Discrete rounded or ovoid groups of epithelial cells, frequently keratinized, found in the lamina propria.

epithelial root sheath   Cervical loop enamel organ cells that proliferate, forming a double layer of cells (Hertwig's) that function in root formation.

epithelium   Cellular avascular layer covering all the free surfaces of the body, internal and external, and the lining of vessels. Consists of cells and small amounts of intercellular substance. *See also* **inner enamel epithelium**.

equatorial plate   The central area of the cell.

equilibrium   Sense of balance controlled by the vestibular organs, which are located in the internal ear.

ER   *See* **endoplasmic reticulum**.

eruption pathway   The altered tissue area of decreased blood vessels and degenerated nerve fibers overlying the teeth, visible as an inverted triangular area.

erythrocytes   The red blood cells.

ethmoid   Cartilaginous nasal capsule.

ethmosphenoid and **sphenoccipital articulations** Interposing bands of cartilage that exist between the ethmoid and sphenoid and the occipital bones in the midline during the period of craniofacial growth.

eustachian tube   Part of the ear that develops from the corresponding first pharyngeal pouch.

excretion   The process of eliminating, shedding, or getting rid of substances by the cells of the body.

exfoliate   To shed or eliminate something from the surface of the body, as in the loss of teeth from the jaws.

exocrine   Denotes glands that release their secretory product(s) into a duct system.

exocytosis   Discharge of secretory product(s) from the cell, preserving the cell membrane through fusion of the secretory vesicles with the cell membrane.

external auditory canal   The canal leading to the middle ear, developed from the deepening of the first pharyngeal groove.

external carotid artery   Main supply of blood to the face, neck, and brain after seven weeks' development.

extracellular phase   Resorption phase in which the mineral is separated from the collagen and is broken into small fragments.

facial sutures   A system of articulations developed between each of the major bones of the face to facilitate growth: categorized as zygomaticomaxillary, frontomaxillary, and zygomaticotemporal.

false denticles   Concentric layers of calcified tissue.

fenestration   The area of alveolar bone loss where an apical root penetrates the bone.

fetal period   The embryo from the eighth prenatal week to birth.

fibroblastoclasts   Those fibroblasts that can both form and destroy collagen fibers.

fibroblasts   Elongated, ovoid, spindle-shaped, or flattened cells found in connective tissue.

filiform papillae   The most numerous papillae appearing on the dorsum of the tongue. These threadlike elevations point dorsally and toward the throat.

fluid   One of the central components of the body, consisting of blood and lymph.

foliate papillae   4 to 11 vertical grooves or furrows containing taste buds on the lateral posterior sides of the tongue.

fontanelle   One of several membrane-covered spaces found in the incompletely ossified skull of the fetus or newborn.

foramen cecum Tissue on the surface of the tongue at the junction of the body and base from which cells arise and migrate ventrally in the throat, creating the thyroid gland.

foramen ovale An opening in the septum between the two atria of the heart.

Fordyce's spots A condition characterized by minute yellowish white papules (sebaceous glands) on the oral mucosa.

forebrain, midbrain, and **hindbrain** The primary brain vesicles formed by closure of the anterior neural tube.

free gingiva The portion of the gingiva that surrounds the tooth and is not directly attached to the tooth surface; the outer wall of the gingival sulcus.

frontal process Covering of the brain from which develops the forehead.

frontal, temporal, and **occipital lobes** Parts of the forebrain formed by the cerebral hemispheres.

frontonasal process Frontal area after the fifth week of prenatal development.

functional eruptive phase Phase in which teeth reach incisal or occlusal contact and then undergo functional eruptive movements, which include compensation for jaw growth and occlusal wear of the enamel.

fundic bone Bone enclosing the apex of the tooth root.

fungiform papillae Minute elevations on the dorsum, tip, and sides of the tongue. The papillae are mushroom shaped, with the top being broader than the base.

G1 phase The reduplication stage of the interphase after mitosis occurs; the initial resting stage in the cell cycle.

G2 phase The quiescent phase of the post-DNA duplication stage of the cell cycle.

ganglion A group of nerve cell bodies located outside the central nervous system.

gap junctions Specialized communicating junction between cells with pores permeable to ions and small molecules.

gastrointestinal tract Tube formed by endodermal cells that eventually becomes pharyngeal pouches, lung buds, liver, gallbladder, pancreas, and urinary bladder.

gene expression Duplication process in which encoded information for different functions is transferred between molecules.

genetic mechanisms Processes that help a cell to develop and maintain a high degree of order.

germinal centers Active sites of lymphocyte formation.

gingiva Soft tissue surrounding the necks of erupted teeth that cover the alveolar process. The gingiva consists of fibrous connective tissue enveloped by mucous membrane. *See also* **attached gingiva**, **free gingiva**, **interdental gingiva**.

gingival fibers Principal fiber group that is located around the necks of the teeth.

gingival sulcus The shallow V-shaped trench around each tooth, bound by the tooth on one surface and the epithelium-lined free margin on the other.

ginglymoarthrodial A type of synovial joint that allows opening and closing, symmetrical protrusion and retrusion, and asymmetrical lateral movement of the mandible.

gland *See* **merocrine gland**.

globular dentin Areas of defective growth with interglobular spaces that underlie the enamel and surface of the root.

glossopalatine glands The minor salivary glands of the tonsillar folds.

gnarled enamel The enamel located at the tips of the cusps, in which the rods or groups of rods are twisted, bent, and intertwined. It is seen ultrastructurally.

Golgi's apparatus or **complex** A continuation of the endoplasmic reticulum. A cuplike structure within cells made up of saccules where carbohydrate side chains of glycoproteins form.

granular layer of Tomes A thin, granular-appearing layer of defective dentin located along the root surface adjacent to the cementum.

granulocyte Any cell containing granules.

growth factors Chemical substances that induce cells to initiate specific cellular processes, including DNA synthesis in a specific temporal and spatial manner.

gubernacular cord A fibrous tissue band connecting the tooth sac with the alveolar mucosa. This cord may function in tooth eruption.

hard palate Anterior part of the palate consisting of the bony palate bound above by the nasal cavity and below by the mouth. It is covered by keratinized stratified squamous epithelium. In addition, the hard palate contains palatine vessels and nerves, adipose tissue, and mucous glands.

haversian bone Compact bone containing tubular channels with blood vessels, nerves, and bone cells surrounded by concentrically located lacunae. These structures are termed the *haversian system*.

haversian canals These nutrient canals are located in cortical bone and extend in the direction of the tooth's long axis.

hemidesmosome Half of a desmosome that forms a site of attachment between epithelial cells and the basal lamina or between epithelial cells (junctional cells) and the tooth's surface.

hemoglobin Complex protein-iron compound in the blood that carries oxygen to the cells from the lungs and carbon dioxide away from the cells to the lungs.

horizontal fiber group Type of fiber within the dentoalveolar fiber group that extends in a horizontal direction from the midroot cementum to the adjacent alveolar bone proper and resists tipping of the teeth.

hormone Chemical substance formed in one organ or part of the body and carried by the bloodstream to another part where it stimulates or depresses activity.

Howship's lacunae Absorption lacunae. Tiny cup-shaped depressions on the resorbing front of any hard tissue, the result of resorptive activity by osteoclasts.

Hunter-Schreger bands Alternating dark and light bands in enamel that result from absorption and reflection of light caused by differences in orientation of adjacent groups of enamel rods originating at the dentinoenamel junction and extending toward the outer enamel surface.

hyaline cartilage A flexible, semitransparent, elastic substance composed of a collagen fibrillar matrix and chondrocytes in lacunae.

hyalinization Effect of compression that is too great or too rapid on the periodontal ligament; the vascularity is excluded, and the ligament appears colorless.

hydrodynamics Science of factors determining the flow of liquids. In dentistry, it refers to a theory that pain conduction through dentin results from odontoblastic movement making contact with nerve endings.

hydroxyapatite An inorganic compound that constitutes bone and teeth.

hyoid Second arch in the development of the face and neck.

IgA A distinct class of immunoglobulins. A protein of animal origin with known antibody activity, synthesized by lymphocytes and plasma cells; found in serum, other body fluids, and tissues.

imbrication lines Also known as *von Ebner's lines*, incremental lines in dentin that run at right angles to the tubules. These lines, which represent the daily growth pattern, indicate layers of dentin that are less calcified and appear darker than adjacent dentin.

impaction Position of a tooth in the alveolus that makes it incapable of eruption into the oral cavity.

implantation The process in which the blastocyst attaches to the wall of the uterus and becomes embedded in its surface.

incisor liability The succession of larger permanent incisors replacing primary ones. The size ratio of the two incisors of the two dentitions.

incisor liability factor The replacement of the smaller primary incisors with larger permanent ones.

increment The amount by which a given quantity is increased. A measurable amount.

incremental deposition Deposition of material in discrete amounts rather than constant deposition. Rhythmic recurrent deposition of enamel, bone, dentin, or cementum.

incremental line An evident line produced through a rhythmic, recurrent deposition of successive layers upon present layers.

incus Cartilage in the first pharyngeal arch that later transforms into bone and functions in the middle ear as hearing bones.

induction The process in which an undifferentiated cell is instructed by specific organizers to produce a morphogenic effect.

inferior parathyroids Resulting organ from the third pharyngeal pouch.

inner enamel epithelium Cells that line the concavity of the enamel organ in the cap and early bell stages of tooth development and differentiate into ameloblasts.

innervation Presence and distribution of nerves within a part or the supply of nerves stimulating a part.

intercalated disks Transverse markings that appear on strands of muscle fiber as the heart tube develops.

intercalated duct Terminal duct that collects secretions from acini.

intercellular tissue Tissue located between or among cells of any structure.

interdental gingiva The soft tissue between adjacent contacting teeth in the same arch.

interdental papilla Gingiva located between the teeth and extending high on the interproximal area of the crowns on the labial and lingual surfaces.

interdental septa Bony partitions that project into the alveoli between the teeth; interalveolar.

interdental zone Zone of gingivae between the two adjacent teeth beneath their contact point.

intermediate cementum A deposition by the epithelial root sheath cells on the root surface formed during root formation. May be termed *enameloid*.

intermediate junction Type of junctional complex found between adjacent odontoblasts.

internal carotid Supply of blood to the face, neck, and brain up to seven weeks' development; afterwards it continues to supply the growing brain.

internasal area The distance between the nostrils.

interradicular bone Bone that forms between the roots of the multirooted teeth.

interradicular fibers Group of fibers that are located between the roots of multirooted teeth, extend perpendicular to the tooth's surface and to the adjacent alveolar bone, and resist vertical and lateral forces.

interstitial growth (endogenous) Growth by expansion of the matrix by cell deposits within the matrix.

interstitial spaces Spaces between groups or bundles of periodontal fibers.

intima Inner lining of vessels within the pulp organ.

intracellular phase Resorption phase in which the osteoclast ingests mineral fragments and continues the dissolution of this mineral.

intralobular duct system System located inside the lobules that contains intercalated and striated ducts.

intramembranous Within a membrane. Bone formation occurring within or among connective tissue fibers. It does not replace cartilage, as does endochondral bone.

intraoral occlusal/incisal movement Fourth event during the prefunctional eruptive phase in which the tooth continues to erupt until clinical contact with the opposing crown occurs.

intratubular or **peritubular dentin** The dentinal matrix that immediately surrounds the dentinal tubule.

junctional epithelium   Epithelial attachment. That epithelium adhering to the tooth surface at the bottom of the gingival crevice and consisting of one or more layers of nonkeratinizing cells.

keratinized   Having developed a horny layer of flattened epithelial cells containing keratin.

keratinized mucosa   Stratified surface of cornified epithelial cells that lack a nucleus and whose cytoplasm is replaced by large amounts of keratohyalin protein.

keratinocytes   Cells of the oral mucosa. These epidermal cells synthesize keratin.

lacunae   The very small cavities in bone that are filled with bone cells. *See* **Howship's lacunae.**

lamella   Thin leaf or plate, as of bone. *See also* **enamel lamellae**.

lamina dura   A thin layer of hard compact bone lining the tooth sockets. Used in radiography to designate a thin radiopaque line.

lamina propria   Layer of connective tissue underlying the epithelium of skin or a mucous membrane.

Langerhans' cells   Clear or dendritic cells found in both superficial and deep layers of the epidermis and oral epithelium.

laryngeal cartilages   Cartilage appearing in the fourth arch.

lateral ligament   Ligament that strengthens the fibers of the capsule enclosing the temporomandibular joint to support the joint and limit excursions of the condyles to the normal range.

lateral nasal process   The tissue lateral to the nasal pits.

lateral palatine processes   Processes that develop from the maxillary tissues laterally and grow to the midline to form the palate.

lateral pterygoid   Muscle of mastication with two heads that function to protrude the mandible and pull the articular disk forward.

leeway space   The difference in the space in the arch required for the two primary molars and the successional permanent premolars replacing them. The leeway space in the maxilla is 1.3 mm and in the mandible is 3.1 mm.

leucocytes   White blood cells.

lingual glands   Mixed salivary glands at the tip of the tongue.

lingual tonsils   Tonsillar tissue on the floor of the mouth.

lingula   The sharp medial boundary of the mandibular foramen, to which is attached the sphenomandibular ligament.

lining mucosa   Nonkeratinized oral mucosa that covers the surface of the cheeks, lips, soft palate, floor of the mouth, and ventral surface of the tongue.

lobes   Groups of salivary gland lobules

lobules   Groups of salivary acini invested in connective tissue.

lymphatic system   System composed of the lymph nodes, the thymus, and the spleen, as well as the vessels that carry the lymph throughout the body; it is the immunological defense of the body.

lymphocytes   Type of agranulocyte originating from stem cells and developing in the bone marrow whose numbers increase in response to infection.

lysosome   Small membrane-bound body that contains a variety of acid hydrolases, which function in breaking down substances both inside and outside the cell. It is visible through electron microscopy.

macroglossia   Enlargement of the tongue that can be caused by muscular hypertrophy.

macrognathia   Excessive size of the jaw.

macrophages   Any of the large mononuclear phagocytic cells found in various tissues and organs of the body. These cells are a normal constituent of the pulp and function in tissue maintenance.

macula adherens   Discoid desmosomes in the oral mucosa.

major glands   Salivary glands that carry their secretion some distance to the oral cavity by means of a main duct.

Malassez's rests   Epithelial cell remnants of Hertwig's sheath in the periodontal ligament. These cell groups appear near the surface of the cementum; they may develop into dental cysts.

malleus   Enlarged bulbous structure signalling the termination of Meckel's cartilages.

mandible   Horseshoe-shaped bone forming the lower jaw and articulating the condyles with the temporal bone on either side. The mandible is composed of the horizontal body and inclined ramus. The body includes the alveolar process, which contains the teeth.

mandibular condyle   The rounded bony projections of the mandible that articulate with the temporal fossa of the temporal bone in the temporomandibular fossa.

mantle dentin   The initially deposited portions of the dentin formed immediately adjacent to the enamel.

masseter muscle   Muscle of mastication, located at the angle of the mandible.

masticatory mucosa   The mucosa that functions in mastication. It tends to be bound to bone and is therefore immovable. This mucosa covers the hard palate and the gingiva.

maturation zone   Zone of cartilage characterized by chondrocyte enlargement.

maxilla   Upper jaw bone, an irregularly shaped bone articulating with the nasal, lacrimal, zygomatic, palatine, ethmoid, sphenoid, and frontal bones of the face and containing teeth.

maxillary processes   Processes that are lateral to the oral pit, from which develop the cheeks.

maxillary sinus   Paired sinus cavities occupying the space beneath the floor of the orbit and above the roots of the posterior maxillary molars.

Meckel's cartilage   The initial skeletal component of the first branchial arch. It is the supporting cartilage of the mandibular arch in the embryo.

medial nasal process   The area of the nose in the embryo. The tissue medial to the naris.

medial pterygoid   Muscle of mastication that protracts and elevates the mandible.

median raphe   The line denoting union of the palatine bones in the midline of the palate. No submucosa is under the palatal mucosa in this area.

meiosis   Process of reduction division of chromosomes in the daughter cell with half as many as in the parent cell.

melanocytes   Cells responsible for synthesis of melanin that provide pigmentation to the skin.

memory cells   Another name for lymphocytes because of their ability to retain coding information for antibody production.

Merkel's cells   Cells located in the basal layer of the gingival epithelium and thought to be epithelial in origin. They function as touch receptors.

merocrine glands   The secreting cells that remain intact during the formation and release of the secretory product. Another name for salivary glands, because the basic mode of product excretion is through membrane vesicles passing to the cell's apex.

mesenchyme   Loose, undifferentiated embryonic connective tissue that is a mixture of mesodermal and neural crest cells. The connective tissues of the body form from this tissue.

mesial drift   General movement of a tooth or teeth anteriorly toward the midline of the jaw.

mesoderm   The third primary germ layer of the embryo to differentiate. It is positioned between the ectoderm and the endoderm. From mesoderm are derived connective tissues, bone, cartilage, muscle, blood and blood vessels, lymphatics, notochord, pleura, and peritoneum.

metaphase   The second stage of mitosis in which chromatids become attached centrally at the equatorial plate to a centromere and split into two sets of chromosomes.

metaphysis   The wider part of the diaphysis adjacent to the epiphyseal line.

microglossia   Smallness of the tongue.

micrognathia   Smallness of the jaw, especially the mandible.

microlamellae   The minute spaces between or around enamel rods and through crystal spaces within rods.

microtubules   Small tubular structures found in the cytoplasm and composed of the protein tubulin. They are cylindrical and hollow.

middle ear   Tissue at the end of the external auditory canal, developing from the corresponding first pharyngeal pouch.

minor glands   Salivary glands that empty their products directly into the mouth by means of short ducts.

mitochondrion   Small spherical organelle that is a membrane-bound structure lying free in the cytoplasm and present in all cells. This structure is the principal site of energy generation in the cell.

mixed dentition   Simultaneous possession of both primary and permanent teeth.

mixed glands   Salivary glands that contain a combination of serous and mucous secretions.

monocyte   Type of agranulocyte.

morula   Mass of blastomeres resulting from the early cleavage divisions of the zygote.

MPD   Myofascial pain dysfunction.

mucin   A glycoprotein that is the primary constituent of mucus.

mucoceles   Retention cysts of the minor salivary gland ducts, which contain mucous secretion. They usually result from rupture of the excretory duct of a minor salivary gland, causing pooling of saliva in the tissues. The resulting vesicular elevation is a mucocele.

mucogingival junction   The separation between attached and free gingiva, and alveolar mucosa.

mucous acinus   Minute saclike secretory portion of a mucous gland. This is the functional unit of the gland.

mucous glands   Glands that produce viscous proteinaceous secretions, such as the sublingual gland and glands of the hard palate.

myoblast   An embryonic cell that becomes a cell of muscle fiber.

myoepithelial cells   Spindle-shaped, contractile epithelial cells with stellate bodies and processes found in salivary and sweat glands. They are located in the terminal portion of the salivary gland acini and are believed to have contractile ability that facilitates movement of the glandular secretion into the ducts.

myofibrils   Fine longitudinal fibrils (parallel to the long axis) found in a muscle fiber. They are composed of numerous myofilaments.

myosin   A protein that is the most abundant in muscle and is partially responsible for the chemical reaction that allows muscular contraction and movement.

myotome   The intermediate mesoderm.

nasal fin   A zone of epithelial contact of the medial nasal and maxillary processes during development.

nasion   A cephalometric landmark located where the intranasal and nasofrontal sutures meet.

nasolacrimal duct   That duct extending from the lacrimal gland of the eye to the internal nasal mucosa.

neonatal line   Accentuated incremental or hesitation line seen in bone, dentin, and enamel, probably caused by changes occurring at or near birth.

nerves   Whitish cords composed of fibers arranged in bundles (fascicles) and held together by a connective tissue sheath, the perineurium. The fascicles are surrounded by epineurium. Nerves transmit stimuli from the central nervous system to the periphery by the efferent motor system or from the periphery to the central nervous system by the afferent sensory system.

neural crest   Ganglionic crest, a band of ectodermal cells that appear along either side of the embryonic neural tube at the time of closure.

neural plate   A plate formed by the ectoderm that gives rise to the neural tube.

neural tube   Tube formed by the lateral boundaries of the neural plate, which will eventually become the brain and spinal cord.

neuroblasts   Primitive nerve cells that develop into adult nerve cells, the neurons. They are the functional cells of the brain, spinal cord, and peripheral nerves.

neurocranium   That part of the skull enclosing the brain, as distinguished from the bones of the face.

neuroglia   The supporting structure of the brain and spinal cord, which is composed of specialized cells and their processes.

neuron   A nerve cell, which is any of the conducting cells of the nervous system, consisting of a cell body and containing the nucleus and its surrounding cytoplasm; the dendrite, which carries impulses to the cell body; and the axon that conducts impulses away from the cell body to the area of synapse.

neutrophils   Type of granulocyte.

nonkeratinized mucosa   Lining mucosa in which the stratified squamous epithelial cells retain their nuclei and cytoplasm. Lining mucosa is found on the inner lips, cheeks, soft palate, vestibular fornix, alveolar mucosa, floor of the mouth, and undersurface of the tongue.

nonkeratinocytes   Cells not producing keratin. Clear or dendritic cells found in oral epithelium, such as pigment cells (melanocytes), Langerhans' cells, Merkel's cells, and inflammatory cells such as lymphocytes.

nuclear envelope   Membrane bounding the nucleus, composed of two phospholipid layers similar to the plasma membrane of the cell.

nuclear pores   Openings in the nuclear envelope associated with the endoplasmic reticulum that forms at the end of each cell division.

nucleolus   A round vacuole-like achromatic body rich in RNA found within the nucleus of a cell.

nucleus   A spheroid body within a cell, containing the genetic matter DNA, organelles, nucleoli, chromatin, linin, and nucleoplasm. It has a thin nuclear membrane vital to protein synthesis.

oblique fiber group   Group of fibers that extend in an oblique direction from the area just above the apical zone of the root upward to the alveolar bone and resist vertical or intrusive masticatory forces.

occlusion   Relation of the functional contact of the maxillary and mandibular teeth during activity of the mandible.

odontoblast   One of a layer of columnar cells with long processes extending into the dentinal tubules and lining the peripheral pulp of a tooth. These cells function in dentin formation and vitalize this tissue.

odontoblastic process   A cytoplasmic extension of the cell body of the odontoblasts, some of which extend from the cell as far as the dentinoenamel junction or the cementoenamel junction.

odontogenic zone   This area is peripherally adjacent to the dentin in both the coronal and radicular pulp. It contains the formative cells of dentin known as odontoblasts.

olfaction   The ability to distinguish odors.

olfactory organ   Process that allows the sense of smell by transmitting olfactory impulses to the brain.

olfactory mucosa   Site of most receptors for the sense of smell. It occupies the superior aspect of the nasal cavity between the superior nasal conchae, roof of the nose, and upper part of the nasal septum.

orbicularis oris   The musculature encircling the mouth.

organelles   Living particles located in the cytoplasm of cells. They include mitochondria, Golgi's complex, centrosomes, lysosomes, ribosomes, centrioles, endoplasmic reticulum, microtubules, and microfilaments.

organic matrix   Formative portion of a tooth or bone as opposed to mineralized hydroxyapatite.

organizer   The part of an embryo that influences another part to direct histological and morphological differentiation.

oro-naso-optic groove   An oblique groove extending from the nostrils to the eyes.

oropharyngeal membrane   Membrane at the deepest extent of the oral pocket that ruptures in the fifth week, opens the oral cavity to the tubular foregut, and soon becomes the oropharynx.

oropharynx   anatomic division of the pharynx arising from the oropharyngeal membrane

osteoblasts   Bone-forming cells derived from mesenchyme. They form the osseous matrix, in which they may become enclosed to become osteocytes.

osteoclasts   Multinucleated cells larger than osteoblasts and derived from monocytes from the bloodstream. Osteoclasts contain abundant acidophilic cytoplasm formed in bone marrow and function in the absorption and removal of osseous tissue.

osteocytes   Cells of the bone located within lacunae, functioning in maintenance and vitality of bone.

osteodentin   Dentin that appears more like bone than dentin because it contains cells.

outer enamel epithelial cells   Cells that cover the enamel organ.

oxytalan fibers   Type of connective tissue fibers chemically different from collagen fibers and found in the periodontal ligament and gingiva. They appear similar to immature elastic fibers. These fibers are believed to support blood vessels and the principal fibers of the ligament.

paciniform (pacinian) corpuscle   Laminated nerve ending that functions in the perception of pressure.

palatal rugae   Transverse ridges located in the mucous membrane of the anterior part of the hard palate. They extend laterally from the incisive papillae and have a core of dense connective tissue.

palatal shelf elevation Process during the eighth prenatal week by which the posterior shelves push together, forcing the tongue forward and down and causing the palatal shelves to slide over the tongue.

palate *See* **primary palate, secondary palate**.

palatine glands The glands of both the posterior hard palate and soft palate.

palatine shelf closure or **fusion** A final growth surge resulting in contact of palatal shelves in the midline.

palatine tonsils Two large oval masses of lymphoid tissue embedded in the lateral wall of the oropharynx and bilaterally located between the pillars of the fauces.

papillae Small protuberances on the tongue that are sensitive eminences, possessing a tactile function.

parasympathetic nervous system The craniosacral portion of the autonomic nervous system, its preganglionic fibers traveling with cranial nerves II, VII, IX, X, and XI and with the second to fourth sacral ventral roots. It innervates the heart, smooth muscle, and glands of the head and neck, and thoracic, abdominal, and pelvic viscera.

parenchyma The functional elements of an organ rather than the supporting framework (stroma) of the organ.

parietal layer Network composed of both myelinated and nonmyelinated axons **(plexus of Raschkow)**

parotid Serous-secreting salivary gland anterior to the ear. It is encapsulated and produces 26% of the secretions of the major salivary glands.

pellicle *See* **acquired pellicle**.

penetration Third event during the prefunctional eruptive phase where the tooth's crown tip moves through the fused epithelial layers and allows entrance of the crown enamel into the oral cavity. Only the organic developmental cuticle (primary), secreted earlier by the ameloblasts, covers the enamel.

perforating fibers (Sharpey's fibers) Penetrating connective tissue fibers by which the tooth is attached to the adjacent alveolar bone. These bundles of collagen fibers penetrate both the cementum and the alveolar bone.

pericytes Cells found in normal pulp that accompany blood cells.

perikaryon The cell body as distinguished from the nucleus and the processes.

perikymata Wavelike transverse grooves and ridges believed to be manifestations of the striae of Retzius on the surface of the enamel. They appear transverse to the long axis of the crown.

perimysium Connective tissue demarcating a fascicle of skeletal muscle fibers.

periodontal ligament Connective tissue ligament that is a mode of attachment of the tooth to the alveolus and that consists of collagenous fiber bundles. Between the bundles are loose connective tissue, blood vessels, and nerves.

periodontium Tissue surrounding and supporting the teeth. The tissue has two distinct components: the gingival unit, composed of the free and attached gingivae and the alveolar mucosa, and the component known as the attachment apparatus of the teeth, which includes the cementum, periodontal ligament, and alveolar bone.

peritubular dentin The zone of dentin forming the wall of the dentinal tubules. This dentin has a 9% higher mineral content than does the remainder of the intertubular dentin.

phagocyte Any cell capable of ingesting particulate matter.

phagocytose To engulf and destroy bacteria and other foreign substances; denoting the action of the phagocytic cells.

pharyngeal arch Tissues that bend around the sides of the pharynx in the shape of bars; each arch is separated by vertical grooves on the lateral sides of the neck at the fifth week.

pharyngeal pouches Grooves that separate each pharyngeal arch.

pharyngeal tonsils A collection of more or less closely aggregated lymphoid cells located superficially in the posterior wall of the nasopharynx, the hypertrophy of which results in the condition called adenoids.

philtrum The vertical groove in the midline of the upper lip.

plaque *See* **dental plaque**.

plasma cells Cells derived from B lymphocytes, which actively synthesize and secrete immunoglobulins from an extensive rough endoplasmic reticulum. Under appropriate conditions, antigen stimulation induces proliferation and morphologic alteration in B lymphocytes to form plasma cells.

plasma membrane or **plasmalemma (cell membrane)** Envelops the entire cell and provides a selective barrier that regulates transport of substances into and out of the cell.

pons That part of the central nervous system lying between the medulla oblongata and the mesencephalon, superior to the cerebellum.

precapillaries Small blood vessels measuring 8 to 12 µm in diameter, present in the peripheral pulp.

predentin Band of newly formed, and as yet unmineralized, matrix of dentin located at the pulpal border of the dentin.

preeruptive phase Developmental stage preparatory to eruption of teeth and characterized by movements of the growing teeth within the alveolar process.

prefunctional eruptive phase Phase of eruption that starts with the initiation of root formation and ends when the teeth reach occlusal contact.

primary cuticle A thin film on the enamel surface of an unerupted tooth. It is the product of the degenerating ameloblasts.

primary palate That part of the palate formed from the median nasal process. The first palate to form is anterior to the secondary palate.

prismless enamel   Enamel formed without any rods or prism pattern.

proliferative period   Time during which cells grow and increase in number by cell division.

prophase   The first stage in cell reduplication.

protective stage   Stage of plaque formation and attachment.

pseudostratified   Epithelium with all cells in contact with the basal lamina but not with the surface.

ptyalin   Synonymous term for salivary amylase, the enzyme in saliva that catalyzes the hydrolysis of starch into water-soluble carbohydrates.

pulmonary circulation   Blood supplied to the lungs by vessels of the sixth arch.

pulpal blood vessels   Characteristic thin-walled blood vessels of the dental pulp.

pulpal stones or **denticles**   Calcified masses of dentinlike substance located within the pulp or embedded in or attached to the dentinal wall. These stones may appear as a result of aging or trauma. They may be free, embedded, or attached to the dentin.

pulp bifurcation   Zone of branching of the pulp organ, as found in multirooted teeth.

pulp organ   Soft tissue within the tooth, consisting of connective tissue, blood vessels, nerves, and lymphatics.

pulp proliferation zone   Zone in the pulp adjacent to the epithelial diaphragm where cellular proliferation occurs.

quiescent stage   A period of inactivity.

radiation   Transmission of rays, such as light rays, short radiowaves, ultraviolet rays, or x-rays.

radicular pulp   The pulp occupying the root canals that extend from the cervical coronal region to the apex of the root.

ramus   General term to designate a smaller structure given off by a larger one or one into which a larger structure divides.

ramus of mandible   Quadrilateral process projecting posteriorly and superiorly from the body of the mandible.

raphe   See **median raphe.**

red blood cell (corpuscle, erythrocyte)   A non-nucleated biconcave hemoglobin that bears cells and is responsible for transport of oxygen to tissues via the circulatory system.

reduced enamel epithelium   The layers of the epithelial enamel organ compacted and remaining on the surface of enamel after its formation is complete.

remodeling   Alteration of the structure by reconstruction. The continuous process of turnover of bone carried out by osteoblasts and osteoclasts.

reparative dentin (tertiary dentin)   Deposited after trauma to the tooth by the original odontoblasts. A defensive reaction whereby hard tissue formation walls off the pulp from the site of injury.

reproduction   Duplication or replication; a vital process carried out by the cells in the body.

RER   See **rough endoplasmic reticulum (RER).**

respiration   Process of molecular exchange of oxygen and carbon dioxide within the body's tissues.

response dentin   Deposited after trauma to the tooth by newly recruited odontoblasts.

reticulum   A system of membrane-bound cavities in the cytoplasm of a cell. It occurs in two types, granular and agranular surfaces.

Retzius' striae   Lines reflecting successive incremental deposition of mineralized enamel.

reversal lines   Lines separating layers of bone or cementum deposited in a resorption site, distinguishing it from the scalloped outline of Howship's lacunae.

ribosomes   Particles that translate genetic codes for proteins and activate mechanisms for their production.

RNA (ribonucleic acid)   Carries information to sites of actual protein synthesis located in the cell cytoplasm.

root canal   Extension of the pulp from the coronal zone to the root apex. *See also* **accessory root canal.**

root formation   First event during the prefunctional eruptive phase involving proliferation of the epithelial root sheath, which in time causes initiation of root dentin and formation of the pulp tissues of the forming root. Root formation also causes an increase in the fibrous tissue of the surrounding dental follicle.

root resorption   Dissolution of the root of a tooth by action of osteoclasts. This may occur anywhere along the surface of the tooth root in response to caries or trauma or during the loss of a primary tooth.

root sheath cells (Hertwig's sheath)   Merged outer and inner epithelial layers of the enamel organ, extending beyond the region of the crown to invest the developing root.

root trunk   The part of the tooth immediately below the crown neck before division into the roots, covered by cementum and fixed in the alveolus.

rotation   Type of tooth movement in which the tooth tends to move about a circular axis.

rough endoplasmic reticulum (RER) (granular)   The ribosomes attached to the endoplasmic reticulum that function in synthesis of secretory protein.

ruffled border   An area enfolding the plasma membrane of the osteoclast that borders the resorptive zone.

saliva   Clear, slightly alkaline, somewhat viscid mixture of secretions of the salivary glands and gingival fluid exudate. It moistens the mucous membranes and food, facilitating speech and mastication. Consists of water and 0.58% solids.

salivary calculi   Calcium phosphate concentrations (salivary stones or sialolithiasis) found within a salivary gland or duct, most commonly in the main excretory duct of the submandibular gland (Wharton's duct).

salivary corpuscle   One of the leukocytes or lymphocytes found in saliva.

salivary glands   Exocrine glands whose secretions flow into the oral cavity.

Schwann's cell   Cell forming the myelin sheath of nerves and seen in association with all nerves of the pulp.

sclerotic (transparent) dentin   Dentin in which the tubules are occluded with mineral. Occurs mostly in elderly people, especially in the roots of the teeth.

sclerotomes   Part of the somite consisting of mesenchymal tissue that develops into vertebrae and ribs.

secondary dentin   Circumpulpal deposition of dentin formed after tooth eruption.

secondary palate   The palate proper formed by fusion of the lateral palatine processes of the maxilla.

sella turcica   A transverse depression in the midline of the sphenoid bone, containing the hypophysis gland.

serous   Relating to, containing, or producing a serum substance with a watery consistency.

serous demilune   Half-moon or crescent-shaped serous cells associated with the terminal external surface or mucous alveoli.

serous glands of tongue (von Ebner's)   Serous glands opening into the bottom of the trough surrounding the circumvallate papillae and functioning in a cleansing action.

serumal calculus   Subgingival calculus, so termed because it results in part from exudation of serum.

Sharpey's fibers   *See* **perforating fibers (Sharpey's fibers)**.

shedding   The loss of the primary dentition caused by the physiologic resorption of the roots, the loss of the bony supporting structure, and therefore the inability of these teeth to withstand the masticatory forces

sialography   Diagnostic x-ray technology used to visualize salivary gland ducts by injection of a radiopaque substance into the main excretory duct.

skeletal or **voluntary muscle**   Type of muscle that allows movement under voluntary control.

smear layer   The fine particles of cut dentinal debris in dentinal tubules that are produced by cavity preparation.

smooth muscle   Nonstriated involuntary muscle.

smooth muscle cells   Cells whose contractility is under control of the autonomic nervous system.

soft palate   Posterior muscular portion of the palate, forming an incomplete septum between the nasopharynx and the oral cavity.

somatic nervous system   System that carries impulses to the voluntary muscles, such as the skeletal muscles, which are under conscious control.

somites   Paired, blocklike masses of mesoderm arranged segmentally along the neural tube in the embryo and forming the dermis, vertebral column, and musculature.

specialized mucosa   Mucosa found on the dorsum of the tongue. It consists of four types of papillae, which are filiform, fungiform, circumvallate, and foliate.

S-Phase   A part of the cell cycle during which DNA is synthesized.

sphenoid   Cartilage that is posterior to the ethmoid. It later forms wings of bone that spread out under the brain laterally.

sphenomandibular ligament   temporomandibular joint ligament that arises superiorly from the spine of the sphenoid bone and extends downward on the medial side of the ramus to insert on the lingual.

spindle fibers   Those fibers not formed between the migrating centrioles during prophase.

spindles   The termination of dentinal tubules in inner enamel.

squamous   Relating to the flat squama, as of the temporal bone.

squamous epithelium   Composed of a single layer of flat scalelike cells, as in the lining of the pulmonary alveoli, or stratified, as in oral epithelium.

stapes   Third body of cartilage within Meckel's cartilages, which later develop into the hearing bones.

stellate reticulum   A network of star-shaped cells in the center of the enamel organ between the outer and inner enamel epithelia.

Stensen's duct   The epithelium-lined duct that drains the parotid gland.

stomodeum   The embryo's future oral cavity, an invagination lined by surface ectoderm.

stratified epithelium   A type of epithelium composed of a series of layers. The cells of each may vary in size and shape, as seen in skin and some mucous membranes.

stratum intermedium   Epithelial cell layer of the enamel organ that lies external and adjacent to the inner enamel epithelium and is attached to it by desmosomes. Stratum intermedium also refers to the intermediate layer of nonkeratinizing epithelia.

stratum superficiale   Third or superficial layer of the epithelium in the lining mucosa, composed of flattened cells, many of which contain small oval nuclei.

striae of Retzius   *See* **Retzius' striae**.

striated duct   An intralobular gland duct that secretes saliva and is involved in ionic transport. The duct is located between the intercalated and interlobular ducts and is named for the basal striations produced by the enfolding of the basal membrane within the cells.

striated voluntary muscles   Groups of muscles with lines across them signifying contraction sites that cause the muscles to function; they supply the dorsal and ventral parts of the limbs and provide both the deep and superficial muscle fibers.

stroma   Supporting framework of a gland, such as the capsule and trabeculae, rather than the functional parenchyma.

stylomandibular ligament   temporomandibular joint ligament that arises from the styloid process and inserts on the posterior border of the ramus.

sublingual   Refers to the area beneath the anterior lower jaw.

sublingual gland   The smallest of the three pairs of major salivary glands. A pure mucous gland located in the anterior floor of the mouth.

submandibular   Refers to the area beneath the angle of the mandible.

submandibular gland   One of the three paired major salivary glands. The submandibular glands contribute 65% of saliva. These bilateral glands are a mixed seromucous type.

submucosa   Layer of tissue that lies beneath the lamina propria underlying the mucous membrane of the lip, cheek, palate, and floor of the mouth.

successional lamina   That portion of the dental lamina lingual to the developing deciduous teeth, which gives rise to the enamel organs of permanent teeth.

superficial temporal artery   One of the main vessels supplying blood to the temporomandibular joint.

superior parathyroids   Organs developing from the fourth pharyngeal pouch.

supporting bone   Bone tissue functionally related to supporting the roots of the teeth. It surrounds, protects, and supports the tooth roots through the alveolar bone proper.

supporting or **sustentacular cells**   Cells that lie in the periphery of the taste bud.

sutures Articulations between each of the major bones of the face (*see* **facial sutures**).

sympathetic nervous system   The thoracolumbar part of the autonomic nervous system. Preganglionic fibers arise from cell bodies in the thoracic and first three lumbar segments of the spinal cord. Postganglionic fibers are distributed to the heart, smooth muscle, and glands of the entire body.

synapse   The region of the junction between two nerve cells where an impulse passes between the axon of one cell and the dendrite of another cell.

synchondrosis   The union of two bones that have been separated by cartilage.

syndesmosis   A type of fibrous joint in which opposing surfaces are united in fibrous connective tissue, as in the union between most facial bones.

synovial membranes   Membranes that line joint cavities and secrete a small amount of transparent alkaline fluid (synovial fluid) in the articular spaces. Synovial fluid acts as a lubricant and nutrient for the avascular tissue cover, that is, the condyle and articular tubercle for the temporomandibular joint.

taste bud   Receptor of taste on the tongue and in the oropharynx. One of several goblet-shaped cells oriented at right angles to the surface by the epithelium. The taste buds consist of supporting and gustatory cells.

taste modality   Process located in cells of the taste buds, which are in the circumvallate papillae on the tongue's posterior dorsal surface.

T cells   Cells, produced by the thymus, that destroy invading microbes and are therefore important to the body's immune system.

telophase   The last of the four stages of mitosis and of the two divisions of meiosis that begins when the chromosomes arrive at the poles of the cell.

temporal and **interoccipital bones**   Membrane bones, including frontal, parietal, and squamous portions, forming the protective covering of the brain.

temporalis   Muscle fibers that originate from the floor of the temporal fossa and temporal fascia and work to elevate and retract the mandible and clench the teeth.

temporomandibular joint (TMJ)   Joint formed between the condyle of the mandible and the mandibular fossa (concavity of the temporal bone).

temporomandibular ligaments   Four ligaments that include the sphenomandibular on the medial surface, the stylomandibular on the posterior surface, the temporomandibular on the lateral surface, and the capsular surrounding the joint.

teratogen   Agent or factor that produces physical defects in the developing embryo.

terminal arterioles   Blood vessels of 10 to 15 μm in diameter present in the pulp organ.

terminal bar apparatus   Localized condensations of cytoplasmic substance associated with the cell membrane of the apical area of the functional ameloblast.

terminal sulcus   V-shaped groove separating the surface of the body and base of the tongue.

tertiary dentin   *See* **reparative dentin**.

thymus   A bilaterally symmetric lymphoid organ consisting of two lobes situated in the anterior superior mediastinum.

thyroglossal cyst   A swelling of the thyroglossal duct due to the presence of infection or a salivary stone.

thyroglossal duct   An epithelial cord by which the thyroid gland remains attached to the tongue while descending to the front of the trachea; later becomes solid and eventually disappears.

thyroglossal fistula   A swelling that has an opening on the surface of the neck.

tipping movement   Pressure applied on a specific point on the tooth that causes compression in a limited area between the root and the bone.

TMJ   *See* **temporomandibular joint**.

Tomes' granular layer   This layer of dentin is found only in the tooth root. It is adjacent to the peripheral zone of hyalinized root dentin as a thin, hypomineralized layer.

Tomes' process   Specialized apical zone of the ameloblasts. Tomes' process is conical and interdigitates with the forming enamel rods.

tonofibrils   Systems of fibrils found in the cytoplasm of epithelial cells, which function with the desmosomal plaque to hold adjacent cells together.

tooth crypt   Space filled by the dental follicle and developing tooth within the alveolar process.

tooth eruption   Process by which teeth emerge into the oral cavity, a stage coordinated with root growth and maturation of tissues surrounding the tooth.

traction bands of the palate   Bundles of collagen fibers that firmly attach the oral mucosa to the underlying bone of the hard palate.

transduction theory   Proposal that odontoblasts are sensory receptors for pain stimuli that are transmitted through the dentin.

transparent dentin   *See* **sclerotic (transparent) dentin**.

transseptal fibers   Fibers that originate in the cervical region of each crown and extend to similar locations on the mesial and distal surfaces of each adjacent tooth. This fiber group functions in resistance to the separation of each tooth.

tuberculum impar   Central tissue of the tongue eventually overgrown by the two lateral tissues.

tuft   *See* **enamel tuft**.

tympanic membrane   The membrane at the depth of the external auditory canal.

ultimobranchial body   Tissues resulting from development of the fifth pharyngeal pouch.

umbilical system   Vascular network connected to the placenta that traverses the umbilical cord and conducts nutrition and oxygen to the embryo while carrying carbon dioxide and wastes to the placenta.

undifferentiated cells   Cells found in normal pulp that accompany blood cells.

vasculature   Refers to the blood vessels and circulating blood system.

vermilion border   The exposed red portion of the lips. This color is due to a thin epithelium with the presence of eleidin in the cells and the superficial position of blood vessels.

vestibular lamina   Lip furrow band located labial and buccal to the dental lamina that forms the oral vestibule between the alveolar portions of the jaws, the lips, and the cheeks.

visceral mesoderm   Part of the embryonic skeleton formed by dermatome cells that supports the endoderm of the gastrointestinal tract.

viscerocranial   Refers to those parts of the facial cranial skeleton originating from the branchial arch.

vitelline vascular system   The blood vascular system of a fertilized egg that overlies the yolk.

Volkmann's canals   "Perforating canals" that enter the bone at right or oblique angles and establish a continuous system that contains the nerves and blood vessels of the bone.

vomer flat   Unpaired bone located in the midline of the face, shaped like a trapezoid, and forming the inferior and posterior portions of the nasal septum. It articulates with the sphenoid, ethmoid, two maxillary, and two palatine bones.

von Ebner's lines   *See* **imbrication lines**.

Waldeyer's ring   A ring of tonsillary tissue surrounding the oropharynx. It is composed of palatine tonsils located laterally, the lingual in the floor of the mouth, and the pharyngeal in the posterior area of the pharynx.

Weil's basal layer   *See* **cell-free zone**.

Wharton's duct   The duct that drains the submandibular gland.

zygoma   The process of the temporal bone that connects with the zygomatic bone.

zygote   The fertilized cell produced by the union of two gametes.

zymogen   An inactive precursor that is activated to an enzyme. Granules in serous cells of enzyme-secreting glands, such as the salivary glands and the pancreas.

INDEX